OPLL

Atsushi Okawa • Morio Matsumoto
Motoki Iwasaki • Yoshiharu Kawaguchi
Editors

OPLL

Ossification of the Posterior Longitudinal Ligament

Third Edition

Springer

Editors
Atsushi Okawa
Department of Orthopaedic Surgery
Tokyo Medical and Dental University
Tokyo
Japan

Morio Matsumoto
Department of Orthopaedic Surgery
Keio University
Shinjyuku-ku, Tokyo
Japan

Motoki Iwasaki
Department of Orthopaedic Surgery
Osaka Rosai Hospital
Sakai, Osaka
Japan

Yoshiharu Kawaguchi
Department of Orthopaedic Surgery
Toyama University Hospital
Sugitani, Toyama
Japan

ISBN 978-981-15-3854-4 ISBN 978-981-15-3855-1 (eBook)
https://doi.org/10.1007/978-981-15-3855-1

This Springer imprint is published by the registered company Springer Nature Singapore Pte Ltd.
The registered company address is: 152 Beach Road, #21-01/04 Gateway East, Singapore 189721, Singapore

Preface

This third edition is dedicated to Keiro Ono, Professor Emeritus of Osaka University Graduate School of Medicine, who was the first editor of this textbook and passed away in 2018.

Aston C. Key first described the ossification of the posterior longitudinal ligament (OPLL) in 1838. Two male patients suffered from bladder disturbance and paraplegia followed by septicemia. Autopsies revealed that they had a narrowed cervical canal due to an ossified posterior longitudinal ligament. In Japan, a similar case was reported in 1960. Since that time, many studies about this disease have been conducted in this country.

In 1975, the government launched a foundation to research this intractable disease, which has continued until the present. Spontaneous OPLL develops over many years, resulting in compression of the spinal cord. Minor trauma can easily cause deterioration of myelopathy or induce spinal cord injury. Although development of ectopic bone formation in the ligamentous tissue has been presumed to be associated with diabetes mellitus or other metabolic diseases, the precise pathogenesis remains unknown.

Cervical OPLL is a common disease, and its prevalence in Japan is approximately 3%. It has been thought that genetic factors are likely to contribute to the etiology of OPLL. Many basic and clinical studies have been conducted on this disease. To propagate this new knowledge to spinal surgeons worldwide, this textbook was first published in 1995 and edited by Professor Keiro Ono. The second version edited by Dr. Kazuo Yonenobu was published in 2011. Since then, research on this disease has progressed, and a new guideline has been prepared that also include thoracic OPLL and ossification of the ligamentum flavum (OLF).

Recent important advancements in basic research for OPLL include genomic studies to precisely determine the genetic factors of spinal ligament ossification. A genome-wide association study was conducted to identify the susceptibility gene(s) for OPLL, which indicated that six loci were susceptible for OPLL. Ectopic ossification of spinal ligaments tends to develop in adults with such genetic factors during middle age. Currently, the functions of some candidate gene are being studied. This marked progression in basic research suggests that a drug can be developed to control the development of ectopic ossification in the near future.

Due to recent advances, whole-spine reconstructions of CAT scan images from the cervical to lumbar spine can be easily obtained in a short time. These whole-spine reconstructed images show that ossification in the thoracic and lumbar spine is more frequently observed in patients with cervical OPLL. Moreover, patients with cervical OPLL are predisposed to have ossification of other spinal ligaments such as the anterior, supraspinal, and yellow ligaments. This imaging technique advancement also allows easy evaluation of ossified bone volume in three-dimensional renderings. Analyses of these data revealed an annual increase in the rate of ossified bone volume and its suppression after fusion surgery. These studies will provide valuable information for future therapeutic methodology.

To date, the mainstream for the treatment for OPLL has been surgery, such as anterior cervical corpectomy and fusion (ACCF) or laminoplasty. Comparative studies between these two types of surgery have indicated that the outcomes do not differ at 2 or 3 years postoperatively, but afterward, neurological symptoms in patients with laminoplasty can deteriorate because of gradual progression of kyphotic alignment or ossification. Concomitant use of posterior instrumentation with laminoplasty was shown to prevent this alignment change and to suppress development of ossification. Fusion operations performed either from the anterior or posterior approach may provide good long-term outcomes for this disease. However, careful use of intraoperative spinal cord monitoring cannot completely prevent neurological complications. Major complications such as airway obstruction, dysphagia, and vertebral artery injury can also occur.

Laminectomy with posterior instrumentation has become popular for thoracic OPLL. Prospective data collection from multiple spine centers nationwide showed that an abnormal wave change occurred in more than 40% cases. Although most of the patients showed spontaneous recovery by the end of the surgery, some remained postoperatively paralyzed. The cause of this critical complication is presumed not to be a technical problem but due to the vulnerability of spinal cords affected by thoracic OPLL.

Recent advancements regarding ossification of spinal ligaments such as those described above were achieved by nationwide multicenter studies in Japan supported by Health, Labour and Welfare Policy Research Grants. Details of these studies are available in this textbook. The research committee was organized by the Japanese Orthopaedic Association. I hope that this textbook will help people who suffer from this intractable disease.

Finally, all authors of this third edition offer special thanks to Professor Yoshiharu Kawaguchi, Professor Morio Matsumoto, and Dr. Motoki Iwasaki, who led our committee and made great efforts to complete this textbook. The ideal therapy for this disease would be to control ossification of ligaments without surgery. We hope that drug therapy can become available before the fourth edition of this textbook is published.

Tokyo, Japan — Atsushi Okawa

Contents

Part I

Introduction

History of Research

1

Atsushi Okawa

Ossification of the posterior longitudinal ligament (OPLL) was first described by Aston C Key [1] in 1838 as a disease that causes paraplegia. Two male patients with OPLL suffered from bladder disturbance and paraplegia, followed by septicemia. The autopsies revealed a narrowed cervical canal due to OPLL. However, the condition then went without notice for a long time. Oppenheimer [2] reported 18 cases of calcification or ossification of the anterior and posterior longitudinal ligaments over 100 years after OPLL was first described by Key. Most of these cases were ossification of the anterior longitudinal ligament. He did not recognize the clinical significance of OPLL.

In Japan, a similar case to Key's was reported in 1960 by Dr. Hirokuni Tsukimoto [3]. A 47-year-old male with finger clumsiness and sensory disturbance in both arms and legs underwent posterior surgery and achieved transient recovery. However, he suffered from pneumonia 3 months after the operation following tetraparesis and pressure sore formation on the sacrum. The autopsy revealed ectopic bone formation adjacent to the vertebral body, which was presumed to have changed from the posterior ligament (Fig. 1.1). The author speculated that the etiology involved repeated minor trauma to the neck, such as whiplash injury, inducing this ectopic bone formation. The author noted that vascular factors are also related to the acceleration of myelopathy. Following this report, many studies have been enthusiastically conducted in Japan.

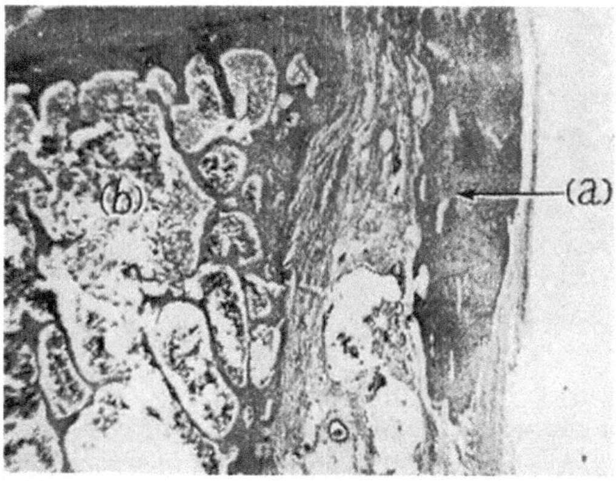

Fig. 1.1 The first reported case of cervical OPLL showed ectopic bone formation (**a**) just behind the vertebral body (**b**). Reprinted with permission from 3)

In 1975, the government launched a research grant to conquer intractable diseases that have continued up to the present. Eight investigation committees have been organized for this disease. Table 1.1 shows the names of the chief researchers of each group and their main topics.

The PLL ossifies spontaneously and increases in length and thickness year by year, resulting in compression of the spinal cord. Minor trauma can easily cause deterioration of paresis or induce spinal cord injury. Although ectopic bone formation

A. Okawa (✉)
Department of Orthopaedic and Spinal Surgery, Tokyo Medical and Dental University, Tokyo, Japan
e-mail: okawa.orth@tmd.ac.jp

A. Okawa et al. (eds.), *OPLL*, https://doi.org/10.1007/978-981-15-3855-1_1

Table 1.1 Names of chief researchers and their main topics in the investigation committee of research groups

Chief researcher (period), affiliation, and main issue of research
Naoichi Tsuyama (1975–1980), Tokyo University
Epidemiology/image diagnosis/pathology
Kazuo Terayama (1981–1987), Shinsyu University
Nationwide family study
Takahide Kurokawa (1988–1991), Tokyo University
Genetics/pathology and pathophysiology/neurology/imaging study
Takashi Sakou (1992–1995), Kagoshima University
Genetics/molecular biology
Seikou Harata (1996–2001) Hirosaki University
Overseas epidemiology/quality of life surveillance
Kozo Nakamura (2002–2007) Tokyo University
Genetics/pathology, pathophysiology/treatment/guideline
Yoshiaki Toyama (2008–2013) Keio University
Genetics (genome wide association study)/spinal cord monitoring
Imaging technique/revise of guild line
Atsushi Okawa (2014–2019) Tokyo Medical and Dental University
Multicenter study/CT study

in ligamentous tissue has been presumed to occur in association with diabetes mellitus or certain foods and other metabolic diseases, the precise mechanism has remained unclear [4, 5].

Although epidemiology, natural history, diagnosis, and treatment were common topics of each period, the development of imaging techniques, such as CT and magnetic resonance imaging, enabled the addition of new information. Reconstructed CT images of the cervical to lumbar spine can be easily obtained within a few minutes. Such whole-spine reconstructed images indicated that ossification of the yellow ligament in the thoracic and lumbar spine was more frequently observed in patients with cervical OPLL than expected. Moreover, cervical OPLL was detected in males three-times more frequently than in females, but thoracic OPLL showed an opposite trend. Additionally, the ossification of other spinal ligaments, such as the anterior, supraspinal, and yellow ligaments, was observed [6–8]. These facts indicate that genetic factors strongly contribute to the development of the ossification of all spinal ligaments. This advancement in imaging also made it easy to evaluate the ossified bone volume in a 3D fashion. Analysis revealed an annual increase in the ossified bone volume and the suppression of ossification after surgical fusion [9, 10]. These studies provide valuable information for the selection of an operative method.

The pathology of ectopic ossification in the spinal ligaments has been studied for a long time. Ossification of the spinal ligaments is ectopic, with hypertrophy of the ligament, proliferation of cartilaginous cells in the ligament, and the release of cytokines related to bone formation (bone morphogenetic protein and transforming growth factor beta) during the ossification process [11]. Recent genetic studies have provided more advanced knowledge of the pathogenesis. A sib-pair study and a genome-wide association study were conducted to identify the susceptibility gene(s) for ectopic bone formation of the spinal ligaments [12, 13]; there were six susceptible loci for OPLL. Ectopic ossification of the spinal ligaments is more likely to develop in middle-aged adults with such genetic factors. The function of some candidate genes has since been studied. This splendid progression in basic research suggests that it is not unreasonable to expect a drug to be available in the future to control the development of ectopic ossification.

Until now, the main treatment for OPLL has been surgery. Many kinds of laminoplasty have been developed in Japan [14, 15]. However, the basic concept of wide and simultaneous decompression of the spinal cord has been mandatory in posterior surgical treatment since the report by Kirita [16]. Anterior cervical corpectomy and fusion (ACCF) is also available for this disease. Yamaura's floating method, in which the ossified ligament is not removed but thinned carefully, has gradually prevailed to avoid intraoperative neurological complications [17]. Comparative studies between these two types of surgery indicated similar outcomes 2 and 3 years postoperatively; however, subsequently, neurological symptoms in patients treated with laminoplasty can deteriorate because of the gradual progression of kyphotic alignment or ossification [18]. The newly proposed K-line is quite useful in the determination of a surgical method. The K-line is defined as the line connecting the midpoints of the spinal canal at the C2 and C7 levels on lateral cervical X-ray examination. When the ossification is large enough to exceed this line toward the spinal cord, anterior surgery will be preferred. The relationship between the ossification and the line depends on the sagittal profile of the cervical spine and the thickness of the ossification [19]. This concept has rapidly prevailed globally in helping to decide on the surgical approach used for each patient.

The concomitant use of posterior instrumentation with laminoplasty was recently proposed to avoid alignment changes [20]. Fusion of the spinal segments may also suppress ossification development. Thus, surgical fusion with either an anterior or posterior approach could help to maintain a good outcome over the long term in the treatment of this disease [21–23].

For thoracic OPLL, laminectomy with posterior instrumentation has become popular [24]. Prospectively collected data from multiple spine centers nationwide have shown that abnormal wave changes occurred in more than 40% of cases. Although most of the patients showed spontaneous recovery until the end of the surgery, some of them remained paralyzed postoperatively. The cause of this critical complication is presumed to be not a technical problem but due to the prone position during surgery [25].

Above all, recent progress in this area has been achieved by great support from governmental research grants. Most of these results were obtained by the collaboration of nationwide spine centers and the research committee organized by the Japanese Orthopaedic Association. Details of the studies are available in this textbook.

References

1. Key GA. On paraplegia depending on the ligament of the spine. Guys Hosp Rep. 1839;3:17–34.
2. Oppenheimer A. Calcification and ossification of vertebral ligaments (spondylitis ossificans ligamentosa): roentgen study of pathogenesis and clinical significance. Radiology. 1942;38:160–73.
3. Tsukimoto H. A case report-autopsy of the syndrome of compression of the spinal cord owing to ossification within the spinal canal of the cervical spine (in Japanese). Nihon Geka Hokan (Arch Jpn Chir). 1960;29:1003–7.
4. Akune T, Ogata N, Seichi A, Ohnishi I, Nakamura K, Kawaguchi H. Insulin secretory response is positively associated with the extent of ossification of the posterior longitudinal ligament of the spine. J Bone Joint Surg Am. 2001;83:1537–44.
5. Okano T, Ishidou Y, Kato M, Imamura T, Yonemori K, Origuchi N, Matsunaga S, Yoshida H, ten Dijke P, Sakou T. Orthotopic ossification of the spinal ligaments of Zucker fatty rats: a possible animal model for ossification of the human posterior longitudinal ligament. J Orthop Res. 1997;15:820–9.
6. Mori K, Imai S, Kasahara T, Nishizawa K, Mimura T, Matsusue Y. Prevalence, distribution, and morphology of thoracic ossification of the posterior longitudinal ligament in Japanese: results of CT-based cross-sectional study. Spine (Phila Pa 1976). 2014;39(5):394–9.
7. Fujimori T, Watabe T, Iwamoto Y, Hamada S, Iwasaki M, Oda T. Prevalence, concomitance, and distribution of ossification of the spinal ligaments: results of whole spine CT scans in 1500 Japanese patients. Spine (Phila Pa 1976). 2016;41(21):1668–76.
8. Hirai T, Yoshii T, Iwanami A, Takeuchi K, Mori K, Yamada T, Wada K, Koda M, Matsuyama Y, Takeshita K, Abematsu M, Haro H, Watanabe M, Watanabe K, Ozawa H, Kanno H, Imagama S, Fujibayashi S, Yamazaki M, Matsumoto M, Nakamura M, Okawa A, Kawaguchi Y. Prevalence and distribution of ossified lesions in the whole spine of patients with cervical ossification of the posterior longitudinal ligament a multicenter study (JOSL CT study). PLoS one. 2016;11(8):e0160117.
9. Katsumi K, Watanabe K, Izumi T, Hirano T, Ohashi M, Mizouchi T, Ito T, Endo N. Natural history of the ossification of cervical posterior longitudinal ligament: a three dimensional analysis. Int Orthop. 2018;42(4):835–42.
10. Ota M, Furuya T, Maki S, Inada T, Kamiya K, Ijima Y, Saito J, Takahashi K, Yamazaki M, Aramomi M, Mannoji C, Koda M. Addition of instrumented fusion after posterior decompression surgery suppresses thickening of ossification of the posterior longitudinal ligament of the cervical spine. J Clin Neurosci. 2016;34:162–5.
11. Kawaguchi H, Kurokawa T, Hoshino Y, Kawahara H, Ogata E, Matsumoto T. Immunohistochemical demonstration of bone morphogenetic protein-2 and transforming growth factor-beta in the ossification of the posterior longitudinal ligament of the cervical spine. Spine (Phila Pa 1976). 1992;17(3 Suppl):S33–6.
12. Karasugi T, Nakajima M, Ikari K, Genetic Study Group of Investigation Committee on Ossification of the Spinal Ligaments, Tsuji T, Matsumoto M, Chiba K, Uchida K, Kawaguchi Y, Mizuta H, Ogata N, Iwasaki M, Maeda S, Numasawa T, Abumi K, Kato T, Ozawa H, Taguchi T, Kaito T, Neo M, Yamazaki M, Tadokoro N, Yoshida M, Nakahara S, Endo K,

Imagama S, Demura S, Sato K, Seichi A, Ichimura S, Watanabe M, Watanabe K, Nakamura Y, Mori K, Baba H, Toyama Y, Ikegawa S. A genome-wide sib-pair linkage analysis of ossification of the posterior longitudinal ligament of the spine. J Bone Miner Metab. 2013;31(2):136–43.
13. Nakajima M, Takahashi A, Tsuji T, Karasugi T, Baba H, Uchida K, Kawabata S, Okawa A, Shindo S, Takeuchi K, Taniguchi Y, Maeda S, Kashii M, Seichi A, Nakajima H, Kawaguchi Y, Fujibayashi S, Takahata M, Tanaka T, Watanabe K, Kida K, Kanchiku T, Ito Z, Mori K, Kaito T, Kobayashi S, Yamada K, Takahashi M, Chiba K, Matsumoto M, Furukawa K, Kubo M, Toyama Y. Genetic Study Group of Investigation Committee on Ossification of the Spinal Ligaments, Ikegawa S. A genome-wide association study identifies susceptibility loci for ossification of the posterior longitudinal ligament of the spine. Nat Genet. 2014;46(9):1012–6.
14. Ogawa Y, Toyama Y, Chiba K, Matsumoto M, Nakamura M, Takaishi H, Hirabayashi H, Hirabayashi K. Long-term results of expansive open-door laminoplasty for ossification of the posterior longitudinal ligament of the cervical spine. J Neurosurg Spine. 2004;1:168–74.
15. Seichi A, Takeshita K, Ohishi I, Kawaguchi H, Akune T, Anamizu Y, Kitagawa T, Nakamura K. Long-term results of double-door laminoplasty for cervical stenotic myelopathy. Spine. 2001;26:479–48.
16. Kirita Y. Posterior decompression for the cervical spondylosis and ossification of the posterior longitudinal ligament in cervical spine (in Japanese). Geka (Surgery). 1976;30:287–302.
17. Yamaura I, Kurosa Y, Matuoka T, Shindo S. Anterior floating method for cervical myelopathy caused by ossification of the posterior longitudinal ligament. Clin Orthop Relat Res. 1999;(359):27–34.
18. Sakai K, Okawa A, Takahashi M, Arai Y, Kawabata S, Enomoto M, Kato T, Hirai T, Shinomiya K. Five-year follow-up evaluation of surgical treatment for cervical myelopathy caused by ossification of the posterior longitudinal ligament: a prospective comparative study of anterior decompression and fusion with floating method versus laminoplasty. Spine (Phila Pa 1976). 2012;37(5):367–76.
19. Fujiyoshi T, Yamazaki M, Kawabe J, Endo T, Furuya T, Koda M, Okawa A, Takahashi K, Konishi H. A new concept for making decisions regarding the surgical approach for cervical ossification of the posterior longitudinal ligament: the K-line. Spine (Phila Pa 1976). 2008;33(26):E990–3.
20. Chen Y, Guo Y, Lu X, Chen D, Song D, Shi J, Yuan W. Surgical strategy for multilevel severe ossification of posterior longitudinal ligament in the cervical spine. (2001). J Spinal Disord Tech. 2011;24(1):24–30.
21. Koda M, Mochizuki M, Konishi H, Aiba A, Kadota R, Inada T, Kamiya K, Ota M, Maki S, Takahashi K, Yamazaki M, Mannoji C, Furuya T. Comparison of clinical outcomes between laminoplasty, posterior decompression with instrumented fusion, and anterior decompression with fusion for K-line (−) cervical ossification of the posterior longitudinal ligament. Eur Spine J. 2016;25(7):2294–301.
22. Yamazaki M, Mochizuki M, Ikeda Y, Sodeyama T, Okawa A, Koda M, Moriya H. Clinical results of surgery for thoracic myelopathy caused by ossification of the posterior longitudinal ligament: operative indication of posterior decompression with instrumented fusion. Spine (Phila Pa 1976). 2006;31(13):1452–60.
23. Yoshii T, Egawa S, Hirai T, Kaito T, Mori K, Koda M, Chikuda H, Hasegawa T, Imagama S, Yoshida M, Iwasaki M, Okawa A, Kawaguchi Y. A systematic review and meta-analysis comparing anterior decompression with fusion and posterior laminoplasty for cervical ossification of the posterior longitudinal ligament. J Orthop Sci. 2020;25(1):58–65. pii: S0949-2658(19)30073-9
24. Matsumoto M, Chiba K, Toyama Y, Takeshita K, Seichi A, Nakamura K, Arimizu J, Fujibayashi S, Hirabayashi S, Hirano T, Iwasaki M, Kaneoka K, Kawaguchi Y, Ijiri K, Maeda T, Matsuyama Y, Mikami Y, Murakami H, Nagashima H, Nagata K, Nakahara S, Nohara Y, Oka S, Sakamoto K, Saruhashi Y, Sasao Y, Shimizu K, Taguchi T, Takahashi M, Tanaka Y, et al. Surgical results and related factors for ossification of posterior longitudinal ligament of the thoracic spine: a multi-institutional retrospective study. Spine. 2008;33(9):1034–41.
25. Imagama S, Ando K, Takeuchi K, Kato S, Murakami H, Aizawa T, Ozawa H, Hasegawa T, Matsuyama Y, Koda M, Yamazaki M, Chikuda H, Shindo S, Nakagawa Y, Kimura A, Takeshita K, Wada K, Katoh H, Watanabe M, Yamada K, Furuya T, Tsuji T, Fujibayashi S, Mori K, Kawaguchi Y, Watanabe K, Matsumoto M, Yoshii T, Okawa A. Perioperative complications after surgery for thoracic ossification of posterior longitudinal ligament: a Nationwide multicenter prospective study. Spine (Phila Pa 1976). 2018;43(23):E1389–97.

Part II

Epidemiology

An Overview of Epidemiology and Genetics

2

Hiroyuki Inose and Atsushi Okawa

Abstract

Ossification of the posterior longitudinal ligament of the spine (OPLL) can cause not only spinal rigidity but also severe paralysis due to compression of the spinal cord by an ectopic ossification of the posterior longitudinal ligament. The prevalence of cervical OPLL is 1.9–6.3% in the Japanese, 0.95–3.6% in other Southeast Asians, and 0.01–1.7% in North American and Europeans. OPLL is ordinarily diagnosed after the age of 50 years. While OPLL can be a secondary complication in patients with monogenic diseases, most clinical cases of OPLL are idiopathic. Idiopathic OPLL is considered to be a multifactorial disease with both genetic and environmental factors contributing to its development and progression. Age, diabetes mellitus, obesity, and mechanical stress have been proposed as clinical and environmental risk factors. On the other hand, OPLL is known to have a strong genetic predisposition. Recently, several genetic studies have demonstrated several genes/loci that link to OPLL susceptibility, but, to date, none of the genes has yet been proven as a functionary gene responsible for the development of OPLL. This chapter reviews the recent progress in the epidemiologic and genomic studies of OPLL.

Keywords

OPLL · Epidemiology · Genetics · Prevalence · Sex ratio

H. Inose · A. Okawa (✉)
Department of Orthopaedic and Spinal Surgery, Tokyo Medical and Dental University, Tokyo, Japan
e-mail: inose.orth@tmd.ac.jp; okawa.orth@tmd.ac.jp

Ossification of the posterior longitudinal ligament (OPLL) was first reported by Key in 1838 [1]. While it has long been known that spinal ligaments can undergo ossification, Forestier was first to define the features of "senile ankylosing hyperostosis of the spine" as hyperostosis of the spinal ligament, spinal rigidity, and advanced age in 1950 [2]. The disease concept of OPLL was established in Japan by Tsukimoto in 1960 in a report on an autopsy examination of a Japanese patient presenting symptoms of severe spinal cord compression due to OPLL [3]. Since then, OPLL has been recognized as a disease that can cause not only spinal rigidity but also severe and irreversible paralysis. It is also a disease of unknown cause and is difficult to treat both conservatively and surgically. Furthermore, in 1976, Resnick et al. coined the term "diffuse idiopathic skeletal hyperostosis" (DISH) for Forestier's disease and recognized ossification of spinal ligaments as a subset of this entity [4].

The Investigation Committee on the OPLL funded by the Japanese Ministry of Health Labour and Welfare (MHLW) has been working on this

A. Okawa et al. (eds.), *OPLL*, https://doi.org/10.1007/978-981-15-3855-1_2

"difficult" disease since 1975. Accordingly, a number of epidemiological and genetic studies regarding OPLL have been performed within the framework of the MHLW study group [5]. This chapter outlines the evidence related to epidemiology and genetics derived from the Japanese guidelines concerning the diagnosis and treatment of OPLL.

The prevalence of cervical OPLL varies among races. Based on the research using plain radiographs, the prevalence of cervical OPLL is 1.9–4.1% in the Japanese [6–8], 0.95–3.6% in other Southeast Asians, and 0.01–1.7% in North American and Europeans [9, 10]. A recent comprehensive study in North America showed that the prevalence of cervical OPLL was 1.3% in Caucasian Americans, 4.8% in Asian Americans, 1.9% in Hispanic Americans, 2.1% in African Americans, and 3.2% in Native Americans [11]. They concluded that the prevalence of cervical OPLL in Asian Americans was significantly higher than that in Caucasian Americans [11]. Prevalence of thoracic OPLL is lower than that of cervical OPLL. The investigation using plain radiographs showed that the prevalence of thoracic OPLL is 0.56–0.8% [12, 13]. In a recent cross-sectional study using whole-spine CT scans, the prevalence was found to be 6.3% in cervical OPLL and 1.6% in thoracic OPLL [14]. Therefore, due to the technological advancement in medical diagnostics, it can be assumed that OPLL is much more common than previously considered.

Regarding the sex ratio of cervical OPLL, most studies suggest the male/female ratio has been 1.6–2.5 [6, 11, 13]. A radiological population study carried out in the Yachiho-mura district showed a male/female ratio of 1.8 about the prevalence of cervical OPLL [13]. A CT-based study showed a prevalence of 8.3% in men and 3.4% in women, with a male/female ratio of 2.4 [11]. In a survey using the data from patients who underwent thyroid CT in Korea, the overall prevalence of cervical OPLL was 5.7% and the prevalence was 8.8% and 4.2% in men and women, respectively, with a male/female ratio of 2.1 [15]. Interestingly, the sex ratio of thoracic OPLL is opposite to that of cervical OPLL. A plain radiograph-based study of thoracic OPLL showed a prevalence of 0.25% for men and 0.74% for women, with a male/female ratio of 0.34 [12]. Moreover, a recent CT-based study showed a prevalence of 1.0% for men and 3.1% for women, with a male/female ratio of 0.32 [16].

Regarding the peak age of the onset of OPLL, cervical OPLL is often seen in people older than 50 years [6]. A CT-based study in Korea showed that age and cervical OPLL prevalence showed a significant positive correlation; the prevalence of cervical OPLL was higher in the 50s, with the over-70s age group having the highest prevalence rate [15]. Regarding thoracic OPLL, a CT-based study revealed that thoracic OPLL was noted after the age of 40 years, with the peak distribution found at the age of 60 years [16].

Several studies have provided evidence revealing the involvement of genetic factors in OPLL development. OPLL can be a secondary complication in patients with monogenic diseases, such as hypophosphatemic rickets, although the incidence is low amongst total OPLL cases. Hereditary hypophosphatemic rickets is caused by a mutation in one of the genes that control renal phosphate reabsorption such as *PHEX*, *FGF23*, *DMP1*, *ENPP1*, and *FAM20C* [17, 18]. Clinically, most cases of OPLL are idiopathic. Idiopathic OPLL is considered to be a multifactorial disease with both genetic and environmental factors contributing to its development and progression. Age [19], diabetes mellitus [20], obesity [19], and mechanical stress [21, 22] have been proposed as clinical and environmental risk factors. On the other hand, OPLL is known to have a strong genetic predisposition because a number of genetic studies, including sibling-pair linkage studies, candidate-gene association studies, and genome-wide association studies (GWAS) have shown several genes/loci that link to OPLL susceptibility [23–25]. There have been several reviews regarding genes associated with OPLL development, such as *FGF2*, *FGFR1*, *BMP2*, *BMP4*, *BMP9*, *VKORC1*, *TGF-beta1*, *ENPP1*, *TGFBR2*, *COL17A1*, *PTCH1*, *BID*, *COL6A1*, *COL11A2*, *IL15RA*, *TLR5*, *20p12*, *RUNX2*, *ACE*, *ESR1*, *ESR2*, *HLA* haplotype, *AHSG*, *RXRB*, *IL-1beta*, *VDR*, and *TGF-beta3* [10, 26–29]. More recently, a GWAS analysis conducted by a MHLW study group identified six

OPLL susceptibility loci [20p12.3 (rs2423294: $P = 1.10 \times 10^{-13}$), 8q23.1 (rs374810: $P = 1.88 \times 10^{-13}$), 12p11.22 (rs1979679: $P = 4.34 \times 10^{-12}$), 12p12.2 (rs11045000: $P = 2.95 \times 10^{-11}$), 8q23.3 (rs13279799: $P = 1.28 \times 10^{-10}$), and 6p21.1 (rs927485: $P = 9.40 \times 10^{-9}$)] [30]. However, to date, none of these genes has yet been proven as a functional gene responsible for the development of OPLL. Therefore, further genetic research is necessary to find specific genes that cause OPLL.

References

1. Key GA. On paraplegia depending on the ligament of the spine. Guys Hosp Rep. 1838;3:17–34.
2. Forestier J, Rotes-Querol J. Senile ankylosing hyperostosis of the spine. Ann Rheum Dis. 1950;9(4):321–30.
3. Tsukimoto H. A case report-autopsy of syndrome of compression spinal cord owing to ossification within spinal canal of cervical spines. Nippon Geka Hokan. 1960;29:1003–7.
4. Resnick D, Shapiro RF, Wiesner KB, Niwayama G, Utsinger PD, Shaul SR. Diffuse idiopathic skeletal hyperostosis (DISH) [ankylosing hyperostosis of forestier and Rotes-Querol]. Semin Arthritis Rheum. 1978;7(3):153–87.
5. Matsunaga S, Sakou T. Overview of epidemiology and genetics. In: Yonenobu K, Nakamura K, Toyama Y, editors. OPLL: ossification of the posterior longitudinal ligament. Tokyo: Springer Japan; 2006. p. 7–9.
6. Yoshimura N, Nagata K, Muraki S, Oka H, Yoshida M, Enyo Y, et al. Prevalence and progression of radiographic ossification of the posterior longitudinal ligament and associated factors in the Japanese population: a 3-year follow-up of the ROAD study. Osteoporos Int. 2014;25(3):1089–98.
7. Shingyouchi Y, Nagahama A, Niida M. Ligamentous ossification of the cervical spine in the late middle-aged Japanese men. Its relation to body mass index and glucose metabolism. Spine (Phila Pa 1976). 1996;21(21):2474–8.
8. Sasaki E, Ono A, Yokoyama T, Wada K, Tanaka T, Kumagai G, et al. Prevalence and symptom of ossification of posterior longitudinal ligaments in the Japanese general population. J Orthop Sci. 2014;19(3):405–11.
9. Inamasu J, Guiot BH, Sachs DC. Ossification of the posterior longitudinal ligament: an update on its biology, epidemiology, and natural history. Neurosurgery. 2006;58(6):1027–39; discussion 39
10. Stapleton CJ, Pham MH, Attenello FJ, Hsieh PC. Ossification of the posterior longitudinal ligament: genetics and pathophysiology. Neurosurg Focus. 2011;30(3):E6.
11. Fujimori T, Le H, Hu SS, Chin C, Pekmezci M, Schairer W, et al. Ossification of the posterior longitudinal ligament of the cervical spine in 3161 patients: a CT-based study. Spine (Phila Pa 1976). 2015;40(7):E394–403.
12. Ono M, Russell WJ, Kudo S, Kuroiwa Y, Takamori M, Motomura S, et al. Ossification of the thoracic posterior longitudinal ligament in a fixed population. Radiological and neurological manifestations. Radiology. 1982;143(2):469–74.
13. Ohtsuka K, Terayama K, Yanagihara M, Wada K, Kasuga K, Machida T, et al. A radiological population study on the ossification of the posterior longitudinal ligament in the spine. Arch Orthop Trauma Surg. 1987;106(2):89–93.
14. Fujimori T, Watabe T, Iwamoto Y, Hamada S, Iwasaki M, Oda T. Prevalence, concomitance, and distribution of ossification of the spinal ligaments: results of whole spine CT scans in 1500 Japanese patients. Spine (Phila Pa 1976). 2016;41(21):1668–76.
15. Sohn S, Chung CK, Yun TJ, Sohn CH. Epidemiological survey of ossification of the posterior longitudinal ligament in an adult Korean population: three-dimensional computed tomographic observation of 3,240 cases. Calcif Tissue Int. 2014;94(6):613–20.
16. Mori K, Imai S, Kasahara T, Nishizawa K, Mimura T, Matsusue Y. Prevalence, distribution, and morphology of thoracic ossification of the posterior longitudinal ligament in Japanese: results of CT-based cross-sectional study. Spine (Phila Pa 1976). 2014;39(5):394–9.
17. Takeyari S, Yamamoto T, Kinoshita Y, Fukumoto S, Glorieux FH, Michigami T, et al. Hypophosphatemic osteomalacia and bone sclerosis caused by a novel homozygous mutation of the FAM20C gene in an elderly man with a mild variant of Raine syndrome. Bone. 2014;67:56–62.
18. Jagtap VS, Sarathi V, Lila AR, Bandgar T, Menon P, Shah NS. Hypophosphatemic rickets. Indian J Endocrinol Metab. 2012;16(2):177–82.
19. Katsumi K, Watanabe K, Izumi T, Hirano T, Ohashi M, Mizouchi T, et al. Natural history of the ossification of cervical posterior longitudinal ligament: a three dimensional analysis. Int Orthop. 2018;42(4):835–42.
20. Akune T, Ogata N, Seichi A, Ohnishi I, Nakamura K, Kawaguchi H. Insulin secretory response is positively associated with the extent of ossification of the posterior longitudinal ligament of the spine. J Bone Joint Surg Am. 2001;83(10):1537–44.
21. Ota M, Furuya T, Maki S, Inada T, Kamiya K, Ijima Y, et al. Addition of instrumented fusion after posterior decompression surgery suppresses thickening of ossification of the posterior longitudinal ligament of the cervical spine. J Clin Neurosci. 2016;34:162–5.
22. Sawada T, Kishiya M, Kanemaru K, Seya K, Yokoyama T, Ueyama K, et al. Possible role of extracellular nucleotides in ectopic ossification of human spinal ligaments. J Pharmacol Sci. 2008;106(1):152–61.

23. Karasugi T, Nakajima M, Ikari K, Tsuji T, Matsumoto M, Chiba K, et al. A genome-wide sib-pair linkage analysis of ossification of the posterior longitudinal ligament of the spine. J Bone Miner Metab. 2013;31(2):136–43.
24. Nakamura I, Ikegawa S, Okawa A, Okuda S, Koshizuka Y, Kawaguchi H, et al. Association of the human NPPS gene with ossification of the posterior longitudinal ligament of the spine (OPLL). Hum Genet. 1999;104(6):492–7.
25. Koga H, Sakou T, Taketomi E, Hayashi K, Numasawa T, Harata S, et al. Genetic mapping of ossification of the posterior longitudinal ligament of the spine. Am J Hum Genet. 1998;62(6):1460–7.
26. Yan L, Gao R, Liu Y, He B, Lv S, Hao D. The pathogenesis of ossification of the posterior longitudinal ligament. Aging Dis. 2017;8(5):570–82.
27. Ikegawa S. Genetics of ossification of the posterior longitudinal ligament of the spine: a mini review. J Bone Metab. 2014;21(2):127–32.
28. Inoue I. Genetic study of ossification of the posterior longitudinal ligament of the spine. Tanpakushitsu kakusan koso. 2001;46(16 Suppl):2289–94.
29. Stetler WR, La Marca F, Park P. The genetics of ossification of the posterior longitudinal ligament. Neurosurg Focus. 2011;30(3):E7.
30. Nakajima M, Takahashi A, Tsuji T, Karasugi T, Baba H, Uchida K, et al. A genome-wide association study identifies susceptibility loci for ossification of the posterior longitudinal ligament of the spine. Nat Genet. 2014;46(9):1012–6.

3 OPLL: Disease Entity, Prevalence, Literature Research, and Growth

Takahito Fujimori

Abstract

Ossification of the spinal ligament is an ectopic bone formation of the spine. This hyperostotic condition was recognized by rheumatologists or radiologists in the nineteenth century. After a report of an autopsy case in 1960, ossification of the posterior longitudinal ligament (OPLL) became to be known as one of the causes of myelopathy. A pathological characteristic of OPLL is endochondral and intramembranous ossification despite mild disc degeneration. Radiographically, cervical OPLL was found from 1.9 to 6.3% in Japanese. Similarly, the prevalence of cervical OPLL was approximately 5% in Korean or Asian Americans. In Caucasian Americans, the prevalence of cervical OPLL was 1.3%. Various types of spinal ossification coexist in patients with hyperostosis. Thirty six percent of the patients with cervical OPLL had diffuse idiopathic skeletal hyperostosis (DISH). In Japanese, the prevalence was from 1.6 to 1.9% for thoracic OPLL, 12% for thoracolumbar DISH, and 23% for ossification of the nuchal ligament.

T. Fujimori (✉)
Department of Orthopedic Surgery, Japan Community Health care Organization, Osaka Hospital, Osaka, Japan

Keywords

OPLL · DISH · Ossification · Prevalence · CT · Japanese · Ethnic · Ligament · Myelopathy · Hyperostosis

3.1 Disease Entity

Compression of nerve tissue by the ossified spinal ligament was first reported by Key in 1838 in Britain [1]. In this literature, Key reported two cases of paraplegia assumed to be caused by ossification of the posterior longitudinal ligament (OPLL). However, this disease entity did not attract much attention until the 1900s.

In 1942, Oppenheimer, an American radiologist, called ossification of the anterior longitudinal ligament (OALL) of the vertebral body as "spondylitis ossificans ligamentosa" [2]. In 1950, Forestier, a French rheumatologist, propounded the concept of "ankylosing hyperostosis of the spine" [3]. Although they mentioned the possibility of OPLL as a cause of nerve disorder, the concept of the disease entity as a cause of myelopathy was not established.

In 1960, Tsukimoto, a Japanese orthopedic surgeon, reported an autopsy case clearly demonstrating that OPLL could compress the spinal cord [4]. After this report, there was a growing recognition of OPLL as a cause of myelopathy among Japanese orthopedic surgeons [5]. As the Asian population commonly has developmental canal

A. Okawa et al. (eds.), *OPLL*, https://doi.org/10.1007/978-981-15-3855-1_3

stenosis, such a bony space occupying lesion in the spinal canal can cause serious neurological damage. That time corresponded to the time when cervical spine surgeries became common in Japan. Various surgeries including laminoplasty were invented to conquer this disease [6, 7]. After establishment of the committee group of the Japanese Ministry of Health and Welfare in 1975, clinical and basic researches have been actively advanced. OPLL became to be recognized globally as one of the causes of myelopathy. The first chairman of the committee group, Tsuyama, classified cervical OPLL into four types: continuous, mixed, segmental, and localized [8]. This radiographic classification has been commonly used.

In this way, ossification of the spinal ligament has been investigated from the perspective of pathology, rheumatology, radiology, and clinical neurology. From the early 1900s, it has been pointed that these ossifications arise not only in the spine but also other joints. Many studies reported that OPLL coexists with ossification of OALL and other spinal ossifications [9–11]. In 1975, Resnick and Niwayama, an American radiologist and pathologist, proposed the concept of diffuse idiopathic skeletal hyperostosis (DISH) [12, 13]. From the perspective of the concept of disease, OPLL can be included in DISH focusing on ossification of the spinal ligament [13]. However, a critical point of OPLL is that OPLL can cause myelopathy. Although dysphagia or vertebral fractures are sometimes problematic in DISH [14], many patients with DISH do not have much disability [12, 13]. In clinical practice, OPLL is generally treated separately from DISH.

3.2 Prevalence

Historically the prevalence of OPLL has been examined in radiography. The prevalence of symptomatic myelopathy due to OPLL has been unknown. Many of the epidemiological studies were performed by Japanese researchers in 1970s. According to these reports, the prevalence of OPLL in the cervical spine found by plain radiograph in Japanese ranged from 1.9 to 4.3% [15–23]. The prevalence of OPLL in non-Japanese was examined in Asia, Europe, and the United States. In Asia, the prevalence of OPLL ranged from 0.8 to 3.0% [24–32]. In Europe or the United States, the prevalence ranged from 0.1 to 1.3% [29, 33–36].

Although plain radiography has advantages of simplicity and low radiation exposure, it has limited ability to detect unclear ossifications. Tsuzuki examined autopsied cervical spine in 376 Japanese patients. He reported that the prevalence of cervical OPLL was 12.5% over 40 years old [37].

Recently, computed tomography (CT) is more commonly used for epidemiological studies. Fujimori et al. examined the prevalence of ossification of the spinal ligament (with thickness ≥2 mm) by using whole body CT in Japan (Fig. 3.1). According to the study, the prevalence of cervical OPLL was 6.3% in Japanese [10]. In other CT-based studies, the prevalence of cervical OPLL was 5.7% in Korean [38] and 4.8% in an Asian Americans [39]. Outside Asian population, the prevalence of OPLL was examined in the United States. The prevalence of cervical OPLL was 1.3% in Caucasian Americans, 1.9% in Hispanic Americans, 2.1% in African Americans, and 3.2% in Native Americans [39] (Table 3.1). Some researchers reported that DISH was also more common in Native Americans than in Caucasian Americans [40, 41].

Thoracic OPLL is much rarer ossification than cervical OPLL. Mori et al. examined the prevalence of thoracic OPLL by using chest CT. The prevalence of thoracic OPLL was 1.9% [42]. Fujimori et al. reported that the prevalence of thoracic OPLL was 1.6% [10]. There is no data about the prevalence of thoracic OPLL in non-Japanese. Speculated from the results of the prevalence of OPLL in the cervical spine, thoracic OPLL would be a very rare disease in Caucasians.

Previous studies reported that men had approximately twice as much cervical OPLL as women [10]. However, as for thoracic OPLL, some studies suggested that women had more thoracic OPLL than men [42]. The nationwide multicenter study of surgical patients for thoracic OPLL included nearly an equal number of male and female patients [43].

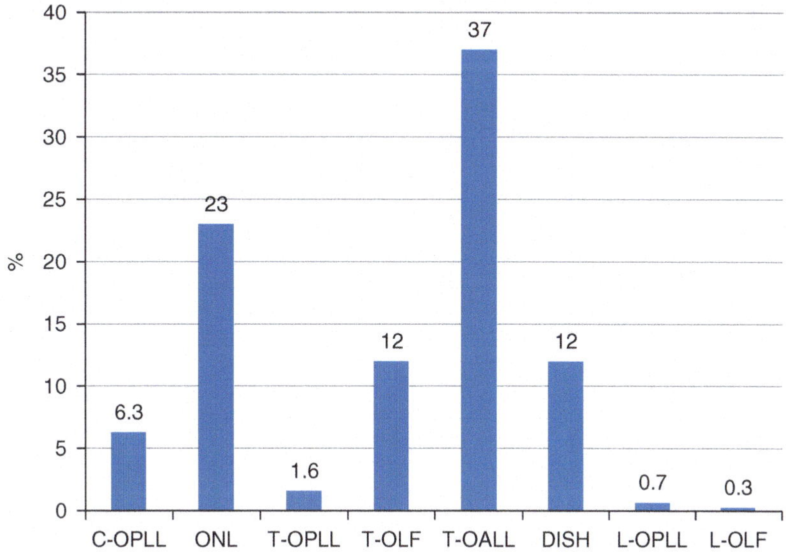

Fig. 3.1 The prevalence of spinal ligament ossification (*C* cervical, *DISH* diffuse idiopathic skeletal hyperostosis, *L* lumbar, *OALL* ossification of the anterior longitudinal ligament, *OLF* ossification of the ligamentum flavum, *ONL* ossification of the nuchal ligament, *OPLL* ossification of the posterior longitudinal ligament, *T* thoracic, *TL* thoracolumbar)

Table 3.1 Prevalence of OPLL by computed tomography

		Total	Male	Female	*N*	Reference
Cervical	Japanese	6.3	8.3	3.4	1500	[10, 39]
	Caucasian American	1.3	1.6	0.8	1593	
	Asian American	4.8	5.8	3.6	624	
	Hispanic American	1.9	1.5	3.1	472	
	African American	2.1	2.2	2	326	
	Native American	3.2	2.8	3.8	62	
	Korean	5.7	6.4	3.6	3240	[38]
Thoracic	Japanese	1.9	1.0	3.0	3013	[10]
	Japanese	1.6	1.4	2	1500	[42]

3.3 Type of OPLL

Generally, small ossifications are more frequently observed than large ossifications. Segmental type was the most common type of ossification. A CT-based study showed that 70% of OPLL found incidentally in general population were segmental types [10]. Continuous type and mixed type only accounted for 17% in total. However, this percentage was different in surgical candidates. In 64 surgically treated patients with a mean occupying ratio of 31%, 28% of the patients had continuous type, 48% had mixed type, and 20% had segmental type [44]. As for massive OPLL with an occupying ratio >60%, continuous type and mixed type accounted for 93% [45].

Recently, a new CT-based classification system was developed [46]. This system classifies OPLL based on three characteristics. Classification A: bridge or non-bridge, Classification B: vertebral or intervertebral, Classification C: central or lateral on axial image.

3.4 Location of OPLL

Cervical OPLL locates most frequently at C5, which is a site subject to degeneration [10, 47]. This distribution tendency suggests that degeneration is related to the onset of OPLL. Thoracic OPLL locates most frequently from T1 to T5 [8, 10, 42, 48] (Fig. 3.2).

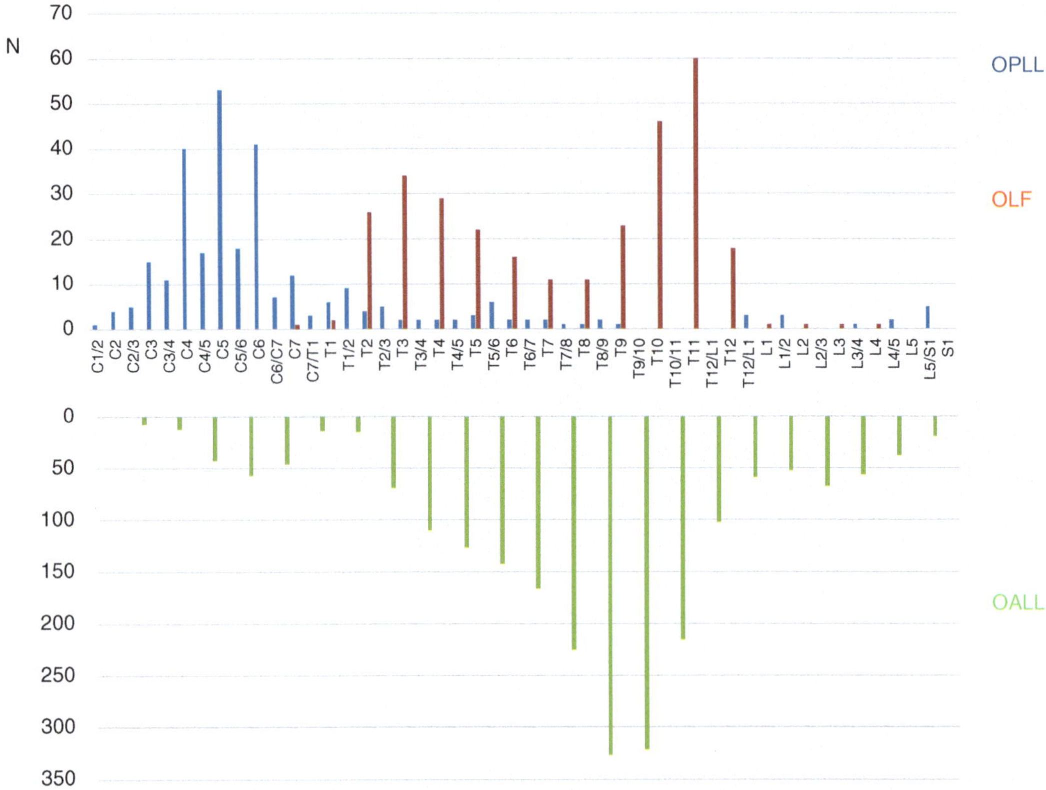

Fig. 3.2 Distribution of the OPLL, OLF, and OALL in the spine (*OALL* ossification of the anterior longitudinal ligament, *OLF* ossification of the ligamentum flavum, *OPLL* ossification of the posterior longitudinal ligament)

Prevalence of other types of ossification of the spinal ligament.

Various types of ossification of the spinal ligament coexist with OPLL [11, 22, 48–51]. A CT-based study in Japanese showed that 13% of cervical OPLL also had thoracic OPLL, 34% of cervical OPLL also had thoracic ossification of the ligamentum flavum, 36% of cervical OPLL also had DISH, and 45% of cervical OPLL also had ossification of the nuchal ligament [10]. According to the study, the prevalence of cervical OALL was 7.5% and that of DISH was 12%. The prevalence of ossification of the nuchal ligament was 23%. Kagotani et al. reported that the prevalence of DISH was 10.8% in Japan by using whole spine radiography [52].

3.5 Literature Review

Patients who need surgical treatment for OPLL usually have neurological symptoms like myelopathy and/or radiculopathy. Myelopathy arises from a complex combination of static compression and dynamic factor. Compression effect is divided into direct compression and ischemia through vascular disturbance [53]. Here, we discuss possible mechanism of ossification process as a cause of compression.

Posterior longitudinal ligament (PLL) is a fibrous connective tissue that connects the vertebral body to other ones. PLL locates in the spinal canal and covers the posterior surfaces of the vertebral bodies and consists of the superficial layer and the deep layer. These ligaments attach to the vertebral body through the enthesis. Ossification of ligament at the enthesis is called enthesophyte [13, 54, 55]. Enthesophyte is a kind of osteophyte that occurs as a physiologic response at the insertion of tendons and ligaments [54, 56, 57]. Endochondral ossification is observed in osteophytes. When a damage occurs at annulus fibrosus or longitudinal ligament, a repair reaction is induced. Transforming growth factor-β1 and basic fibroblast growth factor are related to formation of osteophytes [58]. These osteophytes can be considered to be an adaptive reaction of the intervertebral segment to cope with instability [56, 59, 60]. Osteophytes splint the spine and may play a compensatory role in the redistribution of forces to provide intervertebral protection. When these osteophytes are produced, substantial disc degeneration is usually observed at the segments [61]. However, in patients with OPLL or DISH, disc degeneration is mild despite the large size of ossifications [37, 61]. This tendency is more apparent in patients with continuous type of OPLL or in cases with DISH bridging multiple intervertebral segments. These ossifications cross the intervertebral segment while maintaining disc height. These phenomena suggest that patients with OPLL or DISH have an exaggerated response to stimuli which produce only modest new bone formation in others [12]. Some researchers called these characteristics as "bone formers" [54, 57]. It was reported that patients with spinal ligamentous ossification had higher bone mineral density [62]. Probably because of some abnormality of regulation mechanism, fibrocartilage layer becomes thicker and thicker and a bulky ossified cartilage is formed [63]. In OPLL, endochondral ossification is primarily observed [37, 61, 64, 65]. At the active proliferative site, angiogenesis and intramembranous ossification is also observed [37]. Predisposition to ostosis would be strong in large ossification like the continuous type of OPLL. In these ossifications, the superficial layer of PLL can ossify even skipping the deep layer [37]. On the other hand, in cases with mild-ostosis like the segmental type of OPLL, only the deep layer ossifies [37, 61]. It is sometimes difficult to differentiate these segmental ossifications from degenerative osteophyte because disc degeneration exists at the segment of OPLL. Some researchers advocated that these small segmental type ossifications should be treated differently in clinical practice from large OPLL that can cause myelopathy [37].

3.6 Growth

Although there were several reports about progression of OPLL after surgery [66–70], information about the natural course of progression of OPLL was limited [68, 69, 71]. The reasons for limited information could be: it is difficult to find premature OPLL because patients with premature OPLL have little symptoms. When patients visit clinic, growth may be nearly completed. Patients with large OPLL during the growth are likely to undergo surgery. Previous studies reported the following risk factors about the growth. Younger age [67–69, 72], mixed type or intervertebral segment with motion [70, 72], and surgical invasion especially laminoplasty or laminectomy [67, 73, 74]. It has been known that OPLL rarely grows once the intervertebral segment is fused [67, 70]. Recently, some physicians performed additional fusion surgery to prevent progression [75, 76]. Recent multidetector CT enabled three-dimensional visualization of the growth of OPLL [67, 77].

References

1. Key CA. Paraplegia depending on disease of the ligaments of the spine. Guys Hosp Rep. 1838;3:17–34.
2. Oppenheimer A. Calcification and ossification of vertebral ligaments (spondylitis ossificans ligamentosa). Roentegen study of patogenesis and clinical significance. Radiology. 1942;38:160–4.
3. Forestier J, Rotes-Querol J. Senile ankylosing hyperostosis of the spine. Ann Rheum Dis. 1950;9(4):321–30.
4. Tsukimoto H. A case report: autopsy of sydrome of compression of the spinal cord owing to ossification within cervical spinal canal. Arch Jap Chir. 1960;29:1003–7.
5. Onji Y, Akiyama H, Shimomura Y, Ono K, Hukuda S, Mizuno S. Posterior paravertebral ossification causing cervical myelopathy. A report of eighteen cases. J Bone Joint Surg Am. 1967;49(7):1314–28.
6. Hirabayashi K, Miyakawa J, Satomi K, Maruyama T, Wakano K. Operative results and postoperative pro-

gression of ossification among patients with ossification of cervical posterior longitudinal ligament. Spine (Phila Pa 1976). 1981;6(4):354–64.
7. Hirabayashi K, Toyama Y, Chiba K. Expansive laminoplasty for myelopathy in ossification of the longitudinal ligament. Clin Orthop Relat Res. 1999;359:35–48.
8. Tsuyama N. Ossification of the posterior longitudinal ligament of the spine. Clin Orthop Relat Res. 1984;184:71–84.
9. Kawaguchi Y, Nakano M, Yasuda T, Seki S, Hori T, Kimura T. Ossification of the posterior longitudinal ligament in not only the cervical spine, but also other spinal regions: analysis using multidetector computed tomography of the whole spine. Spine (Phila Pa 1976). 2013;38(23):E1477–82. https://doi.org/10.1097/BRS.0b013e3182a54f00.
10. Fujimori T, Watabe T, Iwamoto Y, Hamada S, Iwasaki M, Oda T. Prevalence, concomitance, and distribution of ossification of the spinal ligaments: results of whole spine CT scans in 1500 japanese patients. Spine (Phila Pa 1976). 2016;41(21):1668–76. https://doi.org/10.1097/BRS.0000000000001643.
11. Nishimura S, Nagoshi N, Iwanami A, Takeuchi A, Hirai T, Yoshii T, Takeuchi K, Mori K, Yamada T, Seki S, Tsuji T, Fujiyoshi K, Furukawa M, Wada K, Koda M, Furuya T, Matsuyama Y, Hasegawa T, Takeshita K, Kimura A, Abematsu M, Haro H, Ohba T, Watanabe M, Katoh H, Watanabe K, Ozawa H, Kanno H, Imagama S, Ando K, Fujibayashi S, Yamazaki M, Watanabe K, Matsumoto M, Nakamura M, Okawa A, Kawaguchi Y, Japanese Organization of the Study for Ossification of Spinal Ligament. Prevalence and distribution of diffuse idiopathic skeletal hyperostosis on whole-spine computed tomography in patients with cervical ossification of the posterior longitudinal ligament: a multicenter study. Clin Spine Surg. 2018;31(9):E460–5. https://doi.org/10.1097/BSD.0000000000000701.
12. Resnick D, Niwayama G. Radiographic and pathologic features of spinal involvement in diffuse idiopathic skeletal hyperostosis (DISH). Radiology. 1976;119(3):559–68. https://doi.org/10.1148/119.3.559.
13. Utsinger PD. Diffuse idiopathic skeletal hyperostosis. Clin Rheum Dis. 1985;11(2):325–51.
14. Paley D, Schwartz M, Cooper P, Harris WR, Levine AM. Fractures of the spine in diffuse idiopathic skeletal hyperostosis. Clin Orthop Relat Res. 1991;267:22–32.
15. Matsunaga S, Sakou T. Ossification of the posterior longitudinal ligament of the cervical spine: etiology and natural history. Spine (Phila Pa 1976). 2012;37(5):E309–14. https://doi.org/10.1097/BRS.0b013e318241ad33.
16. Ikata T, Tezuka S. Epidemiological study on the prevalence of ossification of the posterior longitudinal ligament. In: Investigation comittee report on the ossification of the spinal ligaments of the Japanese Ministry of Public health and Welfare; 1979. p. 24–7.
17. Ohtani K, Higuchi M, Watanabe T, Nakai S, Fujimura S, Manzoku S, Kosaka M, Shibazaki T, Tsubuku M, Saito T. Epidemiological study of ossification of the posterior longitudinal ligament of the cervical spine in Yaeyama Island of Okinawa. In: Investigation comittee report on the ossification of the spinal ligaments of the Japanese Ministry of Public Health and Welfare; 1980. p. 17–8.
18. Yamauchi H, Issei K, Endou A, Kameta I, Kondou A, Yamaguchi T. Comparative study on the prebalence of OPLL by plain X-ray film and heab metal content of hair between Chiba and Yamanashi. In: Investigation comittee report on the ossification of the spinal ligaments of the Japanese Ministry of Public Health and Welfare; 1982. p. 15–9.
19. Sakou T, Morimoto N. Epidemiological study of the cervical OPLL on islands Kagoshima. In: Investigation comittee report on the ossification of the spinal ligaments of the Japanese Ministry of Public Health and Welfare; 1982. p. 20–3.
20. Ohtsuka Y, Terayama K, Wada K, Kasuga K, Matsushima S, Machida T, Furukawa K. Epidemiological study of ossification of the spinal ligament on Yachiho in Nagano Prefecture. In: Investigation comittee report on the ossification of the spinal ligaments of the Japanese Ministry of Public Health and Welfare; 1984. p. 63–7.
21. Ikata T, Takada K, Murase M, Kashiwaguchi S. Epidemiological study on the prevalence of ossification of posterior longitudinal ligament of the cervical spine. In: Investigation comittee report on the ossification of the spinal ligaments of the Japanese Ministry of Public Health and Welfare; 1985. p. 61–5.
22. Ohtsuka K, Yanagihara M. The epidemiology of the hyperostosis of the spine. Seikeigeka MOOK. 1987;50:13–25.
23. Sasaki E, Ono A, Yokoyama T, Wada K, Tanaka T, Kumagai G, Iwasaki H, Takahashi I, Umeda T, Nakaji S, Ishibashi Y. Prevalence and symptom of ossification of posterior longitudinal ligaments in the Japanese general population. J Orthop Sci. 2014;19(3):405–11. https://doi.org/10.1007/s00776-014-0552-0.
24. Kurokawa T. Prevalence of ossification of the posterior longitudinal ligament of the cervical spine in Taiwan, Hong Kong, and Singapore. In: Investigation comittee report on the ossification of the spinal ligaments of the Japanese Ministry of Public Health and Welfare; 1978. p. 8–9.
25. Yamaura I, Kamikozuru M, Shinomiya K. Therapeutic modalities and epidemiological study of ossification of the posterior longitudinal ligament of the cervical spine. In: Investigation comittee report on the ossification of the spinal ligaments of the Japanese Ministry of Public Health and Welfare; 1978. p. 18–20.
26. Yamauchi H. Epidemiological and pathological study of ossification of the posterior longitudinal ligament of the cervical spine. In: Investigation comittee report on the ossification of the spinal ligaments of the Japanese Ministry of Public Health and Welfare; 1978. p. 21–5.

27. Tezuka S. Epidemiological study of ossification of the posterior longitudinal ligament of the cervical spine in Taiwan. In: Investigation comittee report on the ossification of the spinal ligaments of the Japanese Ministry of Public Health and Welfare; 1980. p. 19–23.
28. Lee T, Chacha PB, Khoo J. Ossification of posterior longitudinal ligament of the cervical spine in non-Japanese Asians. Surg Neurol. 1991;35(1):40–4.
29. Izawa K. Comparative roentgenographical study on the incidence of ossification of the posterior longitudinal ligament and other degenerative changes of the cervical spine among Japanese, Koreans, Americans and Germans. Nihon Seikeigeka Gakkai Zasshi. 1980;54(5):461–74.
30. Terayama K, Ohtsuka K, Merlini L, Albisinni U, Gui L. Ossification of the spinal ligament. A radiographic reevaluation in Bologna. Italy Nihon Seikeigeka Gakkai Zasshi. 1987;61(12):1373–8.
31. Harata S, Ueyama K, Ichikawa S, Ito J, Sato T, Mito A, Den I, Yamada S, Tomita T, Sakou T. Epidemiologic study of ossification of the posterior longitudinal ligament of the cervical spine in China. Rinsho Seikeigeka. 1994;29(6):671–6.
32. Liu KC. Epidemiological study on ossification of the posterior longitudinal ligament (OPLL) in the cervical spine—comparison of the prevalency between Japanese and Taiwanese. J Jpn Orthop Ass. 1990;64(5):401–8.
33. Yamauchi H, Izawa K, Sasaki K, Noromoto T, Honda H, Kusue K. Radiological examination by plain film of the cervical spine in West Germany. In: Investigation comittee report on the ossification of the spinal ligaments of the Japanese Ministry of Public Health and Welfare; 1979. p. 22–3.
34. Terayama K, Ohtsuka Y. Epidemiological study of ossification of the posterior longitudinal ligament on Bologna in Italy. In: Investigation comittee report on the ossification of the spinal ligaments of the Japanese Ministry of Public health and Welfare; 1984. p. 55–62.
35. Ijiri K, Sakou T, Taketomi E, Matsunaga S. Epidemiological study of ossification of the posterior longitudinal ligament in Utah. In: Investigation comittee report on the ossification of the spinal ligaments of the Japanese Ministry of Public Health and Welfare; 1996. p. 8–9.
36. Firooznia H, Benjamin VM, Pinto RS, Golimbu C, Rafii M, Leitman BS, McCauley DI. Calcification and ossification of posterior longitudinal ligament of spine: its role in secondary narrowing of spinal canal and cord compression. N Y State J Med. 1982;82(8):1193–8.
37. Tsuzuki N. Ossification of the posterior longitudinal ligament of the cervical spine: its incidence and histopathology. Jpn Dtshc Med Berichte. 1987;32(1):11–22.
38. Sohn S, Chung CK, Yun TJ, Sohn CH. Epidemiological survey of ossification of the posterior longitudinal ligament in an adult Korean population: three-dimensional computed tomographic observation of 3,240 cases. Calcif Tissue Int. 2014;94(6):613–20. https://doi.org/10.1007/s00223-014-9846-7.
39. Fujimori T, Le H, Hu SS, Chin C, Pekmezci M, Schairer W, Tay BK, Hamasaki T, Yoshikawa H, Iwasaki M. Ossification of the posterior longitudinal ligament of the cervical spine in 3161 patients: a CT-based study. Spine (Phila Pa 1976). 2015;40(7):E394–403. https://doi.org/10.1097/BRS.0000000000000791.
40. Henrard JC, Bennett PH. Epidemiological study of vertebral hyperostosis. Survey in an adult population of American Indians. Rev Rhum Mal Osteoartic. 1973;40(10):581–91.
41. Spagnola AM, Bennett PH, Terasaki PI. Vertebral ankylosing hyperostosis (Forestier's disease) and HLA antigens in Pima Indians. Arthritis Rheum. 1978;21(4):467–72.
42. Mori K, Imai S, Kasahara T, Nishizawa K, Mimura T, Matsusue Y. Prevalence, distribution, and morphology of thoracic ossification of the posterior longitudinal ligament in japanese: results of CT-based cross-sectional study. Spine (Phila Pa 1976). 2014;39(5):394–9. https://doi.org/10.1097/BRS.0000000000000153.
43. Imagama S, Ando K, Takeuchi K, Kato S, Murakami H, Aizawa T, Ozawa H, Hasegawa T, Matsuyama Y, Koda M, Yamazaki M, Chikuda H, Shindo S, Nakagawa Y, Kimura A, Takeshita K, Wada K, Katoh H, Watanabe M, Yamada K, Furuya T, Tsuji T, Fujibayashi S, Mori K, Kawaguchi Y, Watanabe K, Matsumoto M, Yoshii T, Okawa A. Perioperative complications after surgery for thoracic ossification of posterior longitudinal ligament: a nationwide multicenter prospective study. Spine (Phila Pa 1976). 2018;43(23):E1389–97. https://doi.org/10.1097/BRS.0000000000002703.
44. Iwasaki M, Kawaguchi Y, Kimura T, Yonenobu K. Long-term results of expansive laminoplasty for ossification of the posterior longitudinal ligament of the cervical spine: more than 10 years follow up. J Neurosurg. 2002;96(2 Suppl):180–9.
45. Fujimori T, Iwasaki M, Okuda S, Takenaka S, Kashii M, Kaito T, Yoshikawa H. Long-term results of cervical myelopathy due to ossification of the posterior longitudinal ligament with an occupying ratio of 60% or more. Spine (Phila Pa 1976). 2014;39(1):58–67. https://doi.org/10.1097/BRS.0000000000000054.
46. Kawaguchi Y, Matsumoto M, Iwasaki M, Izumi T, Okawa A, Matsunaga S, Chiba K, Tsuji T, Yamazaki M, Fujimori T, Yoshii T, Toyama Y. New classification system for ossification of the posterior longitudinal ligament using CT images. J Orthop Sci. 2014;19(4):530–6. https://doi.org/10.1007/s00776-014-0577-4.
47. Hirai T, Yoshii T, Iwanami A, Takeuchi K, Mori K, Yamada T, Wada K, Koda M, Matsuyama Y, Takeshita K, Abematsu M, Haro H, Watanabe M, Watanabe K, Ozawa H, Kanno H, Imagama S, Fujibayashi S, Yamazaki M, Matsumoto M, Nakamura M, Okawa A, Kawaguchi Y. Prevalence and distribution of ossi-

fied lesions in the whole spine of patients with cervical ossification of the posterior longitudinal ligament a multicenter study (JOSL CT study). PLoS One. 2016;11(8):e0160117. https://doi.org/10.1371/journal.pone.0160117.
48. Hirai T, Yoshii T, Nagoshi N, Takeuchi K, Mori K, Ushio S, Iwanami A, Yamada T, Seki S, Tsuji T, Fujiyoshi K, Furukawa M, Nishimura S, Wada K, Furuya T, Matsuyama Y, Hasegawa T, Takeshita K, Kimura A, Abematsu M, Haro H, Ohba T, Watanabe M, Katoh H, Watanabe K, Ozawa H, Kanno H, Imagama S, Ando K, Fujibayashi S, Koda M, Yamazaki M, Matsumoto M, Nakamura M, Okawa A, Kawaguchi Y. Distribution of ossified spinal lesions in patients with severe ossification of the posterior longitudinal ligament and prediction of ossification at each segment based on the cervical OP index classification: a multicenter study (JOSL CT study). BMC Musculoskelet Disord. 2018;19(1):107. https://doi.org/10.1186/s12891-018-2009-7.
49. Yoshii T, Hirai T, Iwanami A, Nagoshi N, Takeuchi K, Mori K, Yamada T, Seki S, Tsuji T, Fujiyoshi K, Furukawa M, Nishimura S, Wada K, Koda M, Furuya T, Matsuyama Y, Hasegawa T, Takeshita K, Kimura A, Abematsu M, Haro H, Ohba T, Watanabe M, Katoh H, Watanabe K, Ozawa H, Kanno H, Imagama S, Ando K, Fujibayashi S, Matsumoto M, Nakamura M, Yamazaki M, Okawa A, Kawaguchi Y. Co-existence of ossification of the nuchal ligament is associated with severity of ossification in the whole spine in patients with cervical ossification of the posterior longitudinal ligament—a multicenter CT study. J Orthop Sci. 2018; https://doi.org/10.1016/j.jos.2018.08.009.
50. Mori K, Yoshii T, Hirai T, Iwanami A, Takeuchi K, Yamada T, Seki S, Tsuji T, Fujiyoshi K, Furukawa M, Nishimura S, Wada K, Koda M, Furuya T, Matsuyama Y, Hasegawa T, Takeshita K, Kimura A, Abematsu M, Haro H, Ohba T, Watanabe M, Katoh H, Watanabe K, Ozawa H, Kanno H, Imagama S, Ito Z, Fujibayashi S, Yamazaki M, Matsumoto M, Nakamura M, Okawa A, Kawaguchi Y. Prevalence and distribution of ossification of the supra/interspinous ligaments in symptomatic patients with cervical ossification of the posterior longitudinal ligament of the spine: a CT-based multicenter cross-sectional study. BMC Musculoskelet Disord. 2016;17(1):492. https://doi.org/10.1186/s12891-016-1350-y.
51. Shingyouchi Y, Nagahama A, Niida M. Ligamentous ossification of the cervical spine in the late middle-aged Japanese men. Its relation to body mass index and glucose metabolism. Spine (Phila Pa 1976). 1996;21(21):2474–8.
52. Kagotani R, Yoshida M, Muraki S, Oka H, Hashizume H, Yamada H, Enyo Y, Nagata K, Ishimoto Y, Teraguchi M, Tanaka S, Nakamura K, Kawaguchi H, Akune T, Yoshimura N. Prevalence of diffuse idiopathic skeletal hyperostosis (DISH) of the whole spine and its association with lumbar spondylosis and knee osteoarthritis: the ROAD study. J Bone Miner Metab. 2015;33(2):221–9. https://doi.org/10.1007/s00774-014-0583-9.
53. Levine DN. Pathogenesis of cervical spondylotic myelopathy. J Neurol Neurosurg Psychiatry. 1997;62(4):334–40.
54. Rogers J, Shepstone L, Dieppe P. Bone formers: osteophyte and enthesophyte formation are positively associated. Ann Rheum Dis. 1997;56(2):85–90.
55. Hotta Y. Anatomical study of the yellow ligament of spine with special reference to its ossification. J Jpn Orthop Ass. 1985;59(3):311–25.
56. Menkes CJ, Lane NE. Are osteophytes good or bad? Osteoarthritis Cartilage. 2004;12(Suppl A):S53–4.
57. Hardcastle SA, Dieppe P, Gregson CL, Arden NK, Spector TD, Hart DJ, Edwards MH, Dennison EM, Cooper C, Williams M, Davey Smith G, Tobias JH. Osteophytes, enthesophytes, and high bone mass: a bone-forming triad with potential relevance in osteoarthritis. Arthritis Rheumatol. 2014;66(9):2429–39. https://doi.org/10.1002/art.38729.
58. Uchino M, Izumi T, Tominaga T, Wakita R, Minehara H, Sekiguchi M, Itoman M. Growth factor expression in the osteophytes of the human femoral head in osteoarthritis. Clin Orthop Relat Res. 2000;377:119–25.
59. Al-Rawahi M, Luo J, Pollintine P, Dolan P, Adams MA. Mechanical function of vertebral body osteophytes, as revealed by experiments on cadaveric spines. Spine (Phila Pa 1976). 2011;36(10):770–7. https://doi.org/10.1097/BRS.0b013e3181df1a70.
60. van der Kraan PM, van den Berg WB. Osteophytes: relevance and biology. Osteoarthr Cartil. 2007;15(3):237–44. https://doi.org/10.1016/j.joca.2006.11.006.
61. Tanaka N. Histopathological studies of the osteophytes and the ossification of the posterior longitudinal ligament in the cervical spine. J Jpn Orthop Ass. 1985;60(3):323–36.
62. Kim KW, Oh YM, Eun JP. Increased prevalence of ossification of posterior longitudinal ligament and increased bone mineral density in patients with ossification of nuchal ligament. Korean J Spine. 2016;13(3):139–43. https://doi.org/10.14245/kjs.2016.13.3.139.
63. Terayama K. Diffuse idiopathic skeletal hyperostosis and ossification of the posterior longitudinal ligament. Bessatsu Seikeigeka. 2004;45:2–6.
64. Ono K, Ota H, Tada K, Hamada H, Takaoka K. Ossified posterior longitudinal ligament: a clinicopathologic study. Spine (Phila Pa 1976). 1977;2(2):126–38.
65. Ono K, Yonenobu K, Miyamoto S, Okada K. Pathology of ossification of the posterior longitudinal ligament and ligamentum flavum. Clin Orthop Relat Res. 1999;359:18–26.
66. Chiba K, Yamamoto I, Hirabayashi H, Iwasaki M, Goto H, Yonenobu K, Toyama Y. Multicenter study investigating the postoperative progression of ossification of the posterior longitudinal ligament in the cervical spine: a new computer-assisted measurement. J Neurosurg Spine. 2005;3(1):17–23. https://doi.org/10.3171/spi.2005.3.1.0017.

67. Fujimori T, Iwasaki M, Nagamoto Y, Ishii T, Sakaura H, Kashii M, Yoshikawa H, Sugamoto K. Three-dimensional measurement of growth of ossification of the posterior longitudinal ligament. J Neurosurg Spine. 2012;16(3):289–95. https://doi.org/10.3171/2011.11.SPINE11502.
68. Hori T, Kawaguchi Y, Kimura T. How does the ossification area of the posterior longitudinal ligament progress after cervical laminoplasty? Spine (Phila Pa 1976). 2006;31(24):2807–12. https://doi.org/10.1097/01.brs.0000245870.97231.65.
69. Hori T, Kawaguchi Y, Kimura T. How does the ossification area of the posterior longitudinal ligament thicken following cervical laminoplasty? Spine (Phila Pa 1976). 2007;32(19):E551–6. https://doi.org/10.1097/BRS.0b013e31814614f3.
70. Lee DH, Cho JH, Kim NH, Kim S, Choi J, Hwang CJ, Lee CS. Radiological risk factors for progression of ossification of posterior longitudinal ligament following laminoplasty. Spine J. 2018;18(7):1116–21. https://doi.org/10.1016/j.spinee.2017.10.069.
71. Katsumi K, Watanabe K, Izumi T, Hirano T, Ohashi M, Mizouchi T, Ito T, Endo N. Natural history of the ossification of cervical posterior longitudinal ligament: a three dimensional analysis. Int Orthop. 2018;42(4):835–42. https://doi.org/10.1007/s00264-017-3667-z.
72. Kawaguchi Y, Kanamori M, Ishihara H, Nakamura H, Sugimori K, Tsuji H, Kimura T. Progression of ossification of the posterior longitudinal ligament following en bloc cervical laminoplasty. J Bone Joint Surg Am. 2001;83-A(12):1798–802.
73. Lee CH, Jahng TA, Hyun SJ, Kim KJ, Kim HJ. Expansive laminoplasty versus laminectomy alone versus laminectomy and fusion for cervical ossification of the posterior longitudinal ligament: is there a difference in the clinical outcome and sagittal alignment? Clin Spine Surg. 2016;29(1):E9–15. https://doi.org/10.1097/BSD.0000000000000058.
74. Lee CH, Sohn MJ, Lee CH, Choi CY, Han SR, Choi BW. Are there differences in the progression of ossification of the posterior longitudinal ligament following laminoplasty versus fusion?: A meta-analysis. Spine (Phila Pa 1976). 2017;42(12):887–94. https://doi.org/10.1097/BRS.0000000000001933.
75. Katsumi K, Izumi T, Ito T, Hirano T, Watanabe K, Ohashi M. Posterior instrumented fusion suppresses the progression of ossification of the posterior longitudinal ligament: a comparison of laminoplasty with and without instrumented fusion by three-dimensional analysis. Eur Spine J. 2016;25(5):1634–40. https://doi.org/10.1007/s00586-015-4328-9.
76. Ota M, Furuya T, Maki S, Inada T, Kamiya K, Ijima Y, Saito J, Takahashi K, Yamazaki M, Aramomi M, Mannoji C, Koda M. Addition of instrumented fusion after posterior decompression surgery suppresses thickening of ossification of the posterior longitudinal ligament of the cervical spine. J Clin Neurosci. 2016;34:162–5. https://doi.org/10.1016/j.jocn.2016.06.013.
77. Izumi T, Hirano T, Watanabe K, Sano A, Ito T, Endo N. Three-dimensional evaluation of volume change in ossification of the posterior longitudinal ligament of the cervical spine using computed tomography. Eur Spine J. 2013;22(11):2569–74. https://doi.org/10.1007/s00586-013-2989-9.

4 Natural History of Ossification of the Posterior Longitudinal Ligament (OPLL)

Shunji Matsunaga

Abstract

Ossification of the posterior longitudinal ligament (OPLL) is an important disease-causing spinal cord symptom. The timing of surgery and indication of preventive surgery have yet to be concluded. The main cause is the lack of research on the natural history of the onset of spinal cord symptoms of this disease. The author will introduce the research results of the single- and the multicenter facilities that have been conducted on the natural history of the clinical symptoms of OPLL and also mention the predictive factors of the onset of neurological symptoms in this disease. The Kaplan–Meier estimate of myelopathy-free survival among patients without myelopathy at the first visit was 71% at 30 years follow-up. The author examined the risk factor for the development of myelopathy in patients with asymptomatic ossification of the posterior longitudinal ligament by a multicenter prospective study. On univariate and multivariate logistic regression analysis, the development of myelopathy was significantly associated with spinal canal stenosis ratio, large range of motion of the cervical spine, and lateral-deviated type OPLL. The knowledge of natural history of this disease is essential for the treatment of this disease and further research in All Japan is desired in the future.

S. Matsunaga (✉)
Department of Orthopaedic Surgery, Imakiire General Hospital, Kagoshima, Japan
e-mail: shunji@imakiire.or.jp

Keywords

Ossification of the posterior longitudinal ligament · Natural history · Risk factor for development of myelopathy

Ossification of the posterior longitudinal ligament (OPLL) is an important disease-causing spinal cord symptom [1–5]. This disease was first reported by Key about 180 years ago [6]. Many reports on the epidemiology, etiology, and treatment of this disease have been published since this report. The epidemiological investigation of this disease is mainly performed in Japan, and the prevalence of OPLL in general Japanese population is reported to be 1.9–4.3% [7], which is not a rare disease. Studies on the etiology of OPLL are known to have a genetic background by family survey and twin survey [8–13]. Several disease candidate genes for OPLL have been discovered in recent genetic analyses performed in All Japan [14–17]. In the near future, the etiology of this disease will be elucidated.

Surgical treatment is selected for patients with severe neurologic deficits due to OPLL. Various surgical procedures have been reported and satisfactory results are obtained. However, the timing of surgery and indication of preventive surgery have yet to be concluded. The main cause is the

A. Okawa et al. (eds.), *OPLL*, https://doi.org/10.1007/978-981-15-3855-1_4

lack of research on the natural history of the onset of spinal cord symptoms of this disease. A huge OPLL may be found in a cervical X-ray taken by chance in a patient who has no neurological symptoms at all. To clarify, the natural history of this disease is essential for determining the timing of surgery and the indication of preventive surgery for this disease. In this chapter, the author will introduce the research results of the single- and the multicenter facilities that have been conducted on the natural history of the clinical symptoms of OPLL and also mention the predictive factors of the onset of neurological symptoms in this disease.

4.1 Clinical Presentation of the First Nationwide Survey in Japan

Several papers on the clinical characteristics of OPLL have been published [4, 5, 18, 19]. The clinical characteristics of patients with OPLL in papers of Japanese and foreign researchers have been similar. Terayama, a previous member of the Investigation Committee on Ossification of the Spinal Ligaments of Japanese Ministry of Public Health and Welfare, performed the first national survey of OPLL in 1975 [19]. Investigators abstracted 880 hospitals, including university hospitals, for this survey, and 2142 OPLL patients were registered. Based on the results of this survey, OPLL typically developed in patients older than 40 years and carried a male predominance of 2:1–3:1. The average age of onset was 51.2 years in men and 48.9 years in women. Sixty-seven percent of patients were 45–65 years old. Ninety-five percent of patients had some clinical symptoms, but 5% of patients were free of symptoms. Initial complaints typically consisted of cervical discomfort in conjunction with numbness of the upper extremity. The typically recognized symptoms of OPLL were as follows: sensory and motor dysfunction of upper and lower extremities, hyperreflexia of tendon reflexes, pathologic reflexes, and bladder dysfunction. As many as 16.8% of patients needed assistance in activities of daily living; 5.4% of patients showed a rapid aggravation of symptoms; and 11.4% of patients showed a chronic aggravation. Symptoms spontaneously appeared and continually progressed. In cases in which quadriparesis had rapidly evolved, sphincteric dysfunction was often also noted. Twenty-three percent of patients had a history of trauma to the cervical region [19]. Trauma in the cervical spine may have precipitated the onset of symptoms, which, in some cases, included quadriparesis [20–22]. However, in the prospective investigation for 368 OPLL patients without myelopathy at the time of initial consultation, only six patients (2%) subsequently develop trauma-induced myelopathy [23]. Patient education to avoid trauma due to falls in patients with this disease is considered important.

OPLL was mostly found at the C4, C5, and C6 levels. The level with the maximal thickness of OPLL was often C5. OPLL in the cervical spine may be radiographically classified into four types [19] based on the findings on a lateral radiograph: continuous, mixed, segmental, and other. When ossification is interrupted at the intervertebral disc levels but is continuous behind the vertebral bodies, this is characterized as segmental type. If ossification is not interrupted, this constitutes the continuous type. The segmental type was recognized in 39%, continuous in 27%, mixed in 26%, and other in 7%. The sagittal diameter of the spinal canal is measured as the distance from the posterior aspect of the vertebral body to the anterior edge of the base of the spinous process on the lateral view. This distance is regarded as the anteroposterior diameter of the cervical canal. The percentage of the thickness of the ossification to the anteroposterior diameter of the spinal canal is then regarded as the maximum spinal canal stenosis rate (Fig. 4.1). The maximum spinal canal stenosis rate, as determined at the thickest point of the ossified area, was 38% on average in cases with myelopathy and 27% in cases without myelopathy. However, the thickness of ossification was not always associated with the degree of neurologic dysfunction, that is, paralysis. Even if ossification is severe within the canal, neurologic symptoms are sometimes mild.

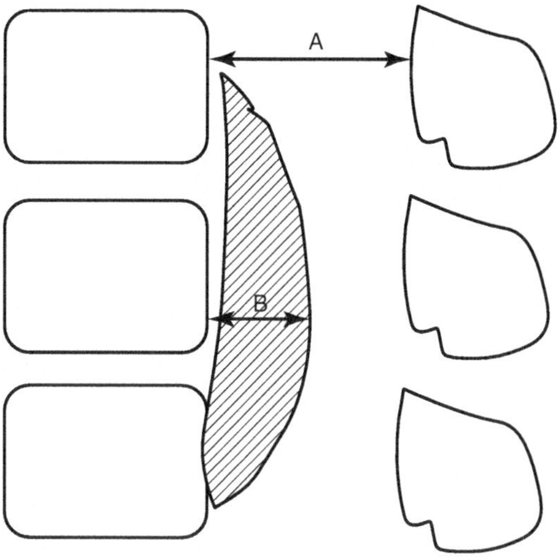

Fig. 4.1 Method of calculation of the maximum canal stenosis ratio by OPLL on a plain roentgenogram (the ratio (%) = B cm/A cm × 100)

OPLL in the cervical spine is often accompanied by ossification in the thoracic or lumbar spine and may be complicated by ossification of the ligamentum flavum in the thoracic spine or ankylosing vertebral hyperostosis [24]. In our private series of 166 cases of OPLL in the cervical spine, 28 (17%) were complicated by thoracic OPLL and 85 (51%) by ossification of the ligamentum flavum in the thoracic or lumbar spine. Sixty-eight cases (41%) had radiographic features of ankylosing vertebral hyperostosis (stage II changes by Forestier classification [24]), affecting more than three vertebral bodies. Furthermore, ligamentous ossification of hip and ankle joints may also be found in these individuals, suggesting that they are indeed systemically predisposed to diffuse ossification of ligaments (DISH) [25, 26].

4.2 Progression of Ossification

Few studies have prospectively evaluated the progression of OPLL. One hundred and twelve patients with OPLL, who had been treated conservatively, were studied (75 men and 37 women) [27]. They ranged in age from 27 to 78 years (mean, 54.5 years), and they were followed for 1–16.9 years. Progression of ossification in length was demonstrated in 24% of patients and in thickness, in 13% of patients in the group followed over 5 years. However, the amount of progression was small. The maximum progression in length was 43 mm over 10 years in one case of continuous OPLL (equivalent to the height of two vertebral bodies), and 3.4 mm in thickness. The type of ossification changed in some instances. The continuous type changed to the mixed type in three cases. The segmental type changed to the mixed type in three cases and to the continuous type in three cases, whereas the mixed type was altered to the continuous type in one instance. In our biomechanical study, progression of OPLL was recognized at the site of increased strain in intervertebral disc [28]. Progression of ossification did not always lead to aggravation of symptoms although there were some instances of worsening. The course of ossification in 94 patients who had surgery was carefully followed [27]. There were 75 men and 19 women included in this cohort, whose ages ranged from 23 to 79 years (mean, 54.8 years). Follow-up periods varied from 8.9 years for anterior decompressions and arthrodesis, 2.5 years for laminoplasties, and 6.6 years after laminectomy. Ossification progressed markedly and at a higher rate in laminectomy-(40%) and in laminoplasty-treated (35%) patients and appeared in relatively shorter intervals after these surgical procedures, that is, earliest within 2 months after surgery and most often within 6 months. The frequency of the ossification progression was shown to be higher in laminectomy- or laminoplasty-treated patients when compared with conservatively treated individuals [29, 30]. Possible explanations include (a) mechanical stress becoming increased in the cervical spine due to destruction of the posterior supportive elements, and (b) biologic stimulation produced by the laminoplasty or laminectomy.

4.3 Natural History of Clinical Symptom of OPLL

The prognosis of patients with OPLL has generally been thought to be disappointing. The author examined the natural course of this disease [31]. In our final follow-up study [32], a total of 450 patients, averaging 72.6 years of age at last evaluation, were prospectively followed for an average of 17.6 years (10–30 years) to discern the natural history of disease progression. Myelopathy was originally recognized in 127 patients, 91 of whom were managed surgically. The remaining 36 myelopathic patients were treated conservatively, and an increase in myelopathy was observed in 23 (65%) of these individuals. For the 323 patients without original myelopathy, 64 (20%) became myelopathic during the follow-up interval. The Kaplan–Meier estimate [33] of myelopathy-free survival among patients without myelopathy at the first visit was 71% at 30 years follow-up (Fig. 4.2). Forty-five patients with more than 60% of the spinal canal compromised by OPLL were all myelopathic. The range of motion of the cervical spine was calculated by dynamic X-rays (Fig. 4.3). The range of motion was significantly larger in patients with myelopathy and with less than 60% of the canal compromised with OPLL (Table 4.1). Although myelopathy was recognized in all patients with more than 60% of the spinal canal compromised by OPLL, small OPLL at first examination rarely developed to large OPLL with more than 60% stenosis during the follow-up. Therefore, one cannot simply say that myelopathy develops with OPLL. Rather, dynamic factors (range of motion) appear to be very important for the evolution of myelopathy in patients with less than 60% of the canal compromised with OPLL. Data from this long-term prospective analysis indicate that prophylactic surgery for non-myelopathic patients with OPLL may not be necessary, particularly because the course of symptomatic progression appears milder than anticipated. However, surgical results for OPLL patients who have trauma-induced myelopathy are far from satisfactory [22]. The study for risk factors for development of myelopathy in patients with OPLL is important.

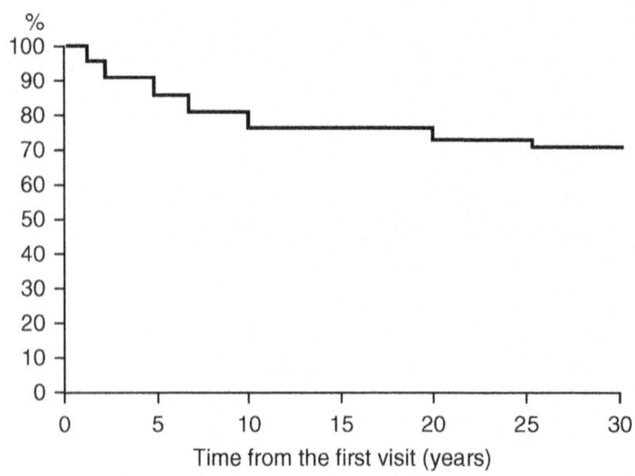

Fig. 4.2 Graph demonstrating results of Kaplan–Meier estimate regarding myelopathy-free rates in patients without myelopathy at initial examination method. Reprinted with permission from Shunji Matsunaga et al. J Neurosurgery (Spine 3) 2004; 100: 245–248

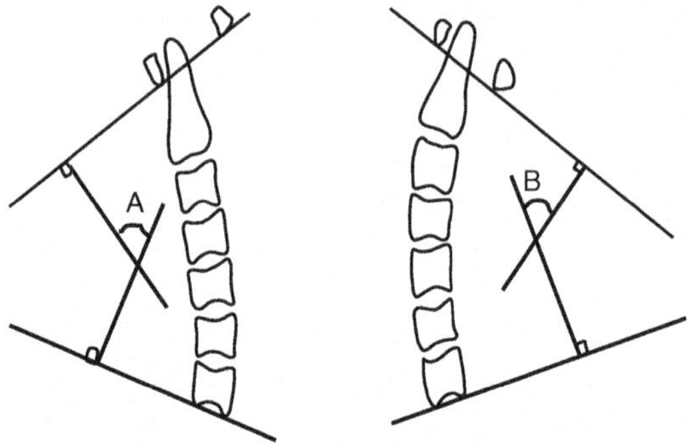

Fig. 4.3 Method of calculation of the range of motion of the cervical spine (α). (**a**) C2/C7 angle on the maximum anterior flexion position. (**b**) C2/C7 angle on the maximum posterior flexion position α = A + B. Reprinted with permission from Shunji Matsunaga et al. J Neurosurgery (Spine 2) 2002; 96: 168–172

Table 4.1 Range of motion of cervical spine of patients with or without myelopathy among patients with less than 60% canal stenosis

	With myelopathy (n = 137)	Without myelopathy (n = 268)	P value
Mean(SD) range of motion of cervical spine (degree)	75.6 (18.3)	36.5 (15.9)	<0.05

Reprinted with permission from Shunji Matsunaga et al. J Neurosurgery (Spine 3) 2004;100:245–248

A multicenter prospective study for development of myelopathy in patients with asymptomatic OPLL by the Investigation Committee on Ossification of the Spinal Ligaments of Japanese Ministry of Public Health and Welfare was performed in 2012 [34]. A total of 109 OPLL patients

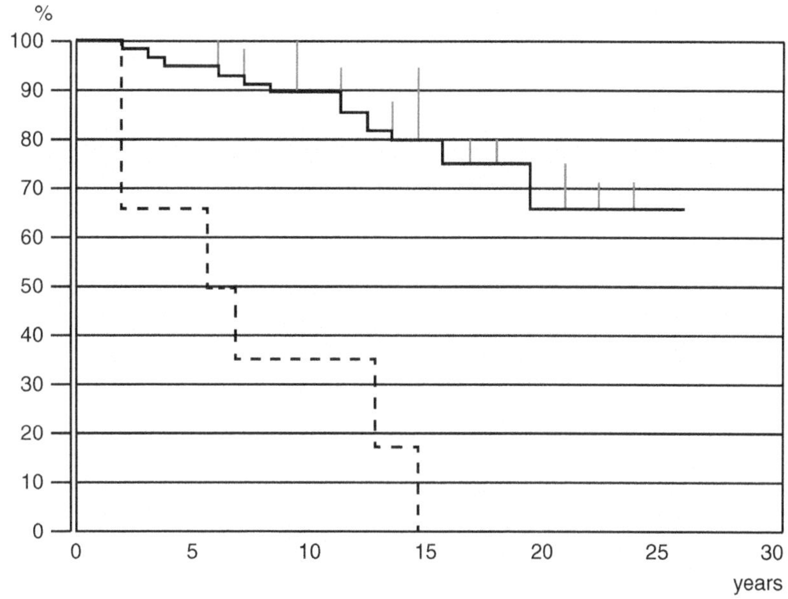

Fig. 4.4 Myelopathy-free rate of asymptomatic subjects with OPLL by Kaplan–Meier method. The bold line indicates the data of subjects with less than 60% spinal canal stenosis. The dotted line indicates the data of subjects with greater than 60% spinal canal stenosis. Reprinted with permission from Shunji Matsunaga et al. J Spine Research 2013; 4:116–122

(66 male and 43 female) from 17 spine institutes nationwide enrolled in this study. All subjects met the following criteria for enrollment: (1) radiographic evidence of OPLL in the cervical spine, (2) asymptomatic OPLL at the initial examination associated with a minimum 5 years follow-up, and (3) agreement from the patients and approval from each institutional review board to use clinical data for this study. The term "asymptomatic" was defined as indicating that the patients did not exhibit apparent myelopathy. Evidence of myelopathy was determined by subjective and objective findings including spastic gait, muscle atrophy, weakness, motor dysfunction of the hand, abnormal tendon reflex of the upper and lower extremities, pathological reflex, clonus, and sensory disturbances by direct examination. All subjects with myelopathy had disabilities affecting their daily lives. Subjects who had stiffness of the neck and a limited range of motion of the cervical spine were included in this study. All subjects had yearly clinical examination at each spine institutes. Age at the first visit of subjects ranged from 41 to 84 with an average of 59.8 years old. OPLL was classified: segmental, 33 cases; continuous, 38 cases; and mixed 38 cases. The follow-up periods ranged from 5 to 26 years (mean 11.3 years). A total of 27/109 (24.8%) subjects developed myelopathy during follow-up. The remaining 82 patients did not exhibit myelopathy throughout the follow-up periods with a minimum of 5 years. All five patients with greater than 60% spinal canal stenosis in the plain X-ray film developed myelopathy within 15 years of follow-up. The myelopathy-free rate was shown by the Kaplan–Meiyer method (Fig. 4.4). The myelopathy-free rate of subjects with less than 60% spinal canal stenosis was 66% at the maximum 26 years of follow-up. Six of 27 subjects who exhibited myelopathy had trauma history. Of the six subjects, five had mixed-type OPLL, and one had segmental-type OPLL. The types of trauma reported included three falls on stairs, two severe whiplash injuries, and one accidental head contusion.

4.4 Risk Factors for Development of Myelopathy

In our personal study, the author had examined the pathogenesis of myelopathy in patients with ossification of the posterior longitudinal ligaments [35]. Furthermore, the author designed a multicenter cohort study to identify the radiographic predictors for the development of myelopathy in patients with OPLL [36]. A total of 156 OPLL patients (104 male and 52 female) from 16 spine institutes nationwide participated in this study. The follow-up periods ranged from 5 to 23 years (mean 10.3 years). Each subject underwent a plain roentgenogram, computed tomography (CT), and magnetic resonance imaging (MRI) of the cervical spine during the follow-up period. OPLL was classified into segmental, 45 cases; continuous, 55 cases; and mixed 56 cases. The trauma history of the cervical spine, maximum percentage of spinal canal stenosis in a plain roentgenogram and CT, range of motion of the cervical spine, and axial ossified pattern in MRI or CT were reviewed in relation to the existence of myelopathy. A total of 90 patients exhibited myelopathy at the initial visit, and 6 patients developed myelopathy during follow-up. The remaining 60 patients did not exhibit myelopathy throughout the follow-up period. All 39 patients with greater than 60% spinal canal stenosis on the plain roentgenogram exhibited myelopathy. Out of 117 patients with less than 60% spinal canal stenosis, 57 (49%) patients exhibited myelopathy. Among the 117 patients with less than 60% spinal canal stenosis, the range of motion of the cervical spine was significantly larger in patients with myelopathy than in those without it (Fig. 4.5). On the basis of CT and MRI, the axial ossified pattern could be classified into two types: central and lateral deviated. The determination of the types is explained as follows. The central type was defined as that in which the most occupied portion of OPLL was located within the middle one third of the width of the vertebral canal on the axial CT or MRI (Fig. 4.6a). The lateral-deviated type was defined as that in which the most occupied portion of OPLL was located outside middle one third of the width (Fig. 4.6b). All 39 patients with greater than 60% spinal canal stenosis of the spinal canal by OPLL on CT exhibited myelopathy. The subjects with less than 60% spinal canal stenosis who developed myelopathy without a cervical trauma history had lateral-deviated type OPLL in 94% (15/16) of the cases. The incidence of myelopathy in patients with less than 60% spinal canal stenosis except for trauma-induced myelopathy cases was significantly higher in the lateral-deviated type group than in the central-type group

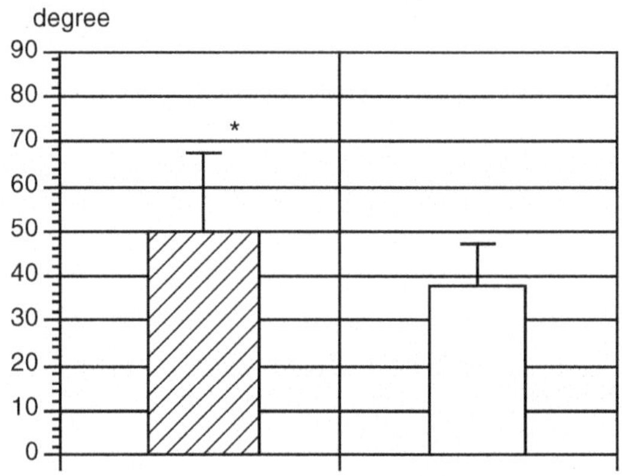

Fig. 4.5 Relationship between ROM and myelopathy in 117 patients with less than 60% maximum stenosis of the spinal canal; data indicate mean ± SE. The grey box indicates patients with myelopathy ($n = 57$). The empty box indicates patients without myelopathy ($n = 60$). The star mark indicates $P < 0.05$

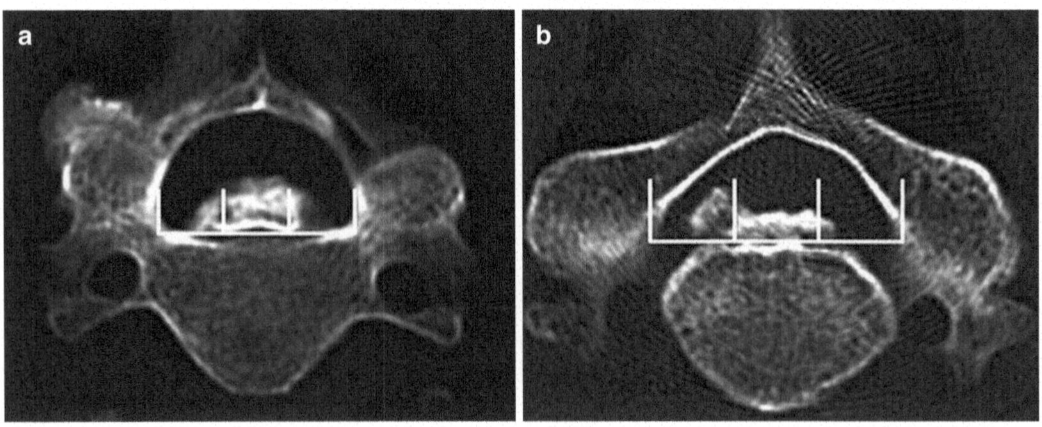

Fig. 4.6 Axial ossified pattern of OPLL on CT or MRI. (**a**) central type, (**b**) lateral-deviated type. Reprinted with permission from Shunji Matsunaga et al. J Spine Research 2013; 4:116–122

(Table 4.2). The sensitivity of lateral-deviated type OPLL for development of myelopathy was 94% and the specificity was 60%. A spinal cord signal change of the T2 weighted MRI was detected in 41 patients. In 36 patients, the presence of spinal cord signal change could not be determined because the patients exhibited severe spinal cord compression by OPLL. The sensitivity of the spinal cord signal change on the development of myelopathy was 87% but the specificity was 66% (Table 4.3). Fifteen patients out the 156 subjects developed trauma-induced myelopathy. Of the 15 patients, 13 had mixed-type OPLL, and 2 had segmental-type OPLL. The author examined the risk factor for development of myelopathy in patients with asymptomatic ossification of the posterior longitudinal ligament by a multicenter prospective study in 2012 [34]. Age at the initial examination, gender, classification of OPLL, history of trauma on the cervical spine, follow-up periods, degree of spinal canal stenosis, range of motion of the cervical spine, and axial ossification type on CT or MRI were analyzed using univariate and multivariate logistic models to determine the correlation with the development of myelopathy in asymptomatic subjects with OPLL. On univariate logistic regression analysis, the development of myelopathy was significantly associated with spinal canal stenosis ratio, large range of motion of the cervical spine, and lateral-deviated type OPLL (Table 4.4). Multivariate logistic regression analysis revealed the same results as univariate analysis (Table 4.5). The knowledge of natural history of this disease is essential for the treatment of this disease and further research in All Japan is desired in the future.

Table 4.2 The relationship between OPLL pattern on CT and myelopathy

	Central-type OPLL	Lateral deviated-type OPLL	*P* value
Percentage of patients with myelopathy (%)	23.5 (12/51)	61.1 (33/54)	0.021

OPLL ossification of the posterior longitudinal ligament

Table 4.3 The correlation between the cord signal change on T2-weighted MRI and myelopathy

	T2-weightedhigh intensity	
	negative	positive
With myelopathy	27	36
Without myeloapthy	52	5

Sensitivity: 36/41 (87%), Specificity: 52/79(66%)
Thirty six (23%) patients were excluded because they could not be determined

Table 4.4 The results of univariate logistic regression analysis of the development of myelopathy

		Development of myelopathy				Crude odds ratio		
Factor		Yes		No		OR	95%Wald CI	Pr > ChiSq
Gender	Male	18	(27.7.)	47	(72.3)			
	Female	9	(20.5)	35	(79.5)	0.671	0.270–1.671	0.3920
Age (years)	<65	18	(32.1)	38	(67.9)			
	≥65	9	(17.0)	44	(83.0)	0.432	0.174–1.073	0.0706
	Mean ± SD	59.6 ± 8.6		61.3 ± 9.1		0.979	0.932–1.028	0.3960
Type of OPLL	Segmental	4	(12.1)	29	(87.9)			
	Mixed	18	(47.4)	20	(52.6)	6.536	1.919–22.222	0.0002
	Continuous	5	(13.2)	33	(86.8)	1.099	0.269–4.484	0.1405
Trauma history	Negative	21	(21.9)	75	(78.1)			
	Positive	6	(46.2)	7	(53.8)	3.062	0.929–10.095	0.0660
ROM (degree)	<50	7	(17.9)	32	(82.1)			
	≥50	20	(28.6)	50	(71.4)	1.829	0.694–4.816	0.2219
	Mean ± SD	55.4 ± 12.9		44.7 ± 12.9		1.082	1.033–1.135	0.0010
Axial OPLL type	Central	8	(14.8)	46	(85.2)			
	Lateral deviated	19	(34.5)	36	(65.5)	3.035	1.192–7.723	0.0198
Maximum canal stenosis (%)	<60	22	(21.2)	82	(78.8)			
	≥60	5	(100.0)	0	(0.0)	–	–	
	Mean ± SD	45.6 ± 11.1		38.4 ± 10.8		1.062	1.018–1.109	0.0054

Reprinted with permission from Shirnji Matsimaga et al. J Spine Reserch 2013;4:116–123

Table 4.5 The results of multivariate logistic regression analysis of the development of myelopathy

Factor		Analysis of maximum likelihood estimates						Odds ratio	
			DF	Estimate	SE	Wald ChiSq	Pr > ChiSq	Estimate	95% Wald CI
Intercept		β_0	1	−17.003	3.682	21.325	<0.0001		
Type of OPLL	Mixed	β_1	1	1.004	0.444	5.108	0.0238	3.863	0.641–23.269
	Continuous	β_2	1	−0.656	0.517	1.614	0.2039	0.734	0.099–5.462
ROM (degree)		β_3	1	0.153	0.040	14.566	0.0001	1.165	1.077–1.260
Axial OPLL type lateral deviated		β_4	1	1.001	0.405	6.119	0.0134	7.396	1.515–36.101
Maximum canal stenosis (%)		β_5	1	0.186	0.047	15.716	<0.0001	1.205	1.099–1.321

Reprinted with permission from Shirnji Matsunaga et al. J Spine Reserch 2013;4:116–123

References

1. Bakay L, Cares HL, Smith RJ. Ossification in the region of the posterior longitudinal ligament as a cause of cervical myelopathy. J Neurol Neurosurg Psychiatry. 1970;33:263–8.
2. Minagi H, Gronner AT. Calcification of the posterior longitudinal ligament: a cause of cervical myelopathy. Am J Roentgenol. 1969;105:365–9.
3. Nagashima C. Cervical myelopathy due to ossification of the posterior longitudinal ligament. J Neurosurg. 1972;37:653–60.
4. Ono K, Ota H, Tada K, et al. Ossified posterior longitudinal ligament. A clinicopathologic study. Spine. 1977;2:126–38.
5. Tsuyama N. Ossification of the posterior longitudinal ligament of the spine. Clin Orthop Relat Res. 1984;184:71–84.
6. Key GA. On paraplegia depending on the ligament of the spine. Guy Hosp Rep. 1838;3:17–34.
7. Matsunaga S, Sakou T. Epidemiology of ossification of the posterior longitudinal ligament. In: Yonenobu K, Sakou T, Ono K, editors. OPLL. Tokyo: Springer; 1997. p. 3–17.
8. Terayama K. Family study of ossification of the posterior longitudinal ligament [in Japanese]. Investigation Committee 1986 report on the ossification of the spinal ligaments of the Japanese Ministry of Public Health and Welfare; 1987. pp. 10–11.
9. Terayama K. Genetic studies on ossification of then posterior longitudinal ligament of the spine. Spine. 1989;14:1184–91.
10. Uehara H, Sakou T, Morimoto N, et al. Familial study of ossification of the posterior longitudinal ligament in the cervical spine [in Japanese]. Seikeigeka to Saigaigeka. 1988;36:800–2.
11. Miura Y, Furusho T, Ibaraki K, et al. Genetic studies for OPLL: analysis of twin [in Japanese]. Investigation Committee 1991 report on the ossification of the spinal ligaments of the Japanese Ministry of Public Health and Welfare; 1992. pp. 5–7.
12. Sakou T, Taketomi E, Matsunaga S, et al. Genetic study of ossification of the posterior longitudinal ligament in the cervical spine with human leukocyte antigen haplotype. Spine. 1991;6:1249–52.
13. Matsunaga S, Yamaguchi M, Hayashi K, et al. Genetic analysis of ossification of the posterior longitudinal ligament. Spine. 1999;24:937–8.
14. Horikoshi T, Maeda K, Kawaguchi Y, et al. A large-scale genetic association study of ossification of the posterior longitudinal ligament of the spine. Hum Genet. 2006;119:611–6.
15. Karasugi T, Nakajima M, Ikari K, et al. A genome-wide sib-pair linkage analysis of ossification of the posterior longitudinal ligament of the spine. J Bone Miner Metab. 2013;31:136–43.
16. Nakajima M, Takahashi A, Tsuji T, et al. A genome-wide association study identifies susceptibility loci for ossification of the posterior longitudinal ligament of the spine. Nat Genet. 2014;46:1012–6.
17. Nakajima M, Kou I, Ohashi H, et al. Identification and functional characterization of RSPO2 as a susceptibility gene for ossification of the posterior longitudinal ligament of the spine. Am J Hum Genet. 2016;99:202–7.
18. Yanagi T. Ossification of the posterior longitudinal ligament. A clinical and radiological analysis of forty-six cases [in Japanese]. Brain Nerve. 1970;22:909–21.
19. Terayama K, Kurokawa T, Seki H. National survey of ossification of the posterior longitudinal ligament [in Japanese]. Investigation Committee 1975 report on the ossification of the spinal ligaments of the Japanese Ministry of Public Health and Welfare; 1976. pp. 8–33.
20. Takeda T, Arima T. A case report of ossification of posterior longitudinal ligament with tetrapalsy by mild trauma [in Japanese]. Rinsho Seikei-geka. 1972;7:949–53.
21. Katoh S, Ikata T, Hirai N, et al. Influence of minor trauma to the neck on the neurological outcome in patients with ossification of the posterior longitudinal ligament (OPLL) of the cervical spine. Paraplegia. 1995;33:330–3.
22. Fujimura Y, Nakamura M, Toyama Y. Influence of minor trauma on surgical results in patients with cervical OPLL. J Spinal Disord. 1998;11:16–20.
23. Matsunaga S, Sakou T, Hayashi K, et al. Trauma-induced myelopathy in patients with ossification of the posterior longitudinal ligament. J Neurosurg. 2002;97:172–5.
24. Forestier J, Lagier R. Ankylosing hyperostosis of the spine. Clin Orthop Relat Res. 1971;74:65–83.
25. Resnick D, Shaul SR, Robinsons JM. Diffuse idiopathic skeletal hyperostosis (DISH): forestier's disease with extraspinal manifestations. Radiology. 1975;115:513–24.
26. Resnick D, Guerra J Jr, Robinson CA, et al. Association of diffuse idiopathic skeletal hyperostosis (DISH) and calcification and ossification of the posterior longitudinal ligament. Am J Roentgenol. 1978;131:1049–53.
27. Taketomi E. Progression of ossification of the posterior longitudinal ligament in the cervical spine. J Jpn Spine Res Soc. 1997;8:359–66.
28. Matsunaga S, Sakou T, Taketomi E, et al. Effects of strain distribution in the intervertebral discs on the progression of ossification of the posterior longitudinal ligaments. Spine. 1996;21:184–9.
29. Ichimoto H, Kawai S, Oda H, et al. Postoperative progression pattern of ossification of the posterior longitudinal ligament in cervical spine [in Japanese]. Investigation Committee 1980 report on the ossification of the spinal ligaments of the Japanese Ministry of Public Health and Welfare; 1981. pp. 199–200.
30. Miyazaki K, Hirofuji E, Onozaki A, et al. Follow-up studies on the development of ossification of the posterior longitudinal ligament in the cervical region

after simultaneous multisegmental laminectomy [in Japanese]. Spine Spinal Cord. 1993;6:905–10.
31. Matsunaga S, Sakou T, Taketomi E, et al. The natural course of myelopathy caused by ossification of the posterior longitudinal ligament in the cervical spine. Clin Orthop Relat Res. 1994;305:168–77.
32. Matsunaga S, Sakou T, Taketomi E, Komiya S. Clinical course of patients with ossification of the posterior longitudinal ligament: a minimum 10-year cohort study. J Neurosurg. 2004;100:245–8.
33. Kaplan EL, Meier P. Nonparametric estimation from incomplete observations. J Am Stat Assoc. 1958;53:457–81.
34. Matsunaga S, Tsuji T, Toyama Y, et al. Risk factors for development of myelopathy in patients with asymptomatic ossification of the posterior longitudinal ligament. J Spine Res. 2013;4:116–22.
35. Matsunaga S, Kukita M, Hayashi K, et al. Pathogenesis of myelopathy on the patients with ossification of the posterior longitudinal ligament. J Neurosurg. 2002;96(Suppl 2):168–72.
36. Matsunaga S, Nakamura K, Seichi A, et al. Radiographic predictors for the development of myelopathy in patients with ossification of the posterior longitudinal ligament: a multicenter cohort study. Spine. 2008;33:2648–50.

Part III

Pathology and Pathogenesis

Overview of Recent Basic Researches on OPLL and OLF

5

Morio Matsumoto

Although extensive basic and clinical researches have been conducted regarding ossification of posterior longitudinal ligament (OPLL) and ossification of ligamentum flavum (OLF), their etiology still remains unclear. However, recently, several breakthroughs in basic researches especially on genetics, biomarkers, stem cells, etc., have taken place. In this chapter, the updates of basic researches are reviewed by frontrunner researchers and the brief summary of these researches is described in this article.

5.1 Genetic Studies on OPLL

Epidemiologic studies and investigations on family history and ancestry have shown that genetic factors play a role in the onset of OPLL, and many genetic studies have been conducted thus far [1–6].

In 2013, Karasugi et al. [7] reported the results of a genome-wide linkage study using 214 Japanese OPLL sib-pairs. They found loci with suggestive linkage on 1p21, 2p22-2p24, 7q22, 16q24, and 20p12.

In 2014, Nakajima et al. [8] conducted the first genome-wide association study (GWAS) on 1130 OPLL patients and 7125 control cases. The DNA samples from more than one thousand OPLL patients were collected by the members of a research group for ossification of the spinal ligament sponsored by the Japanese Ministry of Health, Labor and Welfare (Primary Investigator, Yoshiaki Toyama, Professor of Keio University). They identified six new genomic susceptibility loci related to OPLL and further analyzed gene expression in and around these loci and found several genes involved in the etiology of OPLL. To further clarify the mechanism of the onset of OPLL, a basic study group supported first by the Japanese Ministry of Health, Labour and Welfare and next by the Japan Agency for Medical Research and Development (AMED) was established. Each member of the study group conducted molecular functional analysis of each gene. For example, Nakajima and colleagues [9] investigated the gene, *RSPO2* encoding R-spondin 2 and clarified the functional mechanism of *RSPO2* for the onset of OPLL. In addition to *RSPO2*, other genes susceptible to OPLL including *HAO1*, *CCDC91*, and *CDC5L* were histologically investigated in tissue panels of the posterior longitudinal ligament and the ligamentum flavum from human and rodents (data unpublished) and also in tissues of tiptoe-walking (ttw) mice which are considered as model mice for OPLL.

5.2 Biomarkers Related to OPLL

Metabolites in OPLL and OFL patients have been studied by analysis of blood samples of patients.

M. Matsumoto (✉)
Department of Orthopedic Surgery, Keio University, Tokyo, Japan
e-mail: morio@a5.keio.jp

A. Okawa et al. (eds.), *OPLL*, https://doi.org/10.1007/978-981-15-3855-1_5

Kawaguchi et al. [10] found that highly sensitive C-reactive protein (hs-CRP) was positively correlated with progression of OPLL. Niu et al. [11] reported that serum levels of osteocalcin were high but those of Dickkopf-related protein 1 (DKK1) were lower in AS, DISH, OPLL, and OYL patients than those in the controls. Kashii and colleagues [12] reported that a serum sclerostin level was higher in men with OPLL than in those without, and it was positively correlated with age in men with OPLL and that there was a strong negative correlation between serum sclerostin levels and serum DKK1 levels in men with OPLL.

Tsuji et al. [13] reported the results of analyses on plasma metabolites in 10 patients with cervical OPLL and those in control subjects using capillary electrophoresis time-of-flight mass spectrometry, and lipophilic metabolites were analyzed using liquid chromatograph time-of-flight mass spectrometry. They found six metabolites, acylcarnitine (AC) (14:0), palmitoylcarnitine, AC (18:2), fatty acid (FA) (24:2), thyroxine, and thiaproline, which were significantly larger in the OPLL group than in the control group. Further analyses of these metabolites will be promising to clarify the pathogenesis of OPLL.

5.3 Stem Cell Researches

Mesenchymal stem cells (MSCs) are multipotent stromal cells and they can differentiate into osteoblasts and chondrocytes, both of which may play a role in the onset of OPLL [14]. Asari et al. [15] investigated human spinal ligaments harvested during surgery. They cultured cells isolated from the ligaments using differentiation inducting media and analyzed those cells by flow cytometry and found that phenotypic characteristics of those cells met the criteria of MSCs.

The same research group conducted an immunohistological study on ossified and non-ossified ligamentum flavum harvested during spinal surgery [16]. They found MSCs in the perivascular area and collagenous matrix in spinal ligaments and OLF samples showed a higher accumulation of MSCs around blood vessels and in collagenous matrix than non-OLF samples. MSC markers were also positive in chondrocytes near the ossification front in OLF. Thus, they concluded that MSCs may contribute to the ossification process of OLF through endochondral ossification.

Patient-derived human induced pluripotent stem cells are reported to be useful for the study of the formation of both healthy and pathological bone, [17] and they may be applicable to the study of OPLL and OFL.

5.4 Basic Research on Drug Therapy for OPLL

Several basic researches investigating the effectiveness of candidate agents for treatment of OPLL have been conducted recently. Maeda et al. [18] studied the effectiveness of H2 blocker, famotidine, on progression of OPLL-like ectopic ossification in ttw mice. They found that famotidine was effective to suppress the progression of ectopic ossification as well as to reduce mortality of the mice if it was started as early as 4 weeks of age. Hiratsuka and colleagues [19] investigated the efficacy of a drug therapy targeting the endogenous inhibitor of mineralization, pyrophosphate (PPi), for the treatment of ossification of the spinal ligament in ttw mice. They found that the alkaline phosphatase inhibitor, levamisole (5 mg/kg/day), in combination with exogenous PPi (160 μmol/kg/day) slowed the progression of ossification of the spinal ligament with increase in the serum concentration of PPi.

Although as of present, there is no existing effective drug for OPLL or OFL, further efforts are warranted to develop agents for prevention of the onset and progression of ossification to avoid primary or revision surgery.

5.5 Conclusions

Recent basic researches on OPLL and OFL are overviewed. In the fields of genetics, biomarkers and stem cell, endeavor to clarify pathogenesis and pathophysiology has been made so that treatment options other than surgery, which is currently the only solution for progressive myelopathy due to OPLL and OFL, can be established.

References

1. Terayama K. Genetic studies on ossification of the posterior longitudinal ligament of the spine. Spine (Phila Pa 1976). 1989;14:1184–91.
2. Ikegawa S. Genomic study of ossification of the posterior longitudinal ligament of the spine. Proc Jpn Acad Ser B Phys Biol Sci. 2014;90:405–12.
3. Jekarl DW, Paek CM, An YJ, Kim YJ, Kim M, Kim Y, Lee J, Sung CH. TGFBR2 gene polymorphism is associated with ossification of the posterior longitudinal ligament. J Clin Neurosci. 2013;20:453–6.
4. Kamiya M, Harada A, Mizuno M, Iwata H, Yamada Y. Association between a polymorphism of the transforming growth factor-beta1 gene and genetic susceptibility to ossification of the posterior longitudinal ligament in Japanese patients. Spine (Phila Pa 1976). 2001;26:1264–7.
5. Kawaguchi Y, Furushima K, Sugimori K, Inoue I, Kimura T. Association between polymorphism of the transforming growth factor-beta1 gene with the radiologic characteristic and ossification of the posterior longitudinal ligament. Spine (Phila Pa 1976). 2003;28:1424–6.
6. Wang H, Liu D, Yang Z, Tian B, Li J, Meng X, Wang Z, Yang H, Lin X. Association of bone morphogenetic protein-2 gene polymorphisms with susceptibility to ossification of the posterior longitudinal ligament of the spine and its severity in Chinese patients. Eur Spine J. 2008;17:956–64.
7. Karasugi T, Nakajima M, Ikari K, Genetic Study Group of Investigation Committee on Ossification of the Spinal Ligaments, Tsuji T, Matsumoto M, Chiba K, Uchida K, Kawaguchi Y, Mizuta H, Ogata N, Iwasaki M, Maeda S, Numasawa T, Abumi K, Kato T, Ozawa H, Taguchi T, Kaito T, Neo M, Yamazaki M, Tadokoro N, Yoshida M, Nakahara S, Endo K, Imagama S, Demura S, Sato K, Seichi A, Ichimura S, Watanabe M, Watanabe K, Nakamura Y, Mori K, Baba H, Toyama Y, Ikegawa S. A genome-wide sib-pair linkage analysis of ossification of the posterior longitudinal ligament of the spine. J Bone Miner Metab. 2013;31:136–43.
8. Nakajima M, Takahashi A, Tsuji T, Karasugi T, Baba H, Uchida K, Kawabata S, Okawa A, Shindo S, Takeuchi K, Taniguchi Y, Maeda S, Kashii M, Seichi A, Nakajima H, Kawaguchi Y, Fujibayashi S, Takahata M, Tanaka T, Watanabe K, Kida K, Kanchiku T, Ito Z, Mori K, Kaito T, Kobayashi S, Yamada K, Takahashi M, Chiba K, Matsumoto M, Furukawa K, Kubo M, Toyama Y, Genetic Study Group of Investigation Committee on Ossification of the Spinal Ligaments, Ikegawa S. A genome-wide association study identifies susceptibility loci for ossification of the posterior longitudinal ligament of the spine. Nat Genet. 2014;46:1012–6.
9. Nakajima M, Kou I, Ohashi H, Genetic Study Group of the Investigation Committee on the Ossification of Spinal Ligaments, Ikegawa S. Identification and functional characterization of RSPO2 as a susceptibility gene for ossification of the posterior longitudinal ligament of the spine. Am J Hum Genet. 2016;99:202–7.
10. Kawaguchi Y, Nakano M, Yasuda T, Seki S, Suzuki K, Yahara Y, Makino H, Kitajima I, Kimura T. Serum biomarkers in patients with ossification of the posterior longitudinal ligament (OPLL): inflammation in OPLL. PLoS One. 2017;12:e0174881.
11. Niu CC, Lin SS, Yuan LJ, Chen LH, Yang CY, Chung AN, Lu ML, Tsai TT, Lai PL, Chen WJ. Correlation of blood bone turnover biomarkers and Wnt signaling antagonists with AS, DISH, OPLL, and OYL. BMC Musculoskelet Disord. 2017;18:61.
12. Kashii M, Matuso Y, Sugiura T, Fujimori T, Nagamoto Y, Makino T, Kaito T, Ebina K, Iwasaki M, Yoshikawa H. Circulating sclerostin and dickkopf-1 levels in ossification of the posterior longitudinal ligament of the spine. J Bone Miner Metab. 2016;34:315–24.
13. Tsuji T, Matsumoto M, Nakamura M, Miyamoto T, Yagi M, Fujita N, Okada E, Nagoshi N, Tsuji O, Watanabe K. Metabolite profiling of plasma in patients with ossification of the posterior longitudinal ligament. J Orthop Sci. 2018;23:878–83.
14. Harada Y, Furukawa K, Asari T, Chin S, Ono A, Tanaka T, Mizukami H, Murakami M, Yagihashi S, Motomura S, Ishibashi Y. Osteogenic lineage commitment of mesenchymal stem cells from patients with ossification of the posterior longitudinal ligament. Biochem Biophys Res Commun. 2014;443:1014–20.
15. Asari T, Furukawa K, Tanaka S, Kudo H, Mizukami H, Ono A, Numasawa T, Kumagai G, Motomura S, Yagihashi S, Toh S. Mesenchymal stem cell isolation and characterization from human spinal ligaments. Biochem Biophys Res Commun. 2012;417:1193–9.
16. Chin S, Furukawa K, Ono A, Asari T, Harada Y, Wada K, Tanaka T, Inaba W, Mizukami H, Motomura S, Yagihashi S, Ishibashi Y. Immunohistochemical localization of mesenchymal stem cells in ossified human spinal ligaments. Biochem Biophys Res Commun. 2013;436:698–704.
17. Kawai S, Yoshitomi H, Sunaga J, Alev C, Nagata S, Nishio M, Hada M, Koyama Y, Uemura M, Sekiguchi K, Maekawa H, Ikeya M, Tamaki S, Jin Y, Harada Y, Fukiage K, Adachi T, Matsuda S, Toguchida J. In vitro bone-like nodules generated from patient-derived iPSCs recapitulate pathological bone phenotypes. Nat Biomed Eng. 2019;3:558–70.
18. Maeda Y, Yamamoto K, Yamakawa A, Aini H, Takato T, Chung UI, Ohba S. The H2 blocker famotidine suppresses progression of ossification of the posterior longitudinal ligament in a mouse model. RMD Open. 2015;1:e000068.
19. Hiratsuka S, Takahata M, Shimizu T, Hamano H, Ota M, Sato D, Iwasaki N. Drug therapy targeting pyrophosphate slows the ossification of spinal ligaments in twy mice. J Orthop Res. 2018;36:1256–61.

Histopathological Features of Ossification of the Posterior Longitudinal Ligament

6

Shingo Maeda, Ichiro Kawamura, Hiroyuki Tominaga, and Noboru Taniguchi

Abstract

Ossification of the posterior longitudinal ligament (OPLL) occurs mainly through endochondral ossification. Although researchers have been attempting to elucidate the pathogenesis of OPLL for many years, it remains unclear which cell types in the ligament have chondrogenic capacity. Furthermore, the contribution of direct bone formation without chondrogenesis remains elusive. To characterize the osteochondrogenic potential of the cells around the ossification area of OPLL, we immunohistochemically evaluated a series of proteins specific to endochondral ossification. We found SOX9/type II collagen-positive chondrocytes in the fibrocartilage area, hypertrophic chondrocytes with type X collagen expression, and osteoblastic cells expressing RUNX2, osterix, and bone sialoprotein in the stromal fibrous area (SFA) between the ossified areas, thereby confirming the concept of an endochondral ossification-like process. In addition, the osteoblastic cells and blood vessel cells in the degenerated ligament, as well as the cells in the SFA outside of the ossified area, expressed both osteoblastic markers and SOX9, suggesting that these cells were bipotential osteochondral progenitor cells. Additionally, we revealed that the blood vessel cells and stromal fibrous cells exhibited bipotential osteochondrogenic features. Our observation suggests that any or all of these osteochondral mesenchymal cells may be initiators of OPLL.

Keywords

Endochondral ossification · SOX9 · Type II collagen · Type X collagen · RUNX2 · Osterix · Bone sialoprotein

S. Maeda (✉)
Department of Bone and Joint Medicine, Graduate School of Medical and Dental Sciences, Kagoshima University, Kagoshima, Japan
e-mail: s-maeda@m3.kufm.kagoshima-u.ac.jp; maeda-s@umin.ac.jp

I. Kawamura · H. Tominaga
Department of Orthopaedic Surgery, Graduate School of Medical and Dental Sciences, Kagoshima University, Kagoshima, Japan

N. Taniguchi
Department of Bone and Joint Medicine, Graduate School of Medical and Dental Sciences, Kagoshima University, Kagoshima, Japan

Department of Orthopaedic Surgery, Graduate School of Medical and Dental Sciences, Kagoshima University, Kagoshima, Japan

6.1 Introduction

Histological studies have indicated that ossification of the posterior longitudinal ligament (OPLL) occurs mainly through a process similar to endochondral ossification, because calcified cartilaginous and fibrocartilaginous lesions are observed

A. Okawa et al. (eds.), *OPLL*, https://doi.org/10.1007/978-981-15-3855-1_6

adjacent to the ossification front in the degenerated posterior longitudinal ligament (PLL) [1–4]. Hypertrophy of the PLL had been proposed to be a preliminary step of OPLL [5–7]. Endochondral bone formation is initiated by the chondrogenic master regulator SOX9, which drives the expression of cartilage-specific matrix proteins such as type II collagen (COL II), type XI collagen (COL XI), and aggrecan in chondrocytes [8]. The de novo cartilage enlarges through the proliferation of chondrocytes and matrix synthesis. The chondrocytes then stop proliferating and enlarge to become prehypertrophic chondrocytes that express Indian Hedgehog Homolog (IHH) and continue differentiating into hypertrophic chondrocytes that deposit type X collagen (COL X). Hypertrophic chondrocytes mineralize their surrounding matrix and attract blood vessels and chondroclasts. The chondroclasts then degrade cartilage matrix to provide spaces for osteoblasts, the progenitors of which migrate from blood vessels or adjacent perichondrium to form bone [9]. Osteoblast differentiation is driven by the transcription factors RUNX2 [10] and osterix (OSX) [11], and differentiated osteoblasts produce bone matrix proteins such as bone sialoprotein (BSP) and osteocalcin. The mechanism underlying the initiation of chondrogenesis in PLL remains obscure, and it is unclear which cell types in the PLL gain chondrogenic capacity. In addition, because parts of the ossified area (OA) of OPLL lack a chondrogenic region, a portion of the ossification seems to be formed directly by mesenchymal osteogenic cells [7]; however, it is unclear which of the resident cells of the PLL are responsible for initiating the OPLL. To answer these questions, a systematic immunohistochemical evaluation of the expression of a set of endochondral ossification marker proteins is an option for characterizing the cells. To this end, we investigated the osteochondrogenic differentiation status of the cells in the degenerated PLL, including chondrocyte-like cells, ligament cells, blood vessel cells, and stromal fibrous cells, using immunohistochemistry for the osteoblastic marker proteins RUNX2, OSX, and BSP together with the chondrocyte-specific proteins SOX9, COL II, and COL X in human OPLL specimens. We found that chondrocyte-like cells were positive for SOX9 and COL II in the fibrocartilage area (FCA)

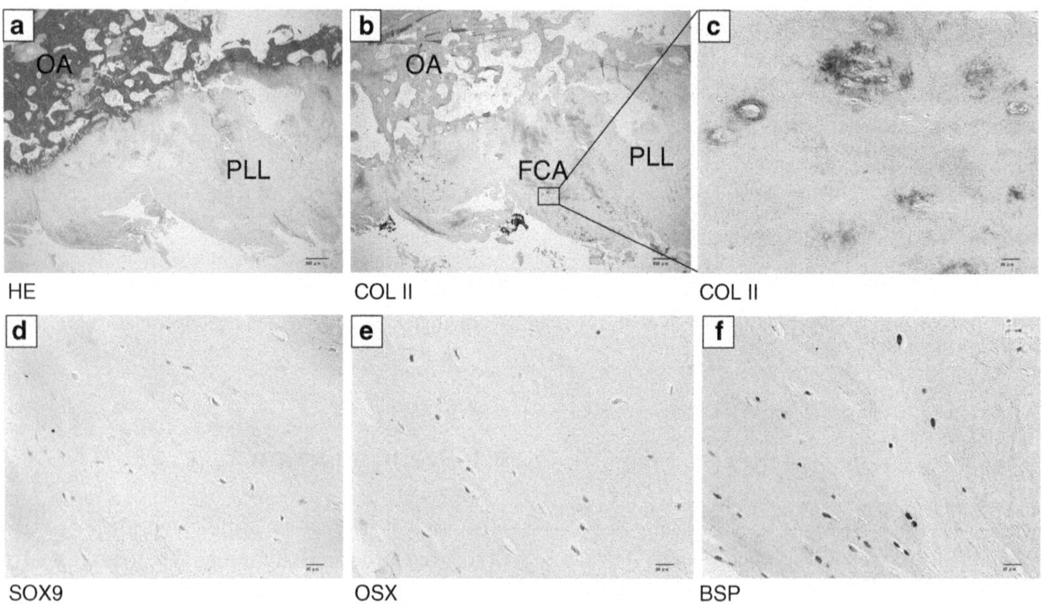

Fig. 6.1 Immunohistochemical evaluation of the fibrocartilage area (FCA) of ossification of the posterior longitudinal ligament (OPLL) (circumscribed type, L4–5) in a 59-year-old man (case 1). (**a**) Hematoxylin and eosin staining of the ossified area (OA) and the FCA in the degenerated PLL. Scale bar = 500 μm. (**b**, **c**) Immunohistochemistry for type II collagen (COL II). Scale bar = 100 μm, 20 μm. (**d**–**f**) Immunohistochemistry using the indicated antibodies. Scale bar = 20 μm

(Fig. 6.1), hypertrophic chondrocytes producing COL X in the hypertrophic chondrocyte area (HCA) (Fig. 6.2), and osteoblastic cells expressing RUNX2, OSX, and BSP in the stromal fibrous area (SFA) between the OA and the margin of the OA (Fig. 6.3). These findings confirm the role of the endochondral ossification-like process in generating OPLL. In addition, we characterized the degenerated ligament area (DLA) containing the osteoblastic cells (Fig. 6.4), blood vessel cells, and stromal cells in the SFA between the PLL and OA (Figs. 6.5 and 6.6). These cells expressed substantial osteoblastic markers and to a lesser extent, SOX9, raising the possibility that OPLL formation, at least in part, is initiated by these bipotential osteochondroprogenitor cells.

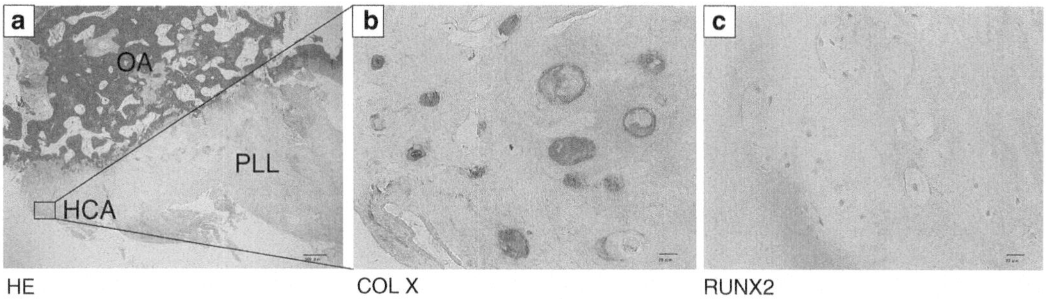

Fig. 6.2 Immunohistochemical evaluation of the hypertrophic cartilage area (HCA) of ossification of the posterior longitudinal ligament (OPLL) in case 1. (**a**) Hematoxylin and eosin staining of the ossified area (OA) and the HCA in the PLL. Scale bar = 500 μm. (**b**, **c**) Immunohistochemistry images of the boxed area in **a** using antibodies against type X collagen (COL X) or RUNX2. Scale bar = 20 μm

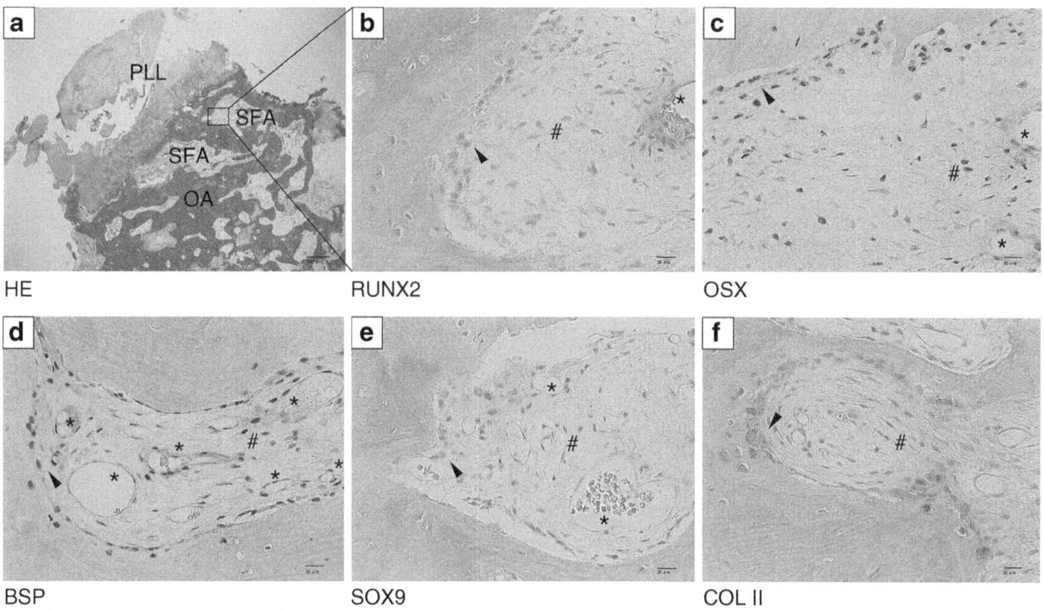

Fig. 6.3 Immunohistochemical evaluation of the stromal fibrous area (SFA) of ossification of the posterior longitudinal ligament (OPLL) in case 1. (**a**) Hematoxylin and eosin staining of the ossified area (OA) and the SFA within the OA close to the degenerated PLL. Scale bar = 500 μm. (**b**–**f**) Immunohistochemistry images of the boxed area in (**a**). Used antibodies are indicated. Scale bar = 20 μm. Blood vessel cells (asterisks), stromal cells (sharps), and lining osteoblasts (arrowheads) are indicated

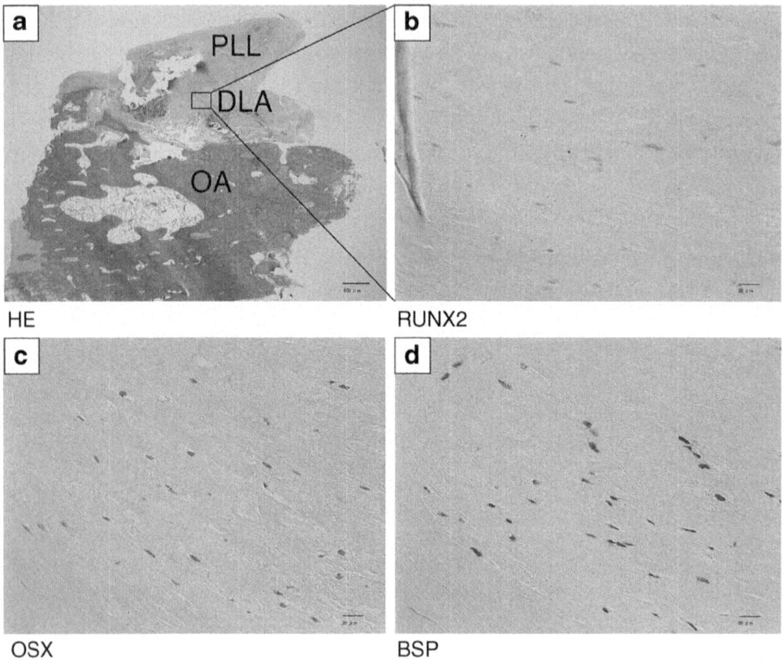

Fig. 6.4 Immunohistochemical evaluation of the degenerated ligament area (DLA) of ossification of the posterior longitudinal ligament (OPLL) (segmental type, C5) in a 48-year-old man (case 2). (**a**) Hematoxylin and eosin staining of the ossified area (OA) and the DLA in the PLL. Scale bar = 500 μm. (**b**–**d**) Immunohistochemistry images of the boxed area in (**a**). Used antibodies are indicated. Scale bar = 20 μm

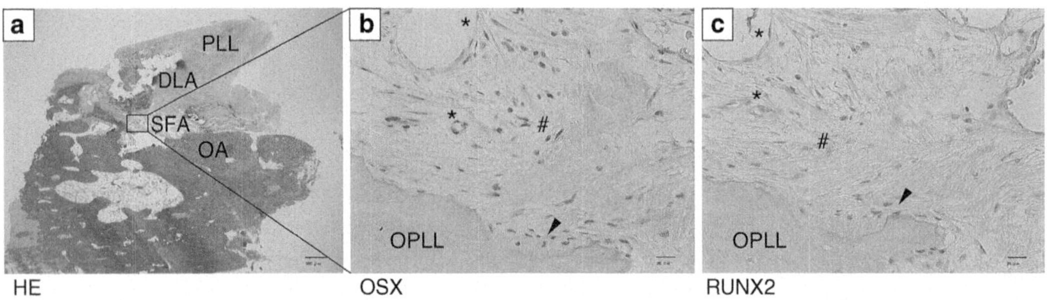

Fig. 6.5 Immunohistochemical evaluation of the stromal fibrous area (SFA) between the degenerated ligament area (DLA) and ossified area (OA): case 2. (**a**) Hematoxylin and eosin staining of the SFA between the DLA and OA. Scale bar = 500 μm. (**b**, **c**) Immunohistochemistry images of the boxed area in (**a**). Used antibodies are indicated. Scale bar = 20 μm. Blood vessel cells (asterisks), stromal cells (sharps), and lining osteoblasts (arrowheads) are indicated

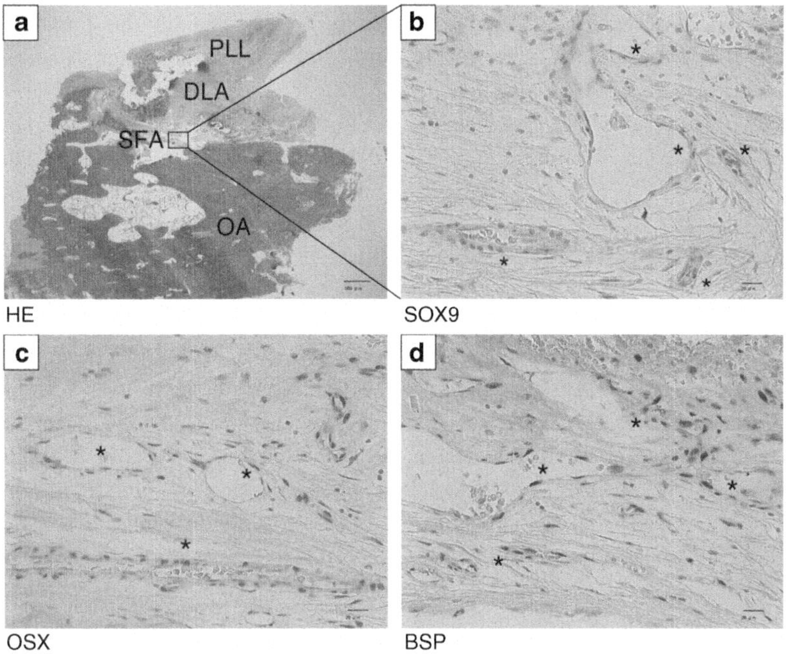

Fig. 6.6 Immunohistochemical evaluation of the blood vessel cells in the stromal fibrous area (SFA) between the degenerated ligament area (DLA) and the ossified area (OA) in a 48-year-old man (case 2). (**a**) Hematoxylin and eosin staining of the SFA between the DLA and the OA. Scale bar = 500 μm. (**b**–**d**) Immunohistochemistry images of the boxed area in (**a**). Used antibodies are indicated. Scale bar = 20 μm. Blood vessel cells (asterisks) are indicated

6.2 The FCA

Previous reports from Baba and colleagues described the presence of the FCA and calcified cartilage area (CCA) at the ossification front of human OPLL [1, 4]. They immunohistochemically demonstrated that chondrocyte-like cells in the FCA expressed SOX9, COL XI, and IHH and that hypertrophic chondrocyte-like cells in the CCA were positive for COL X, whereas mesenchymal cells in the CCA stained positive for SOX9 and COL XI antibodies [4]. These results clearly support the endochondral ossification concept in OPLL formation. Similarly, we also observed round cells expressing SOX9 and COL II, indicating this area to be the FCA (Fig. 6.1). These cells did not produce COL X (not shown), suggesting that these cells were in the early phase of chondrocyte differentiation, which is the initiation step of endochondral ossification. Interestingly, OSX and BSP signals were also detected in these cells, revealing the bipotential features of these ligament cells.

6.3 The HCA

In the degenerated hypertrophied PLL near the OA (Fig. 6.2), greatly enlarged round hypertrophic cells formed clusters to produce COL X in the surrounding matrix (Fig. 6.2a). These cells were negative for SOX9 and COL II (not shown) but were weakly positive for RUNX2 (Fig. 6.2c), suggesting a terminal differentiation state of chondrogenesis, which is the late stage of endochondral ossification.

6.4 The SFA Within the OA

The OA of the OPLL was composed of woven bone and was porous, with pores filled with the SFA. The SFA did not appear like a typical bone marrow because hematopoietic cells were absent although small blood vessels invaded this area (Fig. 6.3, asterisks). The stromal spindle cells roughly filled the space (Fig. 6.3b–f, sharps), and osteoblastic lining cells on the margin of the OA were also evident (Fig. 6.3, arrowheads). The stromal cells, as well as the blood vessel cells, and lining cells were all strongly labeled with OSX and BSP antibodies (Fig. 6.3c–d) and stained mildly for SOX9 and Runx2 (Fig. 6.3b, e), suggesting that these cells possess osteochondral potential. COL II was positive only in the lining cells (Fig. 6.3f). These features of the SFA might represent those of the primary spongiosa observed in the final stage of endochondral ossification.

6.5 Osteoblastic Ligament Cells in the DLA

Spindle-shaped cells in the DLA (Fig. 6.4) showed weak expression of RUNX2, mild expression of OSX, and strong deposition of BSP (Fig. 6.4b–d). Because these cells were found in the deep layer of the PLL, these ligament cells might have directly transdifferentiated into osteoblasts, which were possibly the inducers of direct ossification without chondrogenesis.

6.6 Osteoblastic Cells in the SFA Between the DLA and OA

In the SFA connecting the DLA and OA (Fig. 6.5), the spindle cells roughly filled the SFA and expressed a high degree of OSX and a low level of RUNX2 (Fig. 6.5b–c, sharps), although they were negative for all the chondrocyte markers (not shown), indicating that these cells are osteoblastic. The osteoblastic lining cells on the OPLL margin were confirmed to be osteoblasts because they were stained with antibodies against RUNX2 and OSX (Fig. 6.5b–c, arrowheads). The blood vessels were stained positive for OSX and RUNX2 (Fig. 6.5b–c, asterisks). Blood vessel cells in another field of the SFA (Fig. 6.6) were also positive for OSX and BSP and were determined to be osteoblastic; these cells seemed to expand from the vessel wall to migrate into the PLL matrix (Fig. 6.6c–d, asterisks). Notably, SOX9 was weakly positive in these vessel cells (Fig. 6.6b), indicating that these vessel cells possess osteochondrogenic bipotential features. These results suggest that these bipotential cells might be the source of endochondral ossification and/or direct bone formation of OPLL.

Cardiovascular calcification is a well known osteogenic bone formation process [12, 13] consisting of hydroxyapatite deposited on a bone-like matrix of collagen, osteopontin, and other bone matrix proteins [14, 15], the regulation of which occurs via the activation of specific transcription factors, including RUNX2 [16] and SOX9 [16]. In addition, low-density lipoprotein receptor-related protein 5, the co-receptor of the canonical Wnt pathway, which is important in osteoblast differentiation and regulation of bone mass [17–19], is active in the calcification of arteries [20] and valves [21]. Importantly, the secreted agonistic ligand of Wnt canonical signaling R-spondin 2 was identified as a susceptibility gene for OPLL [22, 23], which inhibits chondrogenesis [23] or promotes osteogenesis [24] by stimulating the Wnt canonical pathway. These findings, together with our immunohistochemical results regarding blood vessels, lead us to speculate that some OPLL formation could be directly initiated by blood vessel cells via a process similar to vascular calcification.

6.7 Conclusions

Our results of a series of immunohistochemical studies demonstrated the following findings in human OPLL:

1. We detected the expression of SOX9 and COL II in chondrocyte-like cells in the FCA and COL X in the matrix around the hypertrophic chondrocytes near the ossification front, confirming the concept of endochondral ossification process in OPLL formation.
2. These "chondrocytes" in the FCA also expressed OSX and BSP, indicating an osteochondral bipotential status (Fig. 6.1).
3. We characterized the blood vessel cells and stromal fibrous cells in the SFA and found that these mesenchymal cells also showed osteochondral bipotential features (Figs. 6.3 and 6.6) and could be initiators, at least in part, of the endochondral or direct ossification of OPLL.
4. The spindle-shaped ligament cells in PLL expressed osteoblast-specific markers (Fig. 6.4), raising the possibility that the ligament cells acquire osteoblastic capacity to directly generate bone under specific degenerative conditions, constituting the direct ossification pathway without chondrogenesis.

References

1. Sato R, Uchida K, Kobayashi S, Yayama T, Kokubo Y, Nakajima H, et al. Ossification of the posterior longitudinal ligament of the cervical spine: histopathological findings around the calcification and ossification front. J Neurosurg Spine. 2007;7(2):174–83.
2. Hashizume Y. Pathological studies on the ossification of the posterior longitudinal ligament (OPLL). Acta Pathol Jpn. 1980;30(2):255–73.
3. Liao CC, Lee ST. Symptomatic ossification of the posterior longitudinal ligament of the lumbar spine. Case report. J Neurosurg. 1999;91(Suppl 2):230–2.
4. Sugita D, Yayama T, Uchida K, Kokubo Y, Nakajima H, Yamagishi A, et al. Indian hedgehog signaling promotes chondrocyte differentiation in enchondral ossification in human cervical ossification of the posterior longitudinal ligament. Spine (Phila Pa 1976). 2013;38(22):E1388–96.
5. Mizuno J, Nakagawa H, Hashizume Y. Analysis of hypertrophy of the posterior longitudinal ligament of the cervical spine, on the basis of clinical and experimental studies. Neurosurgery. 2001;49(5):1091–7. discussion 7–8.
6. Motegi H, Yamazaki M, Goto S, Mikata A, Moriya H. Proliferating cell nuclear antigen in hypertrophied spinal ligaments. Immunohistochemical localization of proliferating cell nuclear antigen in hypertrophied posterior longitudinal ligament of the cervical spine. Spine (Phila Pa 1976). 1998;23(3):305–10.
7. Song J, Mizuno J, Hashizume Y, Nakagawa H. Immunohistochemistry of symptomatic hypertrophy of the posterior longitudinal ligament with special reference to ligamentous ossification. Spinal Cord. 2006;44(9):576–81.
8. Akiyama H, Chaboissier MC, Martin JF, Schedl A, de Crombrugghe B. The transcription factor Sox9 has essential roles in successive steps of the chondrocyte differentiation pathway and is required for expression of Sox5 and Sox6. Genes Dev. 2002;16(21):2813–28.
9. Kronenberg HM. Developmental regulation of the growth plate. Nature. 2003;423(6937):332–6.
10. Komori T, Yagi H, Nomura S, Yamaguchi A, Sasaki K, Deguchi K, et al. Targeted disruption of Cbfa1 results in a complete lack of bone formation owing to maturational arrest of osteoblasts. Cell. 1997;89(5):755–64.
11. Nakashima K, Zhou X, Kunkel G, Zhang Z, Deng JM, Behringer RR, et al. The novel zinc finger-containing transcription factor osterix is required for osteoblast differentiation and bone formation. Cell. 2002;108(1):17–29.
12. Rajamannan NM, Subramaniam M, Rickard D, Stock SR, Donovan J, Springett M, et al. Human aortic valve calcification is associated with an osteoblast phenotype. Circulation. 2003;107(17):2181–4.
13. Demer LL, Tintut Y. Inflammatory, metabolic, and genetic mechanisms of vascular calcification. Arterioscler Thromb Vasc Biol. 2014;34(4):715–23.
14. Mohler ER 3rd, Gannon F, Reynolds C, Zimmerman R, Keane MG, Kaplan FS. Bone formation and inflammation in cardiac valves. Circulation. 2001;103(11):1522–8.
15. Mohler ER 3rd, Adam LP, McClelland P, Graham L, Hathaway DR. Detection of osteopontin in calcified human aortic valves. Arterioscler Thromb Vasc Biol. 1997;17(3):547–52.
16. Caira FC, Stock SR, Gleason TG, McGee EC, Huang J, Bonow RO, et al. Human degenerative valve disease is associated with up-regulation of low-density lipoprotein receptor-related protein 5 receptor-mediated bone formation. J Am Coll Cardiol. 2006;47(8):1707–12.
17. Boyden LM, Mao J, Belsky J, Mitzner L, Farhi A, Mitnick MA, et al. High bone density due to a mutation in LDL-receptor-related protein 5. N Engl J Med. 2002;346(20):1513–21.
18. Gong Y, Slee RB, Fukai N, Rawadi G, Roman-Roman S, Reginato AM, et al. LDL receptor-related protein 5 (LRP5) affects bone accrual and eye development. Cell. 2001;107(4):513–23.
19. Babij P, Zhao W, Small C, Kharode Y, Yaworsky PJ, Bouxsein ML, et al. High bone mass in mice expressing a mutant LRP5 gene. J Bone Miner Res. 2003;18(6):960–74.
20. Awan Z, Denis M, Bailey D, Giaid A, Prat A, Goltzman D, et al. The LDLR deficient mouse as a model for aortic calcification and quantification

by micro-computed tomography. Atherosclerosis. 2011;219(2):455–62.
21. Rajamannan NM. The role of Lrp5/6 in cardiac valve disease: experimental hypercholesterolemia in the ApoE−/− /Lrp5−/− mice. J Cell Biochem. 2011;112(10):2987–91.
22. Nakajima M, Takahashi A, Tsuji T, Karasugi T, Baba H, Uchida K, et al. A genome-wide association study identifies susceptibility loci for ossification of the posterior longitudinal ligament of the spine. Nat Genet. 2014;46(9):1012–6.
23. Nakajima M, Kou I, Ohashi H, Genetic Study Group of the Investigation Committee on the Ossification of Spinal L, Ikegawa S. Identification and functional characterization of RSPO2 as a susceptibility gene for ossification of the posterior longitudinal ligament of the spine. Am J Hum Genet. 2016;99(1):202–7.
24. Knight MN, Karuppaiah K, Lowe M, Mohanty S, Zondervan RL, Bell S, et al. R-spondin-2 is a Wnt agonist that regulates osteoblast activity and bone mass. Bone Res. 2018;6:24.

Ectopic Ossification of Human Spinal Ligaments Caused by Mesenchymal Stem Cell Abnormalities

7

Ken-Ichi Furukawa, Shunfu Chin, Toru Asari, Kanichiro Wada, Gentaro Kumagai, and Yasuyuki Ishibashi

Abstract

Ectopic ossification of the spinal ligament and its progression compresses the spinal cord, resulting in serious neurological deficiencies. Surgery is an established therapy that has had considerable success, but it is often associated with a higher risk of re-progression of ossification followed by neurological complications. Because the detailed mechanism of the onset and development of ectopic ossification have not been clarified, pharmaceutical treatment for this disease has yet to be established. However, a safe and effective treatment is required to improve the quality of life of patients. The disease is thought to be multifactorial, being influenced by both genetic factors and several environmental factors such as mechanical stress. In this review, we discuss recent progress in disease research, with particular focus on what causes initial ossification and which type of abnormality occurs. Mesenchymal stem cells of patients with ossification are thought to misdifferentiate into osteoblasts instead of target ligament cells because they have high osteogenic ability. Elucidation of the genetic and epigenetic transformation of these cells in spinal ligament tissue is crucial to understanding the disease mechanism.

Keywords

Spinal ligament · Ectopic ossification · Mesenchymal stem cells · Mechanical stress · Genetic change · Genome-wide association study · Epigenetic modification · DNA methylation

Abbreviations

CXCR4	C-X-C motif chemokine receptor 4
LF	Ligamentum flavum
MSCs	Mesenchymal stem cells
OLF	Ossification of the ligamentum flavum
OPLL	Ossification of the posterior longitudinal ligament
PLL	Posterior longitudinal ligament
SDF-1	Stromal cell-derived factor

7.1 Introduction

The spine is formed by a series of vertebrae. Multiple longitudinal ligaments connect individual vertebrae longitudinally to stabilize the spine and play an important role in assuring coordinated

K.-I. Furukawa (✉) · S. Chin · T. Asari · K. Wada · G. Kumagai · Y. Ishibashi
Department of Orthopaedic Surgery, Hirosaki University Graduate School of Medicine, Hirosaki, Japan
e-mail: furukawa@hirosaki-u.ac.jp; toru-asari@hirosaki-u.ac.jp; wadak39@hirosaki-u.ac.jp; gen722@hirosaki-u.ac.jp; yasuyuki@hirosaki-u.ac.jp

A. Okawa et al. (eds.), *OPLL*, https://doi.org/10.1007/978-981-15-3855-1_7

movement. Two of the spinal ligaments, the posterior longitudinal ligament (PLL) and the ligamentum flavum (LF) located on the anterior and posterior surfaces of the vertebral canal, respectively, are in contact with the spinal cord running longitudinally in the vertebral foramen. Ossification of the spinal ligament (OPLL and OLF) is a disorder in which the spinal ligament undergoes ectopic ossification. It is possible for ligament tissue to ossify to a small extent because of aging. However, when ossification exceeds a certain amount it compresses the spinal cord, which may lead to numbness of hands and feet and even paralysis [1–4].

There are no established effective preventive methods for the development of spinal ligament ossification, and no treatment option other than spinal surgery which is extremely invasive and burdens the patient [5]. There is also often the possibility of recurrence after surgery. Therefore, to improve the quality of life of patients, the establishment of safe and effective drug treatments is required. For this reason, the determination of disease etiology and pathogenesis is essential.

Because the disorder was found to be hereditary, its cause is presumed to involve genetic factors and the search for causative genes is ongoing [6–10]. Epidemiologically, endocrine and metabolic diseases are considered to be associated with the etiology of spinal ligament ossification [11]. Clinically, the onset and progress of ossification are likely to occur at the ligament site where mechanical stress is applied [11]. Therefore, the ossification of spinal ligaments is considered to be a multifactorial disease caused by a combination of various factors [10, 11]. To clarify the etiology of this disease, we returned to its origin and asked what entity causes the initial ossification and what type of abnormality occurs there. Once the mechanism of onset is clear, the treatment target should also become apparent.

7.2 What Type of Cells Ossify During Ectopic Ossification of the Spinal Ligament?

7.2.1 Ossification of Cells in Ligament Tissue

Advances in cell culture techniques enabled us to isolate cells from spinal ligament tissues and maintain them in vitro [13, 14]. Moreover, with informed patient consent, we also obtained spinal ligament tissue for research purposes that was assigned to be discarded after surgery [15]. From this tissue, ligaments can be digested with enzymes such as collagenase to isolate cells which are cultured to obtain fibroblast-like spinal ligament cells. Long-term culture of these cells, even in normal medium without passaging, results in their gradual calcification from the time point when confluency (uniform covering of cells over the entire surface of the culture dish) has passed. This can be used as an in vitro model system for the ossification of ligament tissue [13–15]. In ligament cells from patients with ossification, calcification progresses more extensively in response to culture medium used to induce ossification compared with cells from patients with no ossification such as those with cervical myelopathy (Fig. 7.1).

When cultured spinal ligament cells are exposed to various stresses such as mechanical stress in the form of repetitive stretch stimuli, which is presumed to be a trigger for ossification, the expression of various ossification-related genes is induced, promoting calcification of the cells [14–18] (Fig. 7.2).

Furthermore, in cells from patients with ossification, the sensitivity of increased expres-

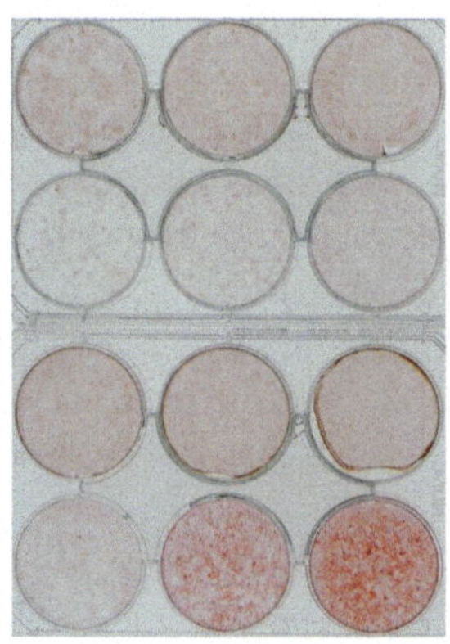

Fig. 7.1 Calcification of spinal ligament cells from ossified and nonossified patients. Ligament cells prepared from ligament tissue of nonossified and ossified patients were cultured for more than 4 weeks, and mineral deposition (calcification) was detected by alizarin red S staining. Marked calcification occurred in cells derived from ossified patients 4 weeks after the initiation of culture

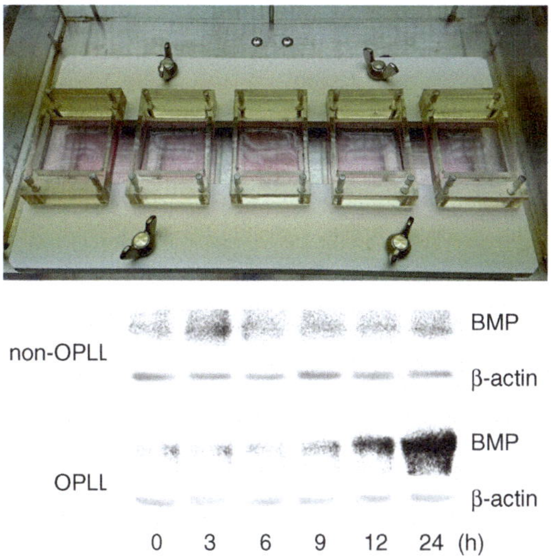

Fig. 7.2 Mechanical stress loading on cultured ligament cells. Ligament cells were cultured in an extensible chamber (upper panel) and subjected to uniaxial cyclic stretch at a constant cycle (120%, 0.5 Hz) to apply mechanical stress for indicated time periods. The production of the osteogenic marker BMP2 was analyzed by western blot (lower panel). β-actin was used as an internal standard of cell proteins. The level of BMP2 expression was enhanced in a time-dependent manner in ligament cells from patients with ossification but not in those from nonossified patients. The figure is reproduced with permission from Bone [13]

sion of ossification-related genes in response to mechanical stress was shown to be much higher than in cells derived from non-ossifying tissues [13–18]. This demonstrated that ligament cells derived from patients with ossification are more likely to be ossified at the isolated cell level, strongly suggesting the following: (1) the main body undergoing ossification is the cell itself which comprises ligament tissue, (2) patient-derived ligament cells undergo some transformation, and (3) the addition of various stresses and environmental factors to a pre-existing abnormality is likely to cause ossification. Based on these findings, we suggest that ligament cells are ossified in the process of repairing the damaged part of the ligament. This is supported by clinical findings that ossification is likely to occur at sites susceptible to mechanical stress, and that it often progresses after spinal surgery [12].

7.2.2 Mesenchymal Stem Cells as Ossifying Entities and their Localization in Ligament Tissue

Previous research used cells obtained by the digestion of ligament tissue with collagenase that were then cultured. Therefore, it is possible that a mixture of cell types had been obtained. Indeed, the calcification of cells in culture vessels is varied, and differences in calcification abilities can be observed among cells. Because the identification of cells with high ossification potentials would likely lead to an understanding of the mechanism of ossification, we hypothesized that cells responsible for the repair of tissue damage are present in ligament tissue but that they carry a mutation enabling them to ossify. Therefore, when tissue repair occurs they behave like osteoblasts rather than ligament cells.

First, we tried to prove that mesenchymal stem cells (MSCs) exist in ligament tissue. Using flow cytometry, we separated cells bearing MSC surface markers (CD73-, CD90-, and CD105-positive, and CD11b-, CD19-, CD34-, CD45-, and human leukocyte antigen-DR-negative) from a cell population obtained by enzymatic digestion of ligament tissue with collagenase [19, 20]. Next, MSCs in ligament tissue were purified by a cell sorter, and shown to have no significant difference in their proliferative potential between ossified and non-ossified patient tissues. Furthermore, MSCs from both tissue types had multilineage (osteogenic, chondrogenic, and adipogenic) differentiation potential. However, the osteogenic potential of MSCs from patients with ossification was significantly higher than those from patients without ossification [21].

Subsequently, when the localization of MSCs was examined by immunohistochemical staining, pericytes around the blood vessels were found to express MSC markers. Additionally, while the tissue of non-ossified patients contained few blood vessels, that of ossified patients contained vascular tissue that extended around the ossification site to the ligament parenchyma. Moreover, MSCs were widely present around blood vessels in the ossification area [22], while hypertrophic chondrocyte-like cells, often found at the ossification junction, expressed MSC markers [19, 22]. This strongly suggested that MSCs participate in ectopic ossification of the ligament by endochondral ossification pathways including angiogenesis, in which changes in MSC localization play an important role. Such changes may involve the MSC regulatory factor stromal cell-derived factor (SDF)-1 and its receptor C-X-C motif chemokine receptor (CXCR)-4 [23]. Osteogenic ligament-derived MSCs showed high expression of SDF-1 and CXCR4 compared with healthy ligaments, together with enhanced motility of MSCs and chemotaxis to SDF-1. This motility and chemotaxis were suppressed by AMD3100, a specific inhibitor of CXCR4 [24], suggesting that MSCs migrating by the SDF-1/CXCR4 system cause ossification (Fig. 7.3).

7.2.3 Endochondral Ossification and MSCs

In the parenchyma of ossified ligament tissue, hypertrophic chondrocytes have been observed near the ossification front [19]. These cells express the chondrocyte-specific connective tissue growth factor [25]. Furthermore, those cells near the ossification front were observed to express MSC markers, indicating that they derive from MSCs [22].

An abundance of blood vessels was reported in the ossified ligament of ossified patients and the amount of blood loss during their spinal surgery was high [26]. This suggests that ligament ossification also follows the pathway of endochondral ossification, which is a normal mechanism of bone metabolism involving conversion to

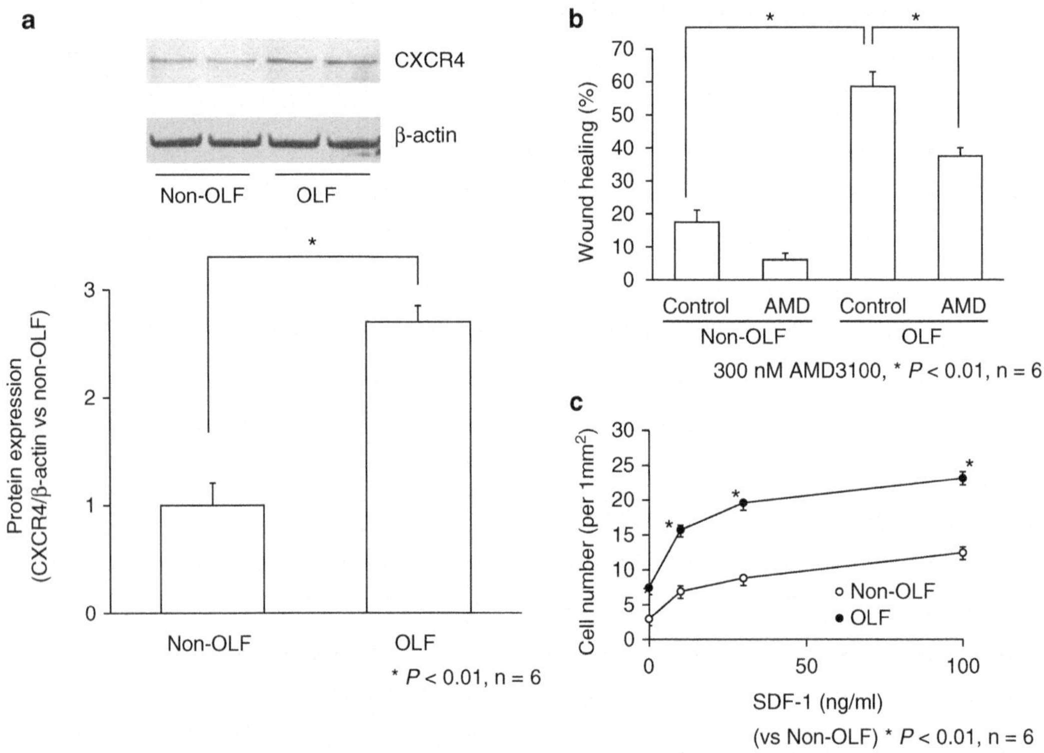

Fig. 7.3 SDF-1 and CXCR4 are expressed in spinal ligament tissue and control the migration activity of MSCs. (**a**) CXCR4 mRNA levels were analyzed by RT-PCR and its protein expression was evaluated by western blotting in MSCs isolated from ossified (OLF) and nonossified (non-OLF) patients. CXCR4 expression was normalized against β-actin as an internal standard. (**b**) The migration activity of MSCs was analyzed by a wound healing assay in the presence of AMD3100, a potent inhibitor of CXCR4. (**c**) MSC migration toward SDF-1 was measured in a chemotaxis chamber containing various concentrations of SDF-1. The figure is reproduced with permission from Journal of Pharmacology and Experimental Therapeutics [21]

bone via cartilage through blood vessel invasion. We observed that chondromodulin-1, a factor expressed in cartilage tissue that suppresses osteogenesis and maintains cartilage tissue [27], is also expressed in MSCs of ligament tissue. Moreover, its expression was significantly reduced in MSCs from patients with ossification compared with those without ossification.

Considering that ligament ossification follows the process of endochondral ossification [27], it is conceivable that decreased expression of chondromodulin-1 permits vascular invasion and promotes ectopic ossification. This mechanism could be used as a target for drug treatment.

7.3 What Determines the Difference Between Healthy and Ossifying MSCs?

7.3.1 Genetic Mechanism

How did MSCs in the spinal ligament tissue of ossified patients acquire (transform) their high ossification capacity? Progressive ossifying fibroplasia (fibrodysplasia ossificans progressiva, FOP) is an example of a genetic disease of ectopic ossification caused by abnormal MSCs [28, 29]. This disease caused by a mutation in the activin receptor-like kinase-2 gene results in the transformation of cells derived from vascular endothelium into mesenchymal cells, leading to ossification. To identify candidate genes responsible for the genetic variation of spinal ligament ossification disease, genome-wide association studies have been carried out by Nakajima et al. [9, 30] and Takegami et al. [31]. They focused on R-spondin 2 as a susceptible gene for ectopic ossification of spinal ligaments. The R-spondin 2 protein is a key player in endochondral ossification that facilitates the differentiation of proliferating chondrocytes into hypertrophic chondrocytes. It is conceivable that its function is altered in patients with ossification, promoting ectopic ossification. However, it is unclear whether only one gene is responsible for disease, so the involvement of mutations in other genes will also need to be considered.

7.3.2 Epigenetic Mechanism

We are tackling this problem using an alternative approach of an epigenetic mechanism, in which transformation occurs by the modification of genomic DNA that is not caused by variation in the nucleic acid sequence. Changes in DNA methylation have been shown to be involved in the pathogenesis of several diseases [32]. For example, Montes et al. reported on the calcification of vascular smooth muscle as an example of ectopic calcification involving an epigenetic mechanism [33]. The calcification of blood vessels in chronic renal failure is presumed to be caused by decreased expression of the vascular smooth muscle specific protein SM22α, resulting in the transformation of vascular smooth muscle cells into osteoblasts. This study found that the decrease was caused by increased methylation of the *SM22α* transcriptional regulatory site. Several epigenetic mechanisms are known, but we focused on the regulation of expression by genomic DNA methylation. This involves a high density of cytosine–guanine nucleotide sequences (CpG) centered on the transcriptional regulatory region of the gene, and the suppression of gene expression by methylation of a CpG island.

The treatment of MSCs with an inhibitor of DNA methylation (5-aza-2′-deoxycytidine, 5AdC) to demethylate DNA resulted in marked changes in the expression of some osteogenic genes [34]. We found that MSCs derived from tissues of both ossified and non-ossified patients were demethylated by 5AdC treatment. Analysis of expression changes in the transcriptome by microarray enabled us to screen genes that are highly expressed through low DNA methylation in MSCs from patients with ossification, and those that are suppressed through high methylation in MSCs from non-ossified patients. This approach identified two candidate genes involved in controlling ossification-related genes: Wnt family member 5A (*WNT5A*) and glial cell line-derived neurotrophic factor (*GDNF*). Treatment of MSCs with small interfering RNA targeting each of these genes significantly suppressed their expression as well as that of osteogenic genes such as alkaline phosphatase, bone morphogenetic protein 2, and Runt-related transcription factor 2. From this, we presumed that *WNT5A* and *GDNF* are involved in the upstream regulation of these osteogenic genes. It also suggested that *WNT5A* and *GDNF* are not suppressed by methylation in MSCs derived from ossified patients, so they are more likely to be ossified. This provided evidence that DNA methylation is involved in ligament ossification. Furthermore, because their expression was suppressed by strong methylation, MSCs deriving from patients with ossification can be used to identify genes contributing to ossification. It has been shown that certain genes involved in angiogenesis are regulated by DNA methylation, and that MSCs deriving from ossified patients have different methylation profiles from those of non-ossified patients (our unpublished observations). In future work, we plan to investigate the abnormal transformation of MSCs by methylation using next-generation sequencing to reveal the profile of genome-wide DNA methylation and its changes related to ossification.

7.4 Summary

The cells responsible for ectopic ossification of the spinal ligament are considered to be MSCs present in the ligament tissue. Their primary role is the repair of damaged tissue which is achieved by differentiation and proliferation through their self-replication ability and multipotency into ligament cells as required. However, the MSCs of patients with ossification are thought to misdifferentiate into osteoblasts instead of target ligament cells because they have high osteogenic ability. We consider epigenetics to be one of the mechanisms responsible for the transformation of patient MSCs (Fig. 7.4). Currently, we are focusing on DNA methylation as a mechanism of epigenetics, but we also intend to analyze other mechanisms such as histone acetylation and regulation by non-coding RNA. The importance of basic research in clinical medicine lies in how the results can be connected to the therapeutics. Therefore, if the mechanism of MSC transformation is elucidated, it will be possible to develop targeted therapies and therapeutic agents.

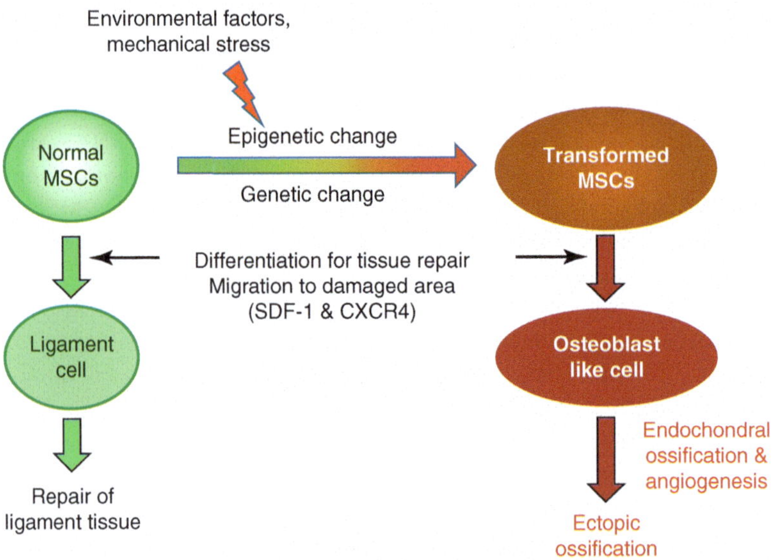

Fig. 7.4 Role of mesenchymal stem cells (MSCs) in the ossification of spinal ligaments. The function of normal MSCs present in ligament tissue is to differentiate and proliferate into ligament cells to repair damage to ligament tissue. In ossified patients, MSCs in the ligament tissue transform in response to a genetic mutation or an epigenetic change caused by several environmental factors or mechanical stresses. Therefore, during tissue repair, they erroneously differentiate into osteoblasts, undergo endochondral ossification and angiogenesis, and ossify ligament tissue

Acknowledgement This research is the result of a joint project with Hirosaki University Graduate School of Medicine Orthopedic Surgery. I would like to express my heartfelt thanks to my collaborators. This work was supported by a Grant-in-Aid from the Practical Research Project for Rare/Intractable Diseases from the Japan Agency for Medical Research and Development (AMED) and a Grant-in-Aid from the Ministry of Education, Culture, Sports, Science and Technology of Japan [Grant 17K10916]. No potential conflicts of interest relevant to this article are reported. We thank Sarah Williams, PhD, from Edanz Group (www.edanzediting.com) for editing a draft of this chapter.

References

1. Resnick D, Shaul SR, Robins JM. Diffuse idiopathic skeletal hyperostosis (DISH). Radiography. 1975;115:513–24.
2. Matsunaga S, Sakou T. In: Yonenobu K, Sakou T, Ono K, editors. Ossification of the posterior longitudinal ligament. Tokyo: Springer; 1997. p. 11–7.
3. Kawaguchi Y, Nakano M, Yasuda T, Seki S, Hori T, Suzuki K, Makino H, Kimura T. Characteristics of ossification of the spinal ligament; incidence of ossification of the ligamentum flavum in patients with cervical ossification of the posterior longitudinal ligament—analysis of the whole spine using multidetector CT. J Orthop Sci. 2016;21:439–45.
4. Tetreault L, Nakashima H, Kato S, Kryshtalskyj M, Nagoshi N, Nouri A, Singh A, Fehlings MG. A systematic review of classification systems for cervical ossification of the posterior longitudinal ligament. Global Spine J. 2019;9:85–103.
5. Joaquim AF, Makhni MC, Riew KD. Post-operative nerve injuries after cervical spine surgery. Int Orthop. 2019;43:791–5.
6. Taketomi E, Sakou T, Matsunaga S, Yamaguchi M. Family study of a twin with ossification of the posterior longitudinal ligament in the cervical spine. Spine. 1992;17:S55–6.
7. Okawa A, Nakamura I, Goto S, Moriya H, Nakamura Y, Ikegawa S. Mutation in Npps in a mouse model of ossification of the posterior longitudinal ligament of the spine. Nat Genet. 1998;19:271–3.
8. Tanaka T, Ikari K, Furushima K, Okada A, Tanaka H, Furukawa K, Yoshida K, Ikeda T, Ikegawa S, Hunt SC, Takeda J, Toh S, Harata S, Nakajima T, Inoue I. Genomewide linkage and linkage disequilibrium analyses identify COL6A1, on chromosome 21, as the locus for ossification of the posterior longitudinal ligament of the spine. Am J Hum Genet. 2003;73:812–22.
9. Nakajima M, Takahashi A, Tsuji T, Karasugi T, Baba H, Uchida K, Kawabata S, Okawa A, Shindo S, Takeuchi K, Taniguchi Y, Maeda S, Kashii M, Seichi A, Nakajima H, Kawaguchi Y, Fujibayashi S, Takahata M, Tanaka T, Watanabe K, Kida K, Kanchiku T, Ito Z, Mori K, Kaito T, Kobayashi S, Yamada K, Takahashi M, Chiba K, Matsumoto M, Furukawa K, Kubo M, Toyama Y, Genetic Study Group of Investigation Committee on Ossification of the Spinal Ligaments, Ikegawa S. A genomewide association study identifies susceptibility loci for ossification of the posterior longitudinal ligament of the spine. Nat Genet. 2014;46:1012–7.
10. Inamasu J, Guiot BH, Sachs DC. Ossification of the posterior longitudinal ligament: an update on its biology, epidemiology, and natural history. Neurosurgery. 2006;58:1027–39.
11. Furukawa KI. Pharmacological aspect of ectopic ossification in spinal ligament tissues. Pharmacol Ther. 2008;118:352–8.
12. Matsunaga S, Sakou T, Taketomi E, Nakanisi K. Effects of strain distribution in the intervertebral discs on the progression of ossification of the posterior longitudinal ligaments. Spine. 1996;21:184–9.
13. Kon T, Yamazaki M, Tagawa M, Goto S, Terakado A, Moriya H, Fujimura S. Bone morphogenetic protein-2 stimulates differentiation of cultured spinal ligament cells from patients with ossification of the posterior longitudinal ligament. Calcif Tissue Int. 1997;60:291–6.
14. Tanaka H, Nagai E, Murata H, Tsubone T, Shirakura Y, Sugiyama T, Taguchi T, Kawai S. Involvement of bone morphogenic protein-2 (BMP-2) in the pathological ossification process of the spinal ligament. Rheumatology (Oxford, England). 2001;40:1163–8.
15. Tanno M, Furukawa KI, Ueyama K, Harata S, Motomura S. Uniaxial cyclic stretch induces osteogenic differentiation and synthesis of bone morphogenetic proteins of spinal ligament cells derived from patients with ossification of the posterior longitudinal ligaments. Bone. 2003;33:475–84.
16. Iwasaki K, Furukawa KI, Tanno M, Kusumi T, Ueyama K, Tanaka M, Kudo H, Toh S, Harata S, Motomura S. Uni-axial cyclic stretch induces Cbfa1 expression in spinal ligament cells derived from patients with ossification of the posterior longitudinal ligament. Calcif Tissue Int. 2004;74:448–57.
17. Iwasawa T, Iwasaki K, Sawada T, Okada A, Ueyama K, Motomura S, Harata S, Inoue I, Toh S, Furukawa KI. Pathophysiological role of endothelin in ectopic ossification of human spinal ligaments induced by mechanical stress. Calcif Tissue Int. 2006;79:422–30.
18. Li JM, Zhang Y, Ren Y, Liu BG, Lin X, Yang J, Zhao HC, Wang YJ, Song L. Uniaxial cyclic stretch promotes osteogenic differentiation and synthesis of BMP2 in the C3H10T1/2 cells with BMP2 gene variant of rs2273073 (T / G). PLoS One. 2014;9:e106598.
19. Asari T, Tanaka S, Kudo H, Mizukami H, Ono A, Numasawa T, Kumagai G, Motomura S, Yagihashi S, Toh S. Mesenchymal stem cell isolation and characterization from human spinal ligaments. Biochem Biophys Res Commun. 2012;417:1193–9.
20. Nancarrow-Lei R, Mafi P, Mafi R, Khan W. A systemic review of adult mesenchymal stem cell sources and their multilineage differentia-

tion potential relevant to musculoskeletal tissue repair and regeneration. Curr Stem Cell Res Ther. 2017;12:601–10.
21. Harada Y, Furukawa KI, Asari T, Chin S, Ono A, Tanaka T, Mizukami H, Yagihashi S, Motomura S, Ishibashi Y. Osteogenic lineage commitment of mesenchymal stem cells from patients with ossification of the posterior longitudinal ligament. Biochem Biophys Res Commun. 2014;443:1014–20.
22. Chin S, Furukawa KI, Ono A, Asari T, Harada Y, Wada K, Tanaka T, Inaba W, Mizukami H, Motomura S, Yagihashi S, Ishibashi Y. Immunohistochemical localization of mesenchymal stem cells in ossified human spinal ligaments. Biochem Biophys Res Commun. 2013;436:698–704.
23. Kucia M, Reca R, Miekus K, Wanzeck J, Wojakowski W, Janowska-Wieczorek A, Ratajczak J, Ratajczak MZ. Trafficking of normal stem cells and metastasis of cancer stem cells involve similar mechanisms pivotal role of the SDF-1-CXCR4 axis. Stem Cells. 2005;23:879–94.
24. Chin S, Furukawa KI, Kurotaki K, Nagasaki S, Wada K, Kumagai G, Motomura S, Ishibashi Y. Facilitation of chemotaxis activity of mesenchymal stem cells via stromal cell-derived factor-1 and its receptor may promote ectopic ossification of human spinal ligaments. J Pharmacol Exp Ther. 2019;369:1–8.
25. Yamamoto Y, Furukawa KI, Ueyama K, Nakanishi T, Takigawa M, Harata S. Possible roles of CTGF/Hcs24 in the initiation and development of ossification of the posterior longitudinal ligament. Spine. 2002;27:1852–7.
26. Kishiya M, Furukawa KI, Yokoyama T, Kudo H, Ono A, Numasawa T, Wada K, Toh S. Comparison of cardiovascular parameters between patients with ossification of posterior longitudinal ligament and patients with cervical spondylotic myelopathy. J Spin Disord Tech. 2009;22:361–6.
27. Hiraki Y, Inoue H, Iyama K, Kamizono A, Ochiai M, Shukunami C, Iijima S, Suzuki F, Kondo J. Identification of chondromodulin I as a novel endothelial cell growth inhibitor. Purification and its localization in the avascular zone of epiphyseal cartilage. J Biol Chem. 1997;272:32419–26.
28. van Dinther M, Visser N, de Gorter DJ, Doorn J, Goumans MJ, de Boer J, ten Dijke P. ALK2 R206H mutation linked to fibrodysplasia ossificans progressiva confers constitutive activity to the BMP type I receptor and sensitizes mesenchymal cells to BMP-induced osteoblast differentiation and bone formation. J Bone Miner Res. 2010;25:1208–15.
29. Medici D, Shore EM, Lounev VY, Kaplan FS, Kalluri R, Olsen BR. Conversion of vascular endothelial cells into multipotent stem-like cells. Nat Med. 2010;16:1400–6.
30. Nakajima M, Kou I, Ohashi H, Genetic Study Group of the Investigation Committee on the Ossification of Spinal Ligaments, Ikegawa S. Identification and functional characterization of RSPO2 as a susceptibility gene for ossification of the posterior longitudinal ligament of the spine. Am J Hum Genet. 2016;99:202–7.
31. Takegami Y, Ohkawara B, Ito M, Masuda A, Nakashima H, Ishiguro N, Ohno K. R-spondin 2 facilitates differentiation of proliferating chondrocytes into hypertrophic chondrocytes by enhancing Wnt/β-catenin signaling in endochondral ossification. Biochem Biophys Res Commun. 2016;473:255–64.
32. Pérez-Campo FM, Riancho JA. Epigenetic mechanisms regulating mesenchymal stem cell differentiation. Curr Genomics. 2015;16:368–83.
33. Montes de Oca A, Madueño JA, Martinez-Moreno JM, Guerrero F, Muñoz-Castañeda J, Rodriguez-Ortiz ME, Mendoza FJ, Almaden Y, Lopez I, Rodriguez M, Aquilera-Tejero E. High-phosphate-induced calcification is related to SM22α promoter methylation in vascular smooth muscle cells. J Bone Miner Res. 2010;25:1996–2005.
34. Chiba N, Furukawa KI, Takayama S, Asari T, Chin S, Harada Y, Kumagai G, Wada K, Tanaka T, Ono A, Motomura S, Ishibashi Y. Decreased DNA methylation in the promoter region of the WNT5A and GDNF genes may promote the osteogenicity of mesenchymal stem cells from patients with ossified spinal ligaments. J Pharmacol Sci. 2015;127:467–73.

A Short History of the Genetic Study of OPLL

8

Shiro Ikegawa

Abstract

This paper briefly reviews the genetic and genomic studies of OPLL in Japan, including linkage, association and model mouse studies.

Keywords

Linkage study · Association study · GWAS R-spondin 2 · *ttw* · Nucleotide pyrophosphatase · Phosphate · Pyrophosphate

8.1 Human Study

8.1.1 Linkage Study

Contribution of genetic factors related to the susceptibility of OPLL has been implicated by the epidemiological studies [1–3]. The modern genetic study for OPLL started with the analysis of HLA (human leukocyte antigen) haplotypes of the sibs [4]. On the basis of the reported association of HLA [5, 6], Koga et al. examined genetic linkage of OPLL using seven microsatellite markers in the HLA region on chromosome 6p in 91 affected sib pairs from 53 families. They found strong linkage on a marker D6S276 ($P = 5.9 \times 10^{-6}$) and reported *COL11A2* as a candidate OPLL susceptibility gene [4].

The same group conducted a genome-wide linkage study for 99 affected sib-pairs from 70 families to identify genetic loci related to OPLL [7]. The best evidence of linkage was detected near the marker D21S1903 on 21q22.3; the linkage region was then extensively investigated for linkage disequilibrium with SNPs covering 20 Mb. Haplotype analysis with three SNPs in *COL6A1* gave a single-point P value of 7×10^{-7}.

To overcome the problem of under-power in the previous linkage studies, Karasugi et al. performed a genome-wide linkage study under the support of the Genetic Study Group of Investigation Committee on Ossification of the Spinal Ligaments supported by a grant from the Ministry of Health and Welfare of Japan (leader: Prof. Yoshiaki Toyama) [8]. The study used 410 cervical OPLL samples (214 affected sib-pairs) from all over Japan and found loci with suggestive linkages on 1p21, 2p22–2p24, 7q22, 16q24, and 20p12. Fine mapping using additional markers detected the highest NPL score (3.43, $P = 2.7 \times 10^{-4}$) at D20S894 on chromosome 20p12 in a subgroup that had no complication of diabetes mellitus.

S. Ikegawa (✉)
Laboratory for Bone and Joint Diseases, Center for Integrative Medical Sciences (IMS), RIKEN, Tokyo, Japan
e-mail: sikegawa@ims.u-tokyo.ac.jp

A. Okawa et al. (eds.), *OPLL*, https://doi.org/10.1007/978-981-15-3855-1_8

8.1.2 Association Study

Because of the low resolution of the linkage study and development of high-throughput genotyping system of single nucleotide polymorphisms (SNPs), genome researchers came to use the association study to map the gene for polygenic genes, which was the case with the genetic study of OPLL. There are many association studies of OPLL; however, almost all are the candidate gene association studies which examined only single variant or gene in less than 500 patients. The largest one is the study by Horikoshi et al. [9] which examined a total of 109 s SNPs in 35 candidate genes in 711 OPLL patients and 896 controls. The result is not remarkable, however. An intronic SNP in *TGFB3* showed the most significant association ($P = 4.0 \times 10^{-4}$). *TGFB3* is located within a genomic region that has been linked with OPLL.

With the support of the Genetic Study Group of Investigation Committee on Ossification of the Spinal Ligaments (project leader: Prof. Yoshiaki Toyama), Nakajima et al. performed a genome-wide association study (GWAS) first in the world. They examined 1112 cases and 6810 controls followed by a replication study using an additional an independent set of 548 Japanese OPLL individuals and 6469 Japanese controls [10]. The GWAS identified six susceptibility OPLL loci with genome-wide significance level of association (Table 8.1). Most of the loci did not contain obvious candidate genes.

8.1.3 R-spondin 2

With a support of Japan Agency for Medical Research and Development (AMED) project lead by Prof. Morio Matsumoto of Keio University, Nakajima et al. performed a post-GWAS in silico and in vitro functional studies for the OPLL loci. Among them, they discovered a candidate functional variant upstream of the R-spondin 2 gene (*RSPO2*) on chromosome 8q23.1 [11]. R-spondin 2 is a member of the R-spondin family of secreted proteins [12]. The R-spondin family consists of four known members (R-spondin 1–4) that share 40–60% amino acid homology and a similar domain organization [12]. R-spondins are identified as ligands of leucine-rich repeat-containing G-protein-coupled receptors (LGRs), including LGR4, 5 and 6 that associate with the Frizzled/low density lipoprotein receptor-related protein (LRP) 5/6-Wnt receptor complex [13]. R-spondin 2 is an agonist of canonical Wnt/β-catenin signaling. Expression of R-spondin 2 was decreased in the early stage of chondrocyte differentiation [11]. R-spondin 2 inhibited expression of early chondrocyte differentiation marker genes by activating Wnt/β-catenin signaling. rs374810, the most significantly associated SNP on chromosome 8q23.1 in the GWAS was located in the chondrocyte promoter region of *RSPO2*. A transcription factor, CCAAT-enhancer-binding protein β (C/EBPβ) specifically bound to the *RSPO2* core promoter region containing rs374810 and increased *RSPO2* expression. The risk allele of rs374810 affected the binding of the promoter with C/EBPβ and decreased the *RSPO2* transcription [11].

8.1.4 Extended GWAS

The GWAS only explains ~2% of the total genetic variance of OPLL. More genetic information is necessary to understand OPLL. With the support of AMED (project leader: Prof. Morio Matsumoto of Keio University), RIKEN group is

Table 8.1 OPLL loci identified by GWAS in Japanese

Lead SNP	Chromosome	Gene in or near the associated region	*P* value	Odds ratio (95% confidence interval)
rs927485	6p21.1	*CDC5L, MIR4642, SUPT3H*	9.40×10^{-9}	1.33 (1.21–1.46)
rs374810	8q23.1	*RSPO2*	1.88×10^{-13}	1.34 (1.24–1.44)
rs13279799	8q23.3	*LINC00536, EIF3H*	1.28×10^{-10}	1.28 (1.19–1.38)
rs1979679	12p11.22	*CCDC91*	4.34×10^{-12}	1.30 (1.21–1.40)
rs11045000	12p12.2	*LOC100506393*	2.95×10^{-11}	1.28 (1.19–1.38)
rs2423294	20p12.3	*HAO1*	1.10×10^{-13}	1.41 (1.29–1.55)

conducting the extended GWAS using more than 1600 OPLL subjects. A meta-analysis of the previous GWAS and the new GWAS would identify additional susceptibility loci for OPLL.

8.2 Mouse Study

8.2.1 ttw

ttw (tiptoe walking; previously called as *twy* (tiptoe walking of Yoshimura)) is an excellent mouse model for ectopic ossification [14, 15]. *ttw* is a naturally occurring mutant that originated from the ICR (*jcl*) strain. The mode of inheritance is autosomal recessive with complete penetrance. Progression of ectopic ossification in the mice is easily monitored by contracture of the limb joints, which leads to characteristic "tiptoe" walking. *ttw* exhibits ossification of various soft tissues. As early as 3 weeks after birth, calcification was observed in tendons, ear cartilage and periarticular tissues. Ectopic calcification is observed in annulus fibrosus at 4 weeks. In the Achilles tendon, it is initially represented as focal calcification in the middle of the tendon (Fig. 8.1a) and then extends longitudinally along the collagen fibers. The calcification progresses along the substance of the tendon and finally merges to the bone (Fig. 8.2). Therefore, the initial event of the ectopic ossification in *ttw* is not enthesopathy (Fig. 8.1b). The ectopic ossification of *ttw* occurs through a mechanism different from enchondral ossification.

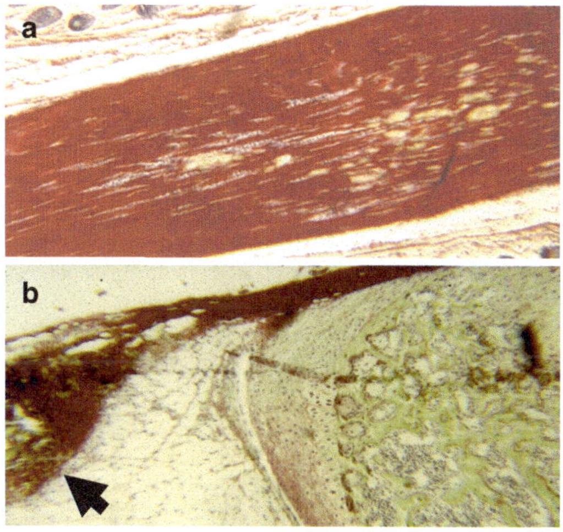

Fig. 8.1 Histology of the Achilles tendon of *ttw*. HE staining. (**a**) The middle portion of the tendon at 4 weeks of age. Focal calcification in the middle of the tendon is the initial lesion. (**b**) The tendon insertion at 6 weeks of age. The ossified lesion (arrow) in the tendon is not continuous to the calcaneus (right)

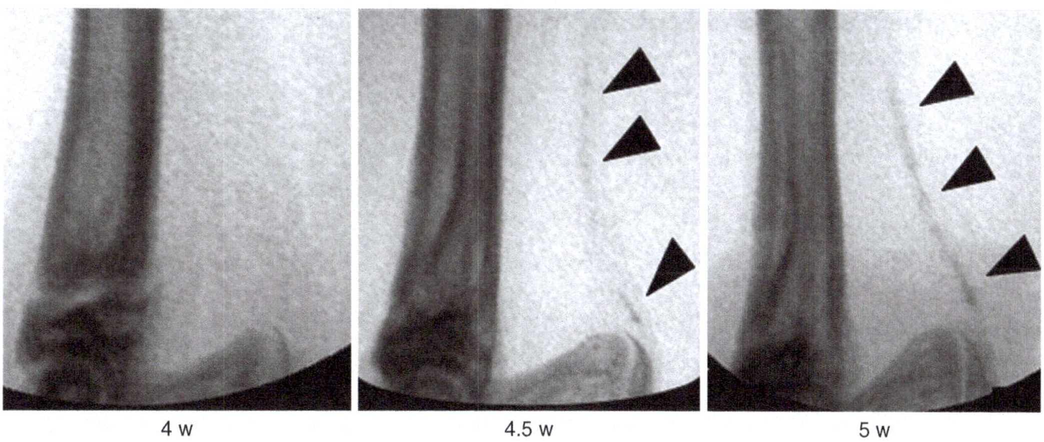

Fig. 8.2 The early stage of ectopic ossification in *ttw*. The lateral radiograph (Soft X-ray) of the Achilles tendon, showing progression of the ectopic ossification (arrow). The lesion progresses along the substance of the tendon and merges to the bone

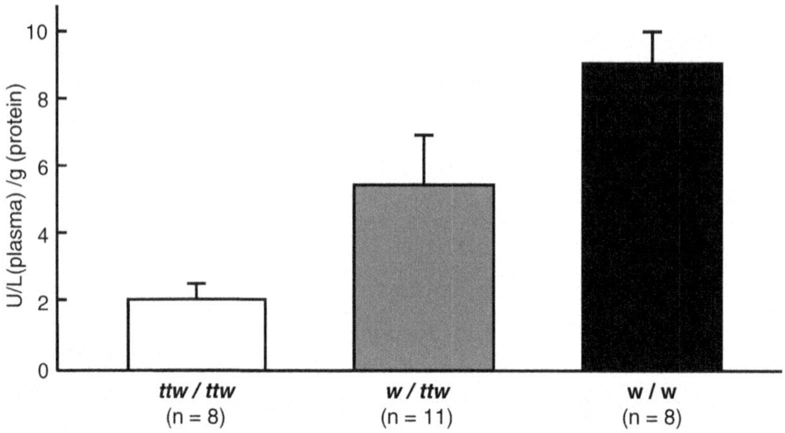

Fig. 8.3 Decreased nucleotide pyrophosphatase (NPPS) activity in *ttw*. The plasma phosphodiesterase activities of *ttw* and its unaffected littermates (w/w and *ttw*/w; w: wild type) were measured by a TMPNP (thymidine monophosphate paranytrophenylester) assay. Absorbance at 405 nm was determined by a BioRad model 550-microtiter reader. Total protein was measured by a protein-assay kit (Biorad). Measurements were done in duplicate. The phosphodiesterase activity is presented as U per plasma per protein. 1 U = phosphodiesterase activity to catalyze a one mole of substrate per hour. The activity is decreased according to the number of the *ttw* allele, being almost absent in *ttw*. Columns indicate the means, and bars standard deviations. The numbers of samples are in parentheses

Table 8.2 Decreased NPPS activity and PPi level in *ttw*

Phenotype	NPPS (p mol/h/mg protein)	PPi (p mol/h/mg protein)
Wild type	363 ± 69	0.15 ± 0.06
ttw	142 ± 22	0.11 ± 0.04

NPPS activity and PPi in vesicles isolated from conditioned media of cultured osteoblastic cells. Wild type mice are littermates of *ttw* with genotypes not homozygous for the *ttw* mutation

8.2.2 Nucleotide Pyrophosphatase and Pyrophosphate

Through a positional cloning using a parametric linkage analysis followed by a candidate gene approach, Ikegawa's group have identified that *ttw* is caused by a nonsense mutation (c.1813G > T; p.Gly568*) of *Enpp1* encoding nucleotide pyrophosphatase (NPPS) [15, 16]. NPPS is a membrane-bound ectoenzyme with both alkaline phosphodiesterase-I and nucleotide pyrophosphatase activities. The *ttw* mutation causes loss of function of NPPS; NPPS activities in serum and osteoblastic cells are significantly decreased in *ttw* (Fig. 8.3, Table 8.2). NPPS generates inorganic phosphate and pyrophosphate (PPi). PPi is a major inhibitor of physiologic and pathologic calcification and ossification. PPi inhibits precipitation of calcium phosphate [17] and organization of hydroxyapatite to bone matrix [18]. These lines of evidence suggest PPi metabolism associated with NPPS play an important role in regulation of ectopic ossification [19]. Notably, *ank* (ankylosis), another mouse model of ectopic ossification, is also caused by abnormal PPi metabolism. It results from the loss of function mutation of the membrane transporter of PPi [7], resulting in decreased extracellular PPi.

8.2.3 Phosphate

The NPPS-PPi metabolism is closely related to phosphate (Pi) metabolism. PPi is degraded to Pi by alkaline phosphatase (ALP). Hypophosphatasia, a heterogenous group of diseases caused by the ALP deficiency presents marked decrease of ossification due to increased PPi. Patients with abnormal Pi metabolism has been implicate in OPLL and associated disease [20, 21]. Patients with hypophosphatemic rickets/osteomalacia

Table 8.3 Novel mouse genes identified by a differential display analysis of *ttw* on high phosphate diet

Gene symbol	Gene name	Expression in high phosphate diet	Human counterpart	Postulated function
Prg4	Proteoglycan 4	Increase	*PRG4*[a]	ECM protein
RNase4	Rnase A family, 4	Increase	*RNASE4*	Ribonuclease
Cst10	Cystatin 10	Increase	(−)	Enzyme inhibitor
Calm4	Calmodulin 4	Decrease	(−)	Intra-Ca regulator
Wrap73[b]	WD repeat containing, antisense to Trp73	Decrease	*WDR8*	Unknown
Etos1	Ectopic ossification 1	Decrease	(−)	ncRNA

[a]Alias: megakaryocyte stimulating factor (MSF) and articular superficial zone protein (SZP)
[b]First reported as *Wdr8*

(MIM #307800) and hypoparathyroidism are frequently complicated by ectopic ossification of the tendons and ligaments of the spine and limbs [22, 23]. Bi-allelic (recessive) loss of function mutations in *ENPP1* cause the autosomal recessive form of hypophosphatemic rickets (MIM #613312) and generalized arterial calcification of infancy-1 (MIM # 208000).

To clarify mechanism of ectopic ossification in *ttw*, Koshizuka et al. examined the effect of dietary Ca and Pi on the *ttw* phenotype. Tests of combination of high or low content of Ca and Pi in the diet showed that a high Pi diet markedly accelerated ectopic ossification [24]. To identify genes involved in ectopic ossification, they examined the expression profile of genes during enhanced ossification in *ttw* on high phosphate diet by differential display method [24]. *ttw* mice were fed by high Ca-high Pi or high Ca-low Pi diet after weaning at 3 weeks of age and serially sacrificed until 2 weeks after the start of the diet. The ear cartilages were subjected to a differential display analysis. They identified nine mouse genes that showed differential expression; six genes were up regulated by high Pi diet, and three down-regulated; six of the nine genes were novel (Table 8.3) [24–26]. Among them is cystatin 10 (also known as carminerin). Yamada et al. reported that carminerin contributes to chondrocyte calcification during endochondral ossification under physiological and pathological conditions through the transcriptional inhibition of NPP1 [27].

Acknowledgement We thank OPLL patients and their families who participated in this study and the OPLL patient network in Japan (Zensekichuren. President, Yasuko Masuda).

References

1. Taketomi E, Sakou T, Matsunaga S, Yamaguchi M. Family study of a twin with ossification of the posterior longitudinal ligament in the cervical spine. Spine. 1992;17:S55–6.
2. Matsunaga S, Sakou T. Epidemiology of ossification of the posterior longitudinal ligament. In: Yonenobu K, Sakou T, Ono K, editors. OPLL. Tokyo: Springer; 1997. p. 11–7.
3. Sakou T, Matsunaga S, Koga H. Recent progress in the study of pathogenesis of ossification of the posterior longitudinal ligament. J Orthop Sci. 2000;5:310–5.
4. Koga H, Sakou T, Taketomi E, Hayashi K, Numasawa T, Harata S, Yone K, Matsunaga S, Otterud B, Inoue I, Leppert M. Genetic mapping of ossification of the posterior longitudinal ligament of the spine. Am J Hum Genet. 1998;62:1460–7.
5. Sakou T, Taketomi E, Matsunaga S, Yamaguchi M, Sonoda S, Yashiki S. Genetic study of ossification of the posterior longitudinal ligament in the cervical spine with human leukocyte antigen haplotype. Spine (Phila Pa 1976). 1991;16:1249–52.
6. Matsunaga S, Yamaguchi M, Hayashi K, Sakou T. Genetic analysis of ossification of the posterior longitudinal ligament. Spine (Phila Pa 1976). 1999;24:937–8.
7. Tanaka T, Ikari K, Furushima K, Okada A, Tanaka H, Furukawa KI, Yoshida K, Ikeda T, Ikegawa S, Hunt SC, Takeda JTS, Harata S, Nakajima T, Inoue I. Genomewide linkage and linkage disequilibrium analyses identify COL6A1, on chromosome 21, as the locus for ossification of the posterior longitudinal ligament of the spine. Am J Hum Genet. 2003;73:812–22.

8. Karasugi T, Nakajima M, Ikari K, Genetic Study Group of Investigation Committee on Ossification of the Spinal Ligaments, Tsuji T, Matsumoto M, Chiba K, Uchida K, Kawaguchi Y, Mizuta H, Ogata N, Iwasaki M, Maeda S, Numasawa T, Abumi K, Kato T, Ozawa H, Taguchi T, Kaito T, Neo M, Yamazaki M, Tadokoro N, Yoshida M, Nakahara S, Endo K, Imagama S, Demura S, Sato K, Seichi A, Ichimura S, Watanabe M, Watanabe K, Nakamura Y, Mori K, Baba H, Toyama Y, Ikegawa S. A genome-wide sib-pair linkage analysis of ossification of the posterior longitudinal ligament of the spine. J Bone Miner Metab. 2013;31:136–43.
9. Horikoshi T, Maeda K, Kawaguchi Y, Chiba K, Mori K, Koshizuka Y, Hirabayashi S, Sugimori K, Matsumoto M, Kawaguchi H, Takahashi M, Inoue H, Kimura T, Matsusue Y, Inoue I, Baba H, Nakamura K, Ikegawa S. A large-scale genetic association study of ossification of the posterior longitudinal ligament of the spine. Hum Genet. 2006;119:611–6.
10. Nakajima M, Takahashi A, Tsuji T, Karasugi T, Baba H, Uchida K, Kawabata S, Okawa A, Shindo S, Takeuchi K, Taniguchi Y, Maeda S, Kashii M, Seichi A, Nakajima H, Kawaguchi Y, Fujibayashi S, Takahata M, Tanaka T, Watanabe K, Kida K, Kanchiku T, Ito Z, Mori K, Kaito T, Kobayashi S, Yamada K, Takahashi M, Chiba K, Matsumoto M, Furukawa K, Kubo M, Toyama Y, Genetic Study Group of Investigation Committee on Ossification of the Spinal Ligaments, Ikegawa S. A genome-wide association study identifies susceptibility loci for ossification of the posterior longitudinal ligament of the spine. Nat Genet. 2014;46:1012–6.
11. Nakajima M, Kou I, Ohashi H, Genetic Study Group of Investigation Committee on the Ossification of Spinal Ligaments, Ikegawa S. Identification and functional characterization of RSPO2 as a susceptibility gene for ossification of the posterior longitudinal ligament of the spine. Am J Hum Genet. 2016;99:202–7.
12. de Lau WB, Snel B, Clevers HC. The R-spondin protein family. Genome Biol. 2012;13:242.
13. de Lau W, Barker N, Low TY, Koo BK, Li VS, Teunissen H, Kujala P, Haegebarth A, Peters PJ, van de Wetering M, Stange DE, van Es JE, Guardavaccaro D, Schasfoort RB, Mohri Y, Nishimori K, Mohammed S, Heck AJ, Clevers H. Lgr5 homologues associate with Wnt receptors and mediate R-spondin signalling. Nature. 2011;476:293–7.
14. Hosoda Y, Yoshimura Y, Higaki SA. New breed of mouse showing multiple osteochondral lesions twy mouse. Ryumachi. 1981;21:157–64.
15. Okawa A, Nakamura I, Goto S, Moriya H, Nakamura Y, Ikegawa S. Mutation in Npps in a mouse model of ossification of the posterior longitudinal ligament of the spine. Nat Genet. 1998a;19:271–3.
16. Okawa A, Ikegawa S, Nakamura I, Goto S, Moriya H, Nakamura Y. Mapping of a gene responsible for twy (tip-toe walking Yoshimura), a mouse model of ossification of the posterior longitudinal ligament of the spine (OPLL). Mamm Genome. 1998b;9:155–6.
17. Fleisch H. Diphosphonates: history and mechanisms of action. Metab Bone Dis Rel Res. 1981;3:279–88.
18. Meyer JL. Can biological calcification occur in the presence of pyrophosphate? Arch Biochem Biophys. 1984;231:1–8.
19. Ho AM, Johnson MD, Kingsley DM. Role of the mouse ank gene in control of tissue calcification and arthritis. Science. 2000;289:265–70.
20. Takuwa Y, Matsumoto T, Kurokawa T, Iizuka M, Hoshino Y, Hata K, Ogata E. Calcium metabolism in paravertebral ligamentous ossification. Acta Endocrinol. 1985;109:428–32.
21. Kawaguchi Y, Nakano M, Yasuda T, Seki S, Suzuki K, Yahara Y, Makino H, Kitajima I, Kimura T. Serum biomarkers in patients with ossification of the posterior longitudinal ligament (OPLL): inflammation in OPLL. PLoS One. 2017;12:e0174881.
22. Yoshikawa S, Shiba M, Suzuki A. Spinal-cord compression in untreated adult cases of vitamin-D resistant rickets. J Bone Joint Surg Am. 1968;50:743–52.
23. Okazaki T, Takuwa Y, Yamamoto M, Matsumoto T, Igarashi T, Kurokawa T, Ogata E. Ossification of the paravertebral ligaments: a frequent complication of hypoparathyroidism. Metabolism. 1984;33:710–3.
24. Koshizuka Y, Ikegawa S, Sano M, Nakamura K, Nakamura Y. Isolation of novel mouse genes associated with ectopic ossification by differential display method using ttw, a mouse model for ectopic ossification. Cytogenet Cell Genet. 2001a;94:163–8.
25. Ikegawa S, Sano M, Koshizuka Y, Nakamura Y. Isolation, characterization and mapping of the mouse and human PRG4 (proteoglycan 4) genes. Cytogenet Cell Genet. 2000;90:291–7.
26. Koshizuka Y, Ikegawa S, Sano M, Nakamura K, Nakamura Y. Isolation, characterization, and mapping of the mouse and human *WDR8* genes, members of a novel wd repeat gene family. Genomics. 2001b;72:252–9.
27. Yamada T, Kawano H, Koshizuka Y, Fukuda T, Yoshimura K, Kamekura S, Saito T, Ikeda T, Kawasaki Y, Azuma Y, Ikegawa S, Hoshi K, Chung UI, Nakamura K, Kato S, Kawaguchi H. Carminerin contributes to chondrocyte calcification during endochondral ossification. Nat Med. 2006;12(6):665–70.

Overview of Possible Roles of OPLL-Associated Genes in OPLL Development

9

Taku Saito

Abstract

In addition to classical genomic studies, a genome-wide association study for ossification of the posterior longitudinal ligament (OPLL) was performed and susceptibility loci and candidate genes were identified. Among them, R-spondin 2 (*RSPO2*) has been focused on as a potent candidate. RSPO2 is a member of the R-spondin secreted protein family and enhances canonical Wnt signaling activity. A recent study showed that RSPO2 suppresses the early-stage differentiation of chondrocytes and that its expression is significantly lower in fibroblasts carrying the risk allele. These findings suggest that RSPO2 may suppress the differentiation of mesenchymal stem cells toward chondrocytes via the inhibition of canonical Wnt signaling. To obtain a deeper understanding of the pathophysiology of OPLL, appropriate experimental animal models and expression analyses of candidate genes in surgical specimens from OPLL patients are necessary.

Keywords

Ossification of the posterior longitudinal ligament (OPLL) · Genome-wide association study (GWAS) · Susceptibility gene

T. Saito (✉)
Sensory and Motor System Medicine, Faculty of Medicine, The University of Tokyo, Tokyo, Japan
e-mail: tasaitou-tky@umin.ac.jp

Many studies aimed at identifying genetic factors associated with the pathogenesis of ossification of the posterior longitudinal ligament (OPLL) have been performed. Previously, affected sib-pair linkage studies and candidate-gene association studies indicated a number of genes or loci associated with susceptibility to this condition: collagen type XI alpha 2 chain (*COL11A2*) [1], retinoid X receptor beta (*RXRB*) [2], ectonucleotide pyrophosphatase/phosphodiesterase 1 (*ENPP1*) [3], transforming growth factor beta 1 (*TGFB1*) [4], interleukin 1 beta (*IL1B*) [5], estrogen receptor 1 (*ESR1*) [5], collagen type VI alpha 1 chain (*COL6A1*) [6], *TGFB3* [7], bone morphogenetic protein 2 (*BMP2*) [8], vitamin D receptor (*VDR*) [9], runt-related transcription factor 2 (*RUNX2*) [10], interleukin 15 receptor subunit alpha (*IL15RA*) [11], and growth differentiation factor 2 (*GDF2*) [12]. Via these strategies, genes related to connective tissue, bone formation, mineral metabolism, and inflammation have been investigated. Recently, Nakajima et al. performed a genome-wide association study (GWAS) for cervical OPLL in ~8000 individuals, followed by a replication study using additional ~7000 individuals [13]. Six susceptibility loci were discovered and several genes located in or near the associated regions were newly identified as candidate genes for OPLL susceptibility, including hydroxyacid oxidase 1 (*HAO1*), R-spondin 2 (*RSPO2*), eukaryotic translation initiation factor 3 subunit E (*EIF3E*), ER membrane protein complex subunit 2 (*EMC2*), and coiled-coil domain

A. Okawa et al. (eds.), *OPLL*, https://doi.org/10.1007/978-981-15-3855-1_9

containing 91 (*CCDC91*) [13]. Notably, the GWAS data indicated that *P*-values for all candidate genes from the affected sib-pair linkage studies and candidate-gene association studies were in the range of 0.0091–0.41, far above the standard significance level in GWAS [14].

In contrast to these achievements by genomic studies, it is still difficult to examine the functional roles of the candidate genes because most of the pathophysiology of OPLL remains unclear. In the ossifying front of OPLL, fibrocartilaginous cell proliferation and matrix hyperplasia are universally observed; however, the ossification process was not always endochondral upon histological examination of specimens, but was instead sometimes membranous [15]. Various kinds of cells may be involved in these complicated processes, such as ligament cells, progenitors, tissue-resident stem cells, fibrocartilaginous cells in entheses, macrophages, and other immune-related cells. To clarify the roles of the candidate genes, we have to search for the responsible cells in which the genes exert their effects. Furthermore, there are no useful experimental animal models for OPLL. These issues make it difficult to investigate the roles of the candidate genes in the pathophysiology of OPLL.

Despite these limitations, *RSPO2* has been focused on as a potent candidate gene conferring susceptibility to OPLL. RSPO2 is a member of the R-spondin family, which consists of four members (RSPO1–4) [16]. The R-spondins are secreted proteins that bind to leucine-rich repeat-containing G-protein-coupled receptors (LRPs). RSPO2 is associated with regulation of the canonical WNT signaling pathway [16–18]. Canonical WNT signaling is one of the major regulators of cartilage and bone development. Wnt signaling should be tightly regulated for normal endochondral ossification, and its loss or gain of function leads to severe impairment of skeletal growth [19–21]. These studies indicate that the canonical WNT signaling inhibits the differentiation of mesenchymal stem cells into chondrocytes, but promotes the hypertrophic differentiation of chondrocytes and osteoblast differentiation [19–21]. Rspo2 expression is observed in the apical ectodermal ridge and spinal column of mouse embryo [22], and activity of the canonical Wnt pathway is decreased in the spinal column of *Rspo2* null mice [23]. *Rspo2* null mice display hypoplasia and deformity in limb and craniofacial regions [23, 24]. Rspo2 promotes osteoblast differentiation and mineralization in the presence of WNT and BMP proteins [25]. Meanwhile, Rspo2 suppresses chondrocyte differentiation and cartilage matrix production [26].

Nakajima et al. performed experimental analyses of RSPO2 and reported its possible roles in the pathophysiology of OPLL [27]. RSPO2 suppresses the early-stage differentiation of chondrocytes, and a single-nucleotide polymorphism (SNP) associated with RSPO2 induction by CCAAT/enhancer binding protein beta (C/EBPβ) has been identified [27]. Notably, RSPO2 expression is significantly lower in fibroblasts carrying the risk allele [27]. From these findings, it was concluded that RSPO2 may suppress the differentiation of mesenchymal stem cells toward chondrocytes via the inhibition of canonical Wnt signaling, and contributes to homeostasis of the posterior longitudinal ligament [27]. Meanwhile, there are no data about the expression pattern of RSPO2 in the posterior longitudinal ligament, nor in human tissue samples with OPLL. A recent study showed that synovial macrophages promote the progression of osteoarthritis partly via the production of Rspo2 [28]. To obtain a comprehensive understanding of the pathophysiology of OPLL, associated inter-cellular interactions and communication should be clarified, and the roles of susceptibility genes including *RSPO2* should be examined in this context.

Acknowledgments I thank Edanz (www.edanzediting.co.jp) for editing the English text of the draft of this manuscript.

References

1. Koga H, Hayashi K, Taketomi E, Matsunaga S, Yashiki S, Fujiyoshi T, et al. Restriction fragment length polymorphism of genes of the alpha 2(XI) collagen, bone morphogenetic protein-2, alkaline phosphatase, and tumor necrosis factor-alpha among patients with ossification of posterior longitudinal ligament and controls from the Japanese population. Spine (Phila Pa 1976). 1996;21(4):469–73.
2. Numasawa T, Koga H, Ueyama K, Maeda S, Sakou T, Harata S, et al. Human retinoic X receptor beta: complete genomic sequence and mutation search for ossification of posterior longitudinal ligament of the spine. J Bone Miner Res. 1999;14(4):500–8.
3. Nakamura I, Ikegawa S, Okawa A, Okuda S, Koshizuka Y, Kawaguchi H, et al. Association of the human NPPS gene with ossification of the posterior longitudinal ligament of the spine (OPLL). Hum Genet. 1999;104(6):492–7.
4. Kamiya M, Harada A, Mizuno M, Iwata H, Yamada Y. Association between a polymorphism of the transforming growth factor-beta1 gene and genetic susceptibility to ossification of the posterior longitudinal ligament in Japanese patients. Spine (Phila Pa 1976). 2001;26(11):1264–6. discussion 6–7.
5. Ogata N, Koshizuka Y, Miura T, Iwasaki M, Hosoi T, Shiraki M, et al. Association of bone metabolism regulatory factor gene polymorphisms with susceptibility to ossification of the posterior longitudinal ligament of the spine and its severity. Spine (Phila Pa 1976). 2002;27(16):1765–71.
6. Tanaka T, Ikari K, Furushima K, Okada A, Tanaka H, Furukawa K, et al. Genomewide linkage and linkage disequilibrium analyses identify COL6A1, on chromosome 21, as the locus for ossification of the posterior longitudinal ligament of the spine. Am J Hum Genet. 2003;73(4):812–22.
7. Horikoshi T, Maeda K, Kawaguchi Y, Chiba K, Mori K, Koshizuka Y, et al. A large-scale genetic association study of ossification of the posterior longitudinal ligament of the spine. Hum Genet. 2006;119(6):611–6.
8. Wang H, Liu D, Yang Z, Tian B, Li J, Meng X, et al. Association of bone morphogenetic protein-2 gene polymorphisms with susceptibility to ossification of the posterior longitudinal ligament of the spine and its severity in Chinese patients. Eur Spine J. 2008;17(7):956–64.
9. Kobashi G, Ohta K, Washio M, Okamoto K, Sasaki S, Yokoyama T, et al. FokI variant of vitamin D receptor gene and factors related to atherosclerosis associated with ossification of the posterior longitudinal ligament of the spine: a multi-hospital case-control study. Spine (Phila Pa 1976). 2008;33(16):E553–8.
10. Liu Y, Zhao Y, Chen Y, Shi G, Yuan W. RUNX2 polymorphisms associated with OPLL and OLF in the Han population. Clin Orthop Relat Res. 2010;468(12):3333–41.
11. Kim DH, Jeong YS, Chon J, Yoo SD, Kim HS, Kang SW, et al. Association between interleukin 15 receptor, alpha (IL15RA) polymorphism and Korean patients with ossification of the posterior longitudinal ligament. Cytokine. 2011;55(3):343–6.
12. Ren Y, Liu ZZ, Feng J, Wan H, Li JH, Wang H, et al. Association of a BMP9 haplotype with ossification of the posterior longitudinal ligament (OPLL) in a Chinese population. PLoS One. 2012;7(7):e40587.
13. Nakajima M, Takahashi A, Tsuji T, Karasugi T, Baba H, Uchida K, et al. A genome-wide association study identifies susceptibility loci for ossification of the posterior longitudinal ligament of the spine. Nat Genet. 2014;46(9):1012–6.
14. Ikegawa S. Genomic study of ossification of the posterior longitudinal ligament of the spine. Proc Jpn Acad Ser B Phys Biol Sci. 2014;90(10):405–12.
15. Ono K, Yonenobu K, Miyamoto S, Okada K. Pathology of ossification of the posterior longitudinal ligament and ligamentum flavum. Clin Orthop Relat Res. 1999;(359):18–26.
16. de Lau WB, Snel B, Clevers HC. The R-spondin protein family. Genome Biol. 2012;13(3):242.
17. Kazanskaya O, Glinka A, del Barco BI, Stannek P, Niehrs C, Wu W. R-Spondin2 is a secreted activator of Wnt/beta-catenin signaling and is required for Xenopus myogenesis. Dev Cell. 2004;7(4):525–34.
18. Kim KA, Wagle M, Tran K, Zhan X, Dixon MA, Liu S, et al. R-Spondin family members regulate the Wnt pathway by a common mechanism. Mol Biol Cell. 2008;19(6):2588–96.
19. Day TF, Guo X, Garrett-Beal L, Yang Y. Wnt/beta-catenin signaling in mesenchymal progenitors controls osteoblast and chondrocyte differentiation during vertebrate skeletogenesis. Dev Cell. 2005;8(5):739–50.
20. Hill TP, Spater D, Taketo MM, Birchmeier W, Hartmann C. Canonical Wnt/beta-catenin signaling prevents osteoblasts from differentiating into chondrocytes. Dev Cell. 2005;8(5):727–38.
21. Tamamura Y, Otani T, Kanatani N, Koyama E, Kitagaki J, Komori T, et al. Developmental regulation of Wnt/beta-catenin signals is required for growth plate assembly, cartilage integrity, and endochondral ossification. J Biol Chem. 2005;280(19):19185–95.
22. Nam JS, Turcotte TJ, Yoon JK. Dynamic expression of R-spondin family genes in mouse development. Gene Expr Patterns. 2007;7(3):306–12.
23. Yamada W, Nagao K, Horikoshi K, Fujikura A, Ikeda E, Inagaki Y, et al. Craniofacial malformation in R-spondin2 knockout mice. Biochem Biophys Res Commun. 2009;381(3):453–8.

24. Aoki M, Kiyonari H, Nakamura H, Okamoto H. R-spondin2 expression in the apical ectodermal ridge is essential for outgrowth and patterning in mouse limb development. Develop Growth Differ. 2008;50(2):85–95.
25. Friedman MS, Oyserman SM, Hankenson KD. Wnt11 promotes osteoblast maturation and mineralization through R-spondin 2. J Biol Chem. 2009;284(21):14117–25.
26. Takegami Y, Ohkawara B, Ito M, Masuda A, Nakashima H, Ishiguro N, et al. R-spondin 2 facilitates differentiation of proliferating chondrocytes into hypertrophic chondrocytes by enhancing Wnt/beta-catenin signaling in endochondral ossification. Biochem Biophys Res Commun. 2016;473(1):255–64.
27. Nakajima M, Kou I, Ohashi H, Ikegawa S. Identification and functional characterization of RSPO2 as a susceptibility gene for ossification of the posterior longitudinal ligament of the spine. Am J Hum Genet. 2016;99(1):202–7.
28. Zhang H, Lin C, Zeng C, Wang Z, Wang H, Lu J, et al. Synovial macrophage M1 polarisation exacerbates experimental osteoarthritis partially through R-spondin-2. Ann Rheum Dis. 2018;77(10):1524–34.

10 Application of iPS Cell Technology for OPLL

Junya Toguchida

Abstract

Ossification of posterior longitudinal ligament (OPLL) is a multifactorial disease with both genetic and acquired factors. Although the current surgical therapies show beneficial results in most of the patients, the high rate of disease progression after surgeries is still a matter to be overcome. To develop pharmaceutical treatments for the prevention of progression, the precise understanding of pathologic mechanisms of ossification is inevitable, for which the identification of genetic factors will be greatly contributed. Patient-derived induced pluripotent stem cells (iPSCs) have been used to recapitulate disease phenotype in vitro and find drugs for monogenic hereditary diseases, and successful results are reported in some diseases. Two approaches are proposed to apply iPSCs for the research of OPLL. One is to use iPSCs established from OPLL patients with multiple affected siblings and analyze the differentiation potential in combination with whole exome analyses to identify candidate variants. The other is to analyze the significance of disease-associated genes identified by genome-wide association study (GWAS). Using the genome editing method, iPSCs with risk and non-risk alleles will be created from an identical clone and compared the differentiation property to investigate the functional role of each gene. Although there are several issues to be overcome, these approaches will facilitate the understanding of OPLL and open the way to discover drugs for this disease.

Keywords

iPSC · Disease recapitulation · GWAS
Genetic factor

10.1 Introduction

Ossification of posterior longitudinal ligament (OPLL) is one of the diseases caused by heterotopic ossification (HO), which is the process of bone tissue formation in soft tissues. Although the diagnosis will be made as an incidental finding in some cases, most of the patients do not notice their disease until they suffer pain and/or neurological disturbances, and therefore when they visit medical treatment ossified tissues are large enough to cause compression of spinal cord or nerves. Because currently there are no ways to extinguish ossified tissues by drugs, the surgical treatment is the only choice to relieve patients' pain and disturbance [1]. With the advancement of preoperative and intraoperative imaging modalities and surgical technique, operations

J. Toguchida (✉)
Institute for Frontier Life and Medical Sciences, Kyoto University, Kyoto, Kyoto, Japan
e-mail: togjun@cira.kyoto-u.ac.jp

A. Okawa et al. (eds.), *OPLL*, https://doi.org/10.1007/978-981-15-3855-1_10

will be performed in safe, and good functionally recovery can be expected in most of the cases [1]. Operations will be either the resection of ossified tissues via anterior approach or resection of posterior elements of spine to decompress the spinal cord leaving ossified tissues as they are. One of the postoperative complications is the recurrence or progression of ossified tissues, which will make long-term results worse, and the incidence of such an event is estimated approximately 30% within 7 years and 70% within 10 years [2]. Pharmaceutical treatment to prevent disease progression will be highly beneficial for patients although there are no effective drugs for this purpose. This is partially due to the limited understanding of pathogenetic mechanisms of this disease. It is well known that OPLL is a multifactorial disease and both genetic and acquired factors are supposed to be involved in the development of this disease [3]. Based on the familial incidence, extensive analyses have been performed to identify the genetic risk factors, and a particular SNP (single nucleotide polymorphism) of a number of genes such as HLA, VDR, or TGFβR, were reported to associate with the occurrence of OPLL [4] although the data were not reproducible and functional significance of them were not demonstrated in any cases. Among the acquired factors, obesity and diabetes mellitus are most frequently associated with OPLL [5] and therefore the involvement of metabolic signals in the development of OPLL is apparent, although the precise mechanism is not yet demonstrated.

In this chapter, I will introduce the strategy of disease modeling and drug discovery using induced pluripotent stem cells (iPSC), and possible applications of iPSCs for the understanding and drug discovery for OPLL.

10.2 Induced Pluripotent Stem Cells

In 2006, Shinya Yamanaka's group announced the establishment of embryonic stem cell-like cells from mouse skin fibroblasts by retrovirally introducing four transcription factors: Oct3/4, Sox2, Klf4, and c-Myc, and designated them as iPSCs [6]. Although the property of this first generation iPSCs was not enough as true pluripotent cells because they failed to contribute adult chimera, Yamanaka's group generated the second-generation mouse iPSCs with germline-competent in 2007, which can make mice completely derived from iPSCs [7] and also they demonstrated that an identical method can create human iPSCs [8]. This astonishing discovery clearly demonstrated the remarkable plasticity of mammalian cells and contributed the developmental and stem cell biology, and therefore awarded with Novel Prize in 2012 entitled "For the discovery that mature cells can be reprogramed to become pluripotent."

10.3 Medical Application of iPSCs

In addition to the contribution of science, the two remarkable properties of iPSCs, proliferating indefinitely and theoretically making any type of cells in our body, have attracted many researchers for medical applications in various clinical fields. One of them is those for the regeneration therapy using iPSC-derived differentiated cells. The general concept is that iPSCs are established from patients' somatic cells such as skin fibroblasts or peripheral blood cells. Then iPSCs are induced for the differentiation toward the target cells, which will be used for cell transplantation. The key technology of this application is the method to induce target cells with appropriate quality as differentiated cells and also without hazardous genetic alterations induced during in vitro culture. In 2014, only 7 years after the discovery of human iPSCs, the first-in-human trial of iPSC-derived cells was done for an eye disease, age-related macular degeneration. In this case, a sheet of retinal pigmented epithelial cells was created from patient-derived iPSCs and transplanted into a patient's eye, and successful results were reported in 2017 [9]. This type of transplantation, autograft transplantation, has no risk for immunological rejection, which is one of the advantages of the use of patient-derived iPSCs. To ensure the safety of cells, however, a considerable amount of time and cost will be required for each case, which is not realistic as a medical treatment for many patients. To facilitate the cell therapy using iPS cell-derived differentiated cells, it is desirable to establish iPSCs for the allogenic transplantation, which can be used for a large number of recipients. HLAs on donor cells, particularly, HLA-A, B, and DR, are key molecules to determine the immunological reaction of the recipient immune system, and mismatches in any single loci elicit immunological rejection. One approach to overcome this issue is to establish iPSCs from donors with homozygous in all three for common haplotype of Japanese population [10]. For example, one iPSC clone with homozygous for major three HLA loci can be transplanted into approximately 16% of Japanese population without immunological rejection in theory, and this approach has already covered approximately 30% of Japanese population [11]. Using these HLA-homo iPSCs, several clinical applications have been done, such as for Parkinson's disease (UMIN000033564) and corneal disease (UMIN000036539). In addition to this HLA-homo approach, researchers have been tackling this issue by creating HLA-modified iPSCs, which are expected to cause minimum immunological response in any donors [12].

The other important application of iPSCs is the disease modeling and drug discovery [13], which I have described in detail in the next section.

10.4 Disease Modeling and Drug Discovery

The general concept of this application is expressed as "Disease in a Dish," which consists of sequential multiple steps to recapitulate the disease phenotype in culture dishes using patients-derived cells (Fig. 10.1). Successful results of this application depend on the important points of each step. The first step is to select disease, which is appropriate for this approach. The ideal disease is a monogenic disorder with a complete penetrance and a homogenous phenotype, of which the modeling in vitro will be amenable. The disease phenotype can be assessed by

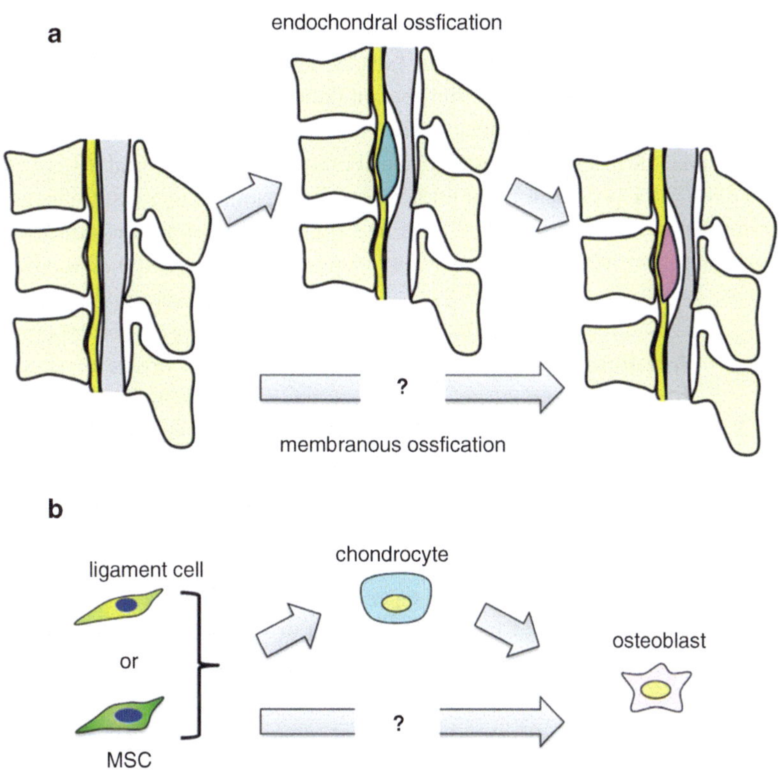

Fig. 10.1 Development of OPLL. (**a**) Possible process of ossification of posterior ligament. Blue and red region represent cartilage and bone tissues, respectively. (**b**) Possible process of cell differentiation during the development of ossification

cellular level and cells responsible for the phenotype are well-defined and inducible in vitro, and the defect of cells, either loss- or gain-of-function can be evaluated by some measurable markers. The second important step is the recruitment of patients with targeted disease, of whom thorough clinical information can be provided to guarantee the clinical diagnosis as will be more important if the targeted disease shows considerable heterogeneity. The third step is the establishment of iPSCs with appropriate qualities and without any genomic alterations. In most of the cases, control iPSCs are required to demonstrate the disease phenotype in vitro and iPSCs established from healthy donors were used for this purpose in early days. However, the genomic information other than the disease-causing gene in such control cells may affect the phenotype, and therefore currently researchers are using genome-edited, mutation-rescued iPSCs for control cells [14]. The last step is the method to induce target cells or tissues from iPSCs, which should be robust and reproducible, and ideally can be performed in a chemically defined condition. The disease phenotype should be accessible by cellular morphology, expression of particular surface markers, increase or decree of soluble factors, and physiological function. Once the recapitulation of disease phenotype is succeeded, researcher should take the drug-screening into consideration and modify the process for that purpose by shortening the differentiation period with less procedures and down-sizing the assay scale.

10.5 Application of iPSCs for a Disease with Heterotopic Ossification

Fibrodysplasia ossificans progressive (FOP) is a rare genetic disease characterized by HO in skeletal muscles, tendons, or ligaments through the endochondral process [15]. HO is periodically initiated by the episode of painful swelling after physical trauma and inflammatory responses, which is called flare-up, and ossified tissues are formed several weeks or months after flare-up. FOP patients harbor a missense mutation in the ACVR1 gene encoding one of the type I receptors for bone morphogenetic protein (BMP) [16]. Because the disease is exaggerated by the flare-up, we expected that the factor produced at the flare-up induces abnormal BMP signal for precursor cells in soft tissues and tried to find the factor by recapitulating this process in vitro using mesenchymal stem cells (MSCs) induced from FOP patients-derived iPSCs [17] (Fig. 10.2). As a result, we successfully identified Activin-A as the HO inducer through mutant ACVR1 [18]. We then performed screening of chemicals, which inhibited the effect of Activin-A, and identified rapamycin (sirolimus), one of the mTOR inhibitors, which effectively inhibited chondrogenesis in vitro and HO in vivo triggered by Activin-A [19]. Because rapamycin is approved for use in Japan for another rare disease, we have started the investigator-initiated clinical trial with rapamycin for FOP patients (UMIN000028429).

10.6 Problems in the Application of iPSC for OPLL

In contrast to the story of FOP, the application of disease-specific iPS cells for the research of OPLL has many difficult issues to be overcome. First, OPLL is not a monogenic disease, but a multifactorial disease. Although epidemiological data suggests the involvement of genetic factors, its contribution of each patient may differ significantly, and therefore selection of suitable patients is not an easy process. The second and may be the most difficult point is that we do not know the cell-of-origin of ossified ligaments. The histological finding of HO in FOP indicated that myofibroblastic cells at the flare-up site differentiated into cartilage cells [20], and therefore we used MSC induced from iPS cells as a precursor of HO and evaluated the process of cartilage differentiation (Fig. 10.2). If this is the case also in OPLL, MSCs in ligamentous tissues will be a possible candidate for target cells, which was demonstrated using primary cultured MSC [21]. Although the published histological data suggested that ossified tissues were developed via endochondral ossification [22], the genetic factor

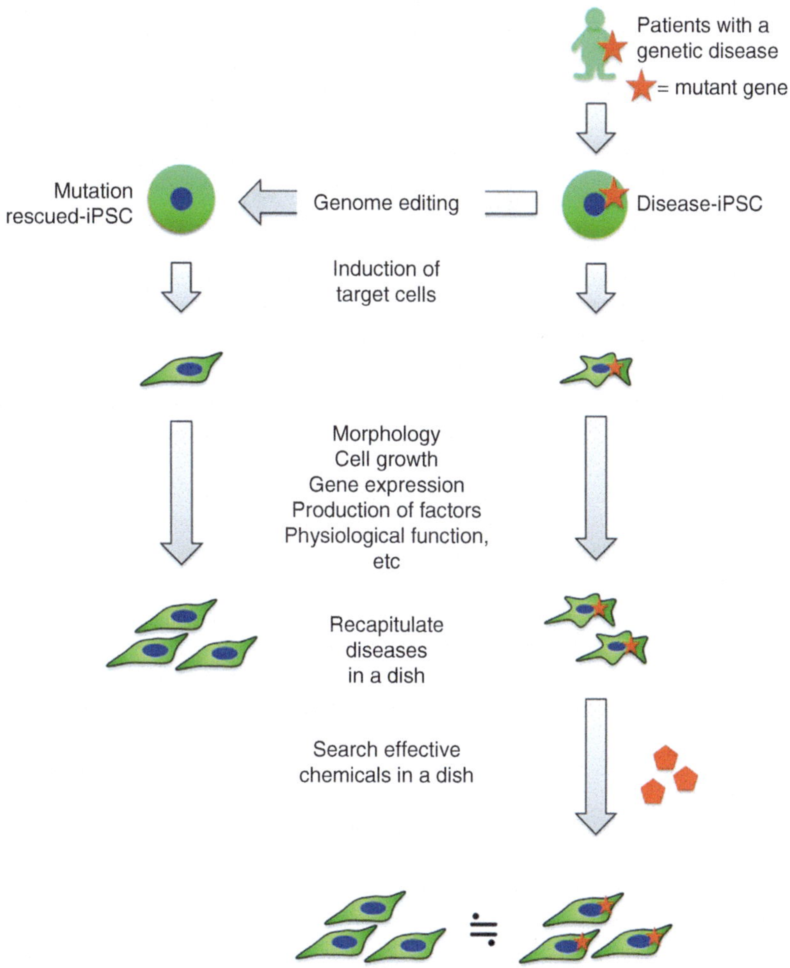

Fig. 10.2 General concept of the application of disease-specific iPSC for disease modeling and drug discovery

might be involved in the process of osteogenesis and therefore we have to investigate both chondrogenesis and osteogenesis of MSC. In addition, the process of trans-differentiation of ligament cells to chondrocytes or osteoblasts is also possible and should be considered. Because the ossification of ligaments takes place preferentially in the spinal ligament such as PLL, anterior longitudinal ligament, and yellow ligament, but not in other ligaments in extremities in most of the cases, local factors specialized in spine may be involved in the process. Therefore, we have to analyze many possible processes including chondrogenic or osteogenic differentiation of MSC or trans-differentiation of ligamentous cells (Fig. 10.3). Finally, even if we identify the candidates of genetic factors, the critical point is how to prove the role of such a candidate in vivo. Currently. Ttw mice is the only mice model for OPLL [23] although the gene responsible for Ttw is not necessarily responsible for human OPLL. The development of ligamentous tissues from iPS cells in vitro may substitute the in vivo experiments in future.

Considering these difficult issues, I will introduce two possible approaches for OPLL using iPSCs.

10.7 Strategy for OPLL-Familial Cases

The first approach is to identify the genetic factors using patients with multiple affected siblings, in whom the contribution of genetic factors may be much stronger than in sporadic OPLL

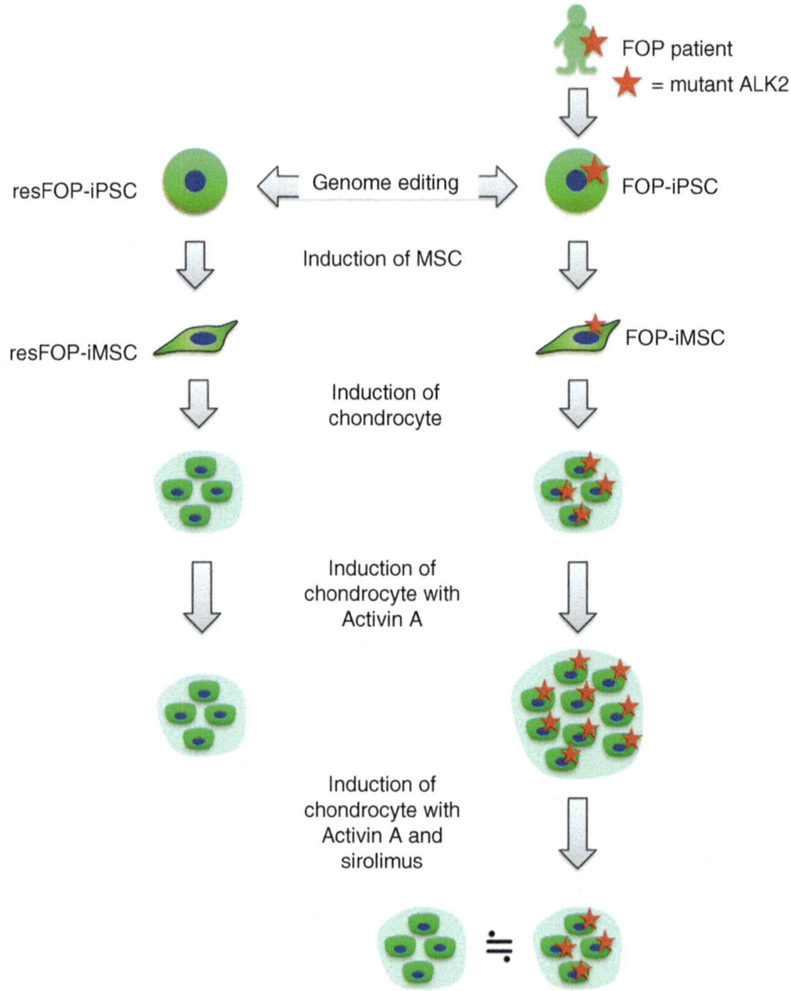

Fig. 10.3 Application of disease-specific iPSC for drug discovery of fibrodysplasia ossificans progresssiva

patients (Fig. 10.4). The first and the most important step in this strategy is the selection of patients. Our current criteria for the proband are those who have more than two affected siblings and patients with an early onset without acquired factors such as diabetes mellitus will be ideal. iPSCs established not only from affected siblings but also from unaffected members will be extremely useful although the definition of "unaffected" might be difficult because of the relatively late onset of this disease. MSCs will be induced from iPSC and chondrogenic and osteogenic differentiation properties will be investigated. In addition to iPSCs established from healthy donors, those from unaffected siblings will be used as a control. At the same time, genome analyses such as whole exome analyses will be performed to identify genome variants associated with OPLL. The candidate genomic variants will be a rare SNP without previous characterization, common in all affected members but not in unaffected members. The information of tissue expression will be used to narrow down the candidates, which will be obtained by immunostaining of ossified tissues in vivo and also confirmed in vitro by the induction of each type of cells from iPSCs. The functional significance of candidate gene will be analyzed by loss-of-function or gain-of-function experiments. If the biochemical function of the candidate gene is known, loss-of-function experiments will be performed by specific inhibitors, and if not, siRNA experiments should be considered. Gain-of-function experiments will be performed by the transfection of an expression

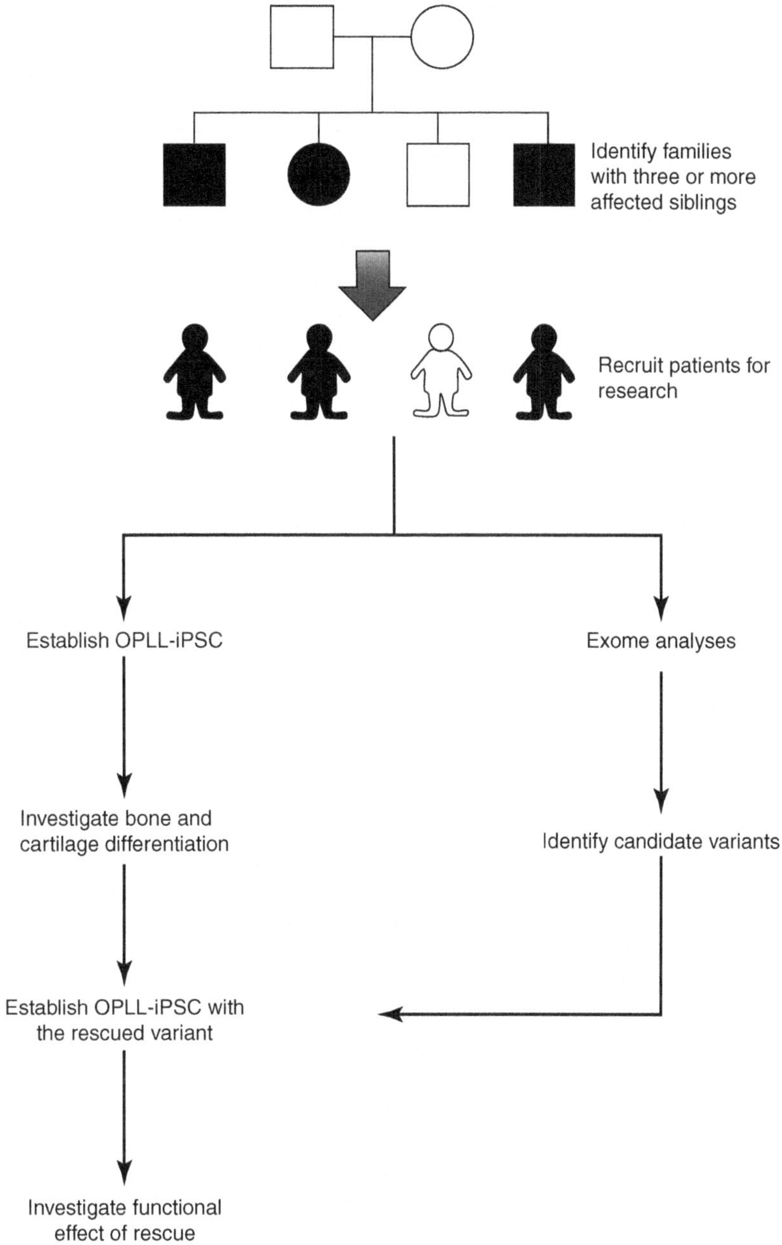

Fig. 10.4 Strategy for OPLL–Familial cases. Schematic presentation of the flow chart of sequential analyses

vector. In both types of experiments, the read-out will be an in vitro phenotype relating ossification process such as cartilage matrix formation or alizarin-red bone-like nodule formation. Finally, iPSC carrying the candidate variants will be modified by gene-editing and rescued iPSC will be established and the functional effect of rescue will be investigated to confirm the significance of variants for the development of OPLL.

10.8 Strategy for OPLL–GWAS

The second approach is to use the information of Genome-Wide Association Study (GWAS). GWAS is one of the approaches for dissecting the genetic factors for multifactorial diseases [24]. Combining the data of a large number of SNPs in the whole genome and a large number of patients with solid clinical information, Shiro Ikegawa's

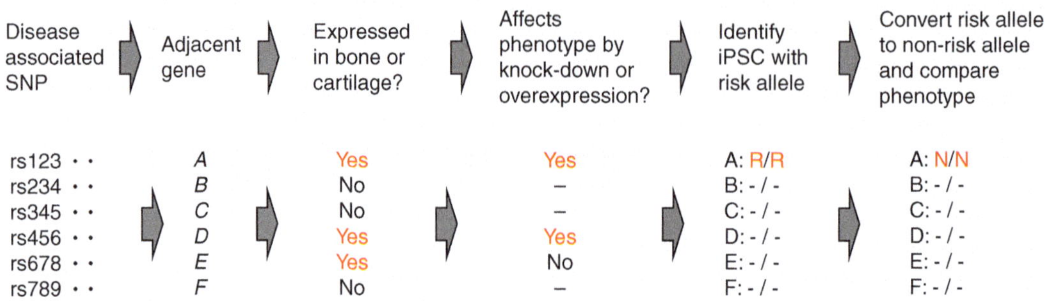

Fig. 10.5 Strategy for OPLL–GWAS. Flow chart of sequential analyses. Starting from the information of disease-associated SNP, appropriate genes are selected by tissue expression and function and then iPSCs with homozygous for the risk allele of the selected gene is identified among the standard iPSCs. Finally, the risk is converted to a non-risk allele and the phenotype is compared with parental clone

group successfully identified six SNPs with the incidence of OPLL [25]. The next step is to validate the functional significance of each SNP for the development of OPLL, which is not an easy process, and we are now challenging this issue using iPSCs (Fig. 10.5). The first step is to select genes associated with each SNP. Some SNPs are located nearby the coding region, but others may locate in the middle of intron or even intergenic region and work as an enhancer element. The next step is to obtain the information of protein expression of each gene in bone or cartilage as described in the previous section. Because some risk genes may indirectly affect the process of ossification such as the inorganic phosphate metabolism in the kidney, which should be analyzed by a differentiate strategy. The next step is the loss-of-function or gain-of-function experiments, which are also described in the previous section. If we find such genes the next step is whether SNP really affects such a phenotype or not. For this purpose, it is not rational to simply compare the phenotype of one iPSC with a risk allele and the other with a non-risk allele because the genomic background in each iPSC may affect the phenotype and make the effect of SNP unclear. To overcome this issue, iPSCs with a non-risk allele will be made from those with a risk allele by genome editing. The phenotypic difference will be solely due to the difference of SNP. Further interesting experiments will be to examine whether the accumulation of multiple risk SNPs demonstrate additive or synergistic effects, and this will be feasible by sequential genome editing from single iPSCs.

10.9 Conclusion

There are still many puzzles in OPLL pathology, and the application of iPSCs for this disease is a challenging issue. Further investigation will require considerations of additional factors, such as mechanistic effect or metabolomic effect such as glucose concentration.

References

1. Abiola R, Rubery P, Mesfin A. Ossification of the posterior longitudinal ligament: etiology, diagnosis, and outcomes of nonoperative and operative management. Global Spine J. 2016;6:195–204.
2. Iwasaki M, Kawaguchi Y, Kimura T, et al. Long-term results of expansive laminoplasty for ossification of the posterior longitudinal ligament of the cervical spine: more than 10 years follow up. J Neurosurg. 2002;96:180–9.
3. Matsunaga S, Sakou T. Ossification of the posterior longitudinal ligament of the cervical spine. Etiology and natural history. SPINE. 2014;37:E309–14.
4. Wilson JR, Patel AA, Brodt ED, et al. Genetics and heritability of cervical spondylotic myelopathy and ossification of the posterior longitudinal ligament. Results of a systematic review. SPINE. 2013;38:S123–46.

5. Nam DC, Lee HJ, Lee CJ, et al. Molecular pathophysiology of ossification of the posterior longitudinal ligament (OPLL). Biomol Ther (Seoul). 2019;27:342–8.
6. Takahashi K, Yamanaka S. Induction of pluripotent stem cells from mouse embryonic and adult fibroblast cultures by defined factors. Cell. 2006;126:663–76.
7. Okita K, Ichisaka T, Yamanaka S. Generation of germline-competent induced pluripotent stem cells. Nature. 2007;448:313–7.
8. Takahashi K, Tanabe K, Ohnuki M, et al. Induction of pluripotent stem cells from adult human fibroblasts by defined factors. Cell. 2007;131:861–72.
9. Mandai M, Watanabe A, Kurimoto Y, et al. Autologous induced stem-cell-derived retinal cells for macular degeneration. N Engl J Med. 2017;376:1038–46.
10. Okita K, Matsumura Y, Sato Y, et al. A more efficient method to generate integration- free human iPS cells. Nat Methods. 2011;8:409–12.
11. Umekage M, Sato Y, Takasu N. Overview: an iPS cell stock at CiRA. Inflamm Regen. 2019;39:17.
12. Xu H, Wang B, Ono M, et al. Targeted disruption of HLA genes via CRISPR-Cas9 generates iPSCs with enhanced immune compatibility. Cell Stem Cell. 2019;24:566–78.
13. Grskovic M, Javaherian A, Strulovici B, et al. Induced pluripotent stem cells—opportunities for disease modeling and drug discovery. Nat Rev Drug Discov. 2011;10:915–29.
14. Jang YY, Ye Z. Gene correction in patient-specific iPSCs for therapy development and disease modeling. Hum Genet. 2016;135:1041–58.
15. Kaplan FS, Glaser DL, Shore EM, et al. The phenotype of fibrodysplasia ossificans progressiva. Clin Rev Bone Mineral Metabo. 2005;3:183–8.
16. Shore EM, Xu M, Feldman GJ, et al. A recurrent mutation in the BMP type I receptor ACVR1 causes inherited and sporadic fibrodysplasia ossificans progressiva. Nat Genet. 2006;38:525–7.
17. Matsumoto Y, Ikeya M, Hino K, et al. New protocol to optimize ips cells for genome analysis of fibrodysplasia ossificans progressiva. Stem Cells. 2015;33:1730–42.
18. Hino K, Ikeya M, Horigome K, et al. Neofunction of ACVR1 in fibrodysplasia ossificans progressiva. Proc Natl Acad Sci U S A. 2015;112:15438–43.
19. Hino K, Horigome K, Nishio M, et al. Enhanced mTOR signaling triggered by Activin-A in chondrogenesis of fibrodysplasia ossificans progressiva (FOP). J Clin Invest. 2017;127:3339–52.
20. Pignolo RJ, Suda RK, Kaplan FS. The fibrodysplasia ossificans progressiva lesion. Clin Rev Bone Miner Metab. 2005;3:195–200.
21. Asari T, Furukawa KI, Tanaka S, et al. Mesenchymal stem cell isolation and characterization from human spinal ligament. Biochem Biophys Res Commun. 2012;417:1193–9.
22. Yonemori K, Imamura T, Ishidou Y, et al. Bone morphogenetic protein receptors and activin receptors are highly expressed in ossified ligament tissues of patients with ossification of the posterior longitudinal ligament. Am J Pathol. 1997;150:1335–47.
23. Okawa A, Nakamura I, Goto S, et al. Mutation in Npps in a mouse model of ossification of the posterior longitudinal ligament of the spine. Nat Genet. 1998;19:271–3.
24. Ikegawa S. A short history of the genome-wide association study: where we were and where we are going. Genom Inform. 2012;10:220–5.
25. Nakajima M, Takahashi A, Tsuji T, et al. A genome-wide association study identifies susceptibility loci for ossification of the posterior longitudinal ligament of the spine. Nat Genet. 2014;46:1012–6.

11 Mechanisms Underlying OPLL Development in Tiptoe Walking (ttw) Mice

Takeshi Miyamoto

Abstract

Ossification of the posterior longitudinal ligament (OPLL) is a disease characterized by an ectopic ossification in a spinal ligament, leading to several neurological deficits due to canal stenosis or nerve compression by ectopically ossified tissues. Since OPLL is a rare disease and mechanisms underlying it are not clear, treatment strategies aimed at preventing ectopic ossification or slowing its progression have not been developed. Previously, tiptoe walking (ttw) mice were shown to exhibit ectopic ossification in several tissues, including Achilles tendon and the PLL, making these mice an OPLL model. Ttw mice were subsequently shown to harbor a loss of function mutation in the *Ectonucleotide pyrophosphatase/phosphodiesterase 1* (*Enpp1*) gene. Recently, mechanisms underlying ectopic ossifications due to Enpp1 dysfunction have been clarified and shown to involve excessive vitamin D signaling.

Keywords

Ossification of the posterior longitudinal ligament (OPLL) · Tip toe walking (ttw) mouse · Ectonucleotide pyrophosphatase/phosphodiesterase 1 (Enpp1) · Vitamin D Vitamin D receptor (VDR) · FGF23 · Klotho Aging · Phosphate metabolism

11.1 Background

Ossification of the posterior longitudinal ligament (OPLL) phenotypes were identified in tiptoe walking (ttw) mice, which were shown to harbor a homozygous G to T substitution at nucleotide 1813 of the *Ectonucleotide pyrophosphatase/phosphodiesterase 1* (*Enpp1*) gene, which changed a glycine codon at residue 568 to a stop codon [1]. Enpp1 functions is required for generation of extracellular pyrophosphate (PPi), which inhibits hydroxyapatite crystal deposition [2]. Therefore, ectopic ossification seen in ttw mice may be due to loss of the inhibitory function of hydroxyapatite crystal deposition, although precise mechanisms remain unknown. *ENPP1* muta-

T. Miyamoto (✉)
Department of Orthopaedic Surgery, Keio University School of Medicine, Tokyo, Japan

Department of Advanced Therapy for Musculoskeletal Disorders, Keio University School of Medicine, Tokyo, Japan

Department of Musculoskeletal Reconstruction and Regeneration Surgery, Keio University School of Medicine, Tokyo, Japan

Department of Orthopaedic Surgery, Faculty of Life Science, Kumamoto University, Kumamoto, Japan

Center for Metabolic Regulation of Healthy Aging, Faculty of Life Science, Kumamoto University, Kumamoto, Japan
e-mail: miyamoto.takeshi@kuh.kumamoto-u.ac.jp

A. Okawa et al. (eds.), *OPLL*, https://doi.org/10.1007/978-981-15-3855-1_11

tions are also seen in patients with OPLL [3–5], and thus ttw mice are considered animal models of the disease. Human *ENPP1* mutations are also known to cause autosomal recessive hypophosphatemic rickets (ARHR) or Generalized Arterial Calcification of Infancy (GACI) [6–9]. The $Enpp1^{asj/asj}$ mouse, a different *Enpp1* mutant, reportedly exhibits GACI-like phenotypes [10].

11.2 OPLL Phenotypes Worsen in ttw Mice Fed with a High Phosphate Diet

In agreement with phenotypes associated with hypophosphatemic rickets, ttw mice exhibit significantly lower serum phosphate (Pi) levels relative to controls [11]. Relatively low serum Pi levels are also seen in patients with OPLL [12]. Interestingly, in ttw mice, feeding a high phosphate diet (HPD) does not elevate serum Pi levels but instead promotes deterioration of OPLL phenotypes [11]. A different study reported that ectopic ossification in the ear is accelerated by feeding ttw mice a HPD [13], while ectopic calcification in kidney and aorta is reported in ttw mice fed with a HPD [11]. In that study, ttw mice became inactive and marantic and died within 3 weeks of initiation of HPD feeding [11]. Finally, ttw mice fed with a HPD exhibit reduced bone mass and skin atrophy, phenotypes resembling human aging and also seen in mice with mutations in the *Klotho* gene (*kl/kl* mice), models of human aging [11, 14].

11.3 Ttw Mice Fed with a HPD Show Concomitant Elevation of FGF23 and Active Vitamin D3, $1,25(OH)_2D_3$, in Sera

Both FGF23 and vitamin D3 are key regulators of phosphate metabolism. Active vitamin D3, $1,25(OH)_2D_3$, promotes intestinal phosphate absorption, and elevated serum Pi stimulates FGF23 expression in osteocytes of bones (Fig. 11.1). Complex formation of the FGF receptor (FGFR) and Klotho is required to transduce the FGF23 signals. FGF23 binds to the FGFR and the Klotho complex to inhibit expression of Cyp27b1, an enzyme that converts 25(OH)D, an inactive form of vitamin D3, to active vitamin D3, $1,25(OH)_2D_3$, in kidney (Fig. 11.1). Thus, elevated serum FGF23 levels result in decreased $1,25(OH)_2D_3$ levels and down-regulate Pi absorption from the intestine via

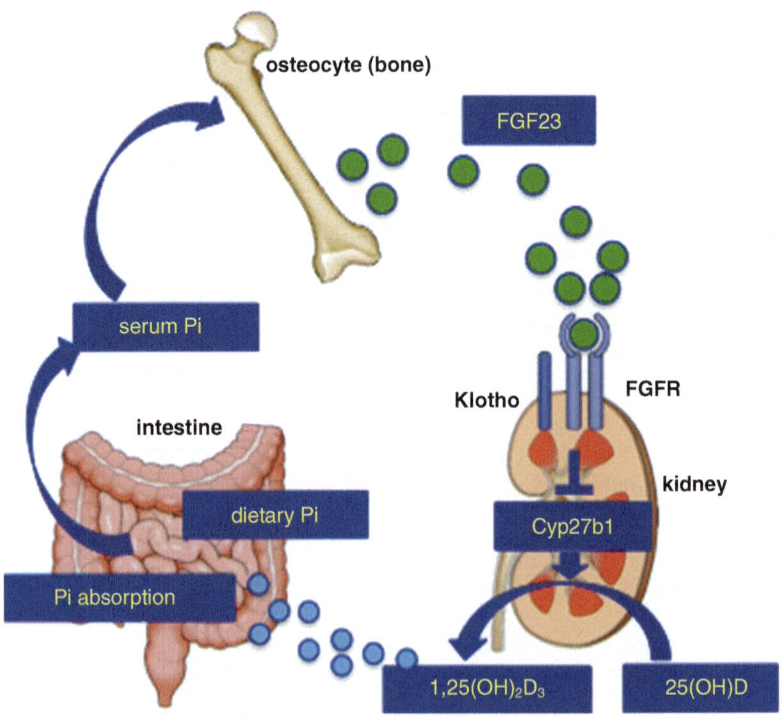

Fig. 11.1 Regulation of phosphate levels by Klotho and active vitamin D3. Dietary phosphate (Pi) is absorbed from the intestine, and elevated levels of serum Pi stimulate FGF23 expression in osteocytes. FGF23 secreted from bones binds to the Klotho/FGF receptor (FGFR) complex in kidney and inhibits expression of Cyp27b1, which catalyzes conversion of 25(OH)D to active vitamin D3, $1,25(OH)_2D_3$, which promotes Pi absorption from the intestine, in a negative feedback manner

a negative feedback mechanism. Accordingly, in normal conditions, FGF23 and 1,25(OH)$_2$D$_3$ levels cannot be concomitantly elevated. However, concomitant elevation of both is seen in sera of ttw mice fed with a HPD [11]. In agreement, *Cyp27b1* expression in kidney is significantly elevated in ttw mice fed with a HPD compared to either ttw mice fed with a normal diet or WT mice fed with a HPD [11].

11.4 Klotho Is Down-Regulated in ttw Mice Fed with a HPD

As noted, phenotypes seen in ttw mice fed with a HPD resemble those seen in Klotho-deficient *kl/kl* mice, and indeed, *Klotho* expression in kidney significantly decreases in ttw mice fed with a HPD compared to either ttw mice fed with a normal diet or WT mice fed with a HPD [11]. Crossing transgenic Klotho-overexpressing mice with ttw mice partially rescues phenotypes seen in ttw mice [11], suggesting that those phenotypes are due to Klotho downregulation. Accordingly, OPLL phenotypes are also seen in *kl/kl* mice [11].

FGF23-deficient mice reportedly exhibit aging-related phenotypes similar to *kl/kl* mice [15]. Tumoral calcinosis characterized by ectopic vascular calcifications is caused by loss-of-function mutations in either *KLOTHO* or *FGF23* [16, 17]. Thus, Klotho and FGF23 likely cooperate to inhibit ectopic calcification. Aging-associated phenotypes in either *kl/kl* or FGF23-deficient mice are abrogated by blocking the function of the vitamin D receptor (VDR) [18–20], suggesting that excessive vitamin D signaling promotes ectopic calcification due to either Klotho or FGF23 loss of function.

11.5 Decreases in Vitamin D Signaling Rescue OPLL Progression in ttw Mice

As described above, phenotypes seen in ttw mice fed with a HPD and *kl/kl* mice are similar, *kl/kl* mouse phenotypes are abrogated by VDR inhibition, and phenotypes in ttw mice fed with a HPD are hypothesized to be rescued by inhibiting VDR. Indeed, feeding ttw mice a high phosphate low vitamin D diet (HPLD) rescues phenotypes seen in ttw mice, even under phosphate overload conditions [11]. Moreover, crossing ttw with VDR-deficient mice completely abrogates phenotypes seen in ttw mice fed with a HPD. Taken together, these results indicate that development of OPLL in ttw mice under phosphate overload conditions is due to reduced Klotho expression in kidney (Fig. 11.2). Klotho down-regulation

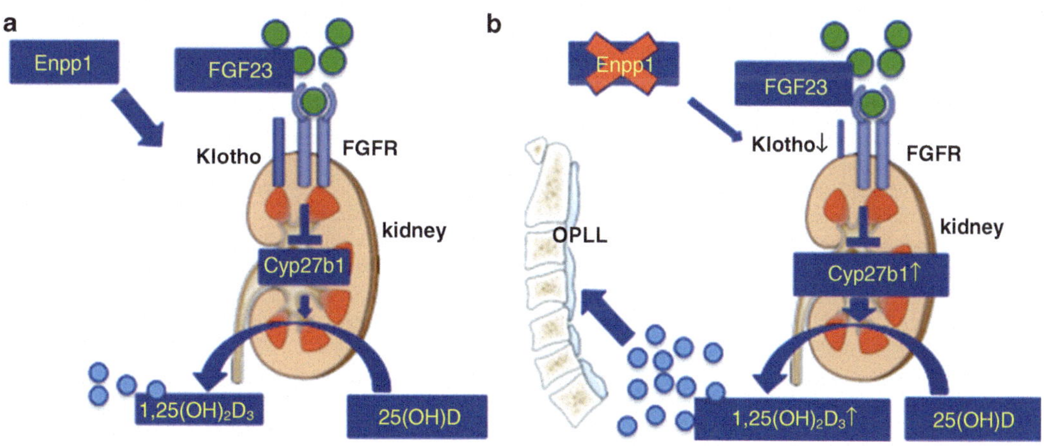

Fig. 11.2 Enpp1 is required for Klotho expression and maintenance of phosphate homeostasis in phosphate overload conditions. (**a**) In dietary phosphate overload conditions, Enpp1 is required for maintaining renal Klotho expression to inhibit Cyp27b1 expression by FGF23, and subsequent suppression of active vitamin D3 levels. Since the active form of vitamin D3, 1,25(OH)$_2$D$_3$, stimulates intestinal phosphate absorption, Enpp1 is required for negative feedback regulation of phosphate levels. (**b**) Ennp1 loss significantly down-regulates renal Klotho expression under dietary phosphate overload conditions. Thus FGF23 cannot transduce signals required to inhibit Cyp27b1 expression, leading to 1,25(OH)$_2$D$_3$ overproduction and ectopic ossification

results in elevated Cyp27 expression and $1,25(OH)_2D_3$ levels [11]. We propose that Enpp1 is required to maintain Klotho expression in kidney under phosphate overload conditions (Fig. 11.2).

11.6 Future Aspects

Based on the analysis of ttw mice, excessive VDR signaling could constitute a therapeutic target to prevent OPLL progression. Although *Enpp1* gene mutations are reported in OPLL patients, it is now critical to determine if the system seen in ttw mice is applicable to human OPLL patients. Since vitamin D3 is required for bone health, and low vitamin D3 levels are reportedly associated with fragile fractures in elderly [21–24], VDR signals should be manipulated with care to balance effects on ectopic ossification in PLL with proper maintenance of bone homeostasis.

References

1. Okawa A, Nakamura I, Goto S, Moriya H, Nakamura Y, Ikegawa S. Mutation in Npps in a mouse model of ossification of the posterior longitudinal ligament of the spine. Nat Genet. 1998 Jul;19(3):271–3.
2. Johnson KA, Hessle L, Vaingankar S, Wennberg C, Mauro S, Narisawa S, Goding JW, Sano K, Millan JL, Terkeltaub R. Osteoblast tissue-nonspecific alkaline phosphatase antagonizes and regulates PC-1. Am J Physiol Regul Integr Comp Physiol. 2000;279(4):R1365–77.
3. Nakamura I, Ikegawa S, Okawa A, Okuda S, Koshizuka Y, Kawaguchi H, Nakamura K, Koyama T, Goto S, Toguchida J, Matsushita M, Ochi T, Takaoka K, Nakamura Y. Association of the human NPPS gene with ossification of the posterior longitudinal ligament of the spine (OPLL). Hum Genet. 1999;104(6):492–7.
4. Koshizuka Y, Kawaguchi H, Ogata N, Ikeda T, Mabuchi A, Seichi A, Nakamura Y, Nakamura K, Ikegawa S. Nucleotide pyrophosphatase gene polymorphism associated with ossification of the posterior longitudinal ligament of the spine. J Bone Miner Res. 2002;17(1):138–44.
5. Tahara M, Aiba A, Yamazaki M, Ikeda Y, Goto S, Moriya H, Okawa A. The extent of ossification of posterior longitudinal ligament of the spine associated with nucleotide pyrophosphatase gene and leptin receptor gene polymorphisms. Spine (Phila Pa 1976). 2005;30(8):877–80. discussion 881.
6. Rutsch F, Ruf N, Vaingankar S, Toliat MR, Suk A, Höhne W, Schauer G, Lehmann M, Roscioli T, Schnabel D, Epplen JT, Knisely A, Superti-Furga A, McGill J, Filippone M, Sinaiko AR, Vallance H, Hinrichs B, Smith W, Ferre M, Terkeltaub R, Nürnberg P. Mutations in ENPP1 are associated with 'idiopathic' infantile arterial calcification. Nat Genet. 2003;34(4):379–81.
7. Rutsch F, Vaingankar S, Johnson K, Goldfine I, Maddux B, Schauerte P, Kalhoff H, Sano K, Boisvert WA, Superti-Furga A, Terkeltaub R. PC-1 nucleoside triphosphate pyrophosphohydrolase deficiency in idiopathic infantile arterial calcification. Am J Pathol. 2001;158(2):543–54.
8. Lorenz-Depiereux B, Schnabel D, Tiosano D, Häusler G, Strom TM. Loss-of-function ENPP1 mutations cause both generalized arterial calcification of infancy and autosomal-recessive hypophosphatemic rickets. Am J Hum Genet. 2010;86(2):267–72.
9. Levy-Litan V, Hershkovitz E, Avizov L, Leventhal N, Bercovich D, Chalifa-Caspi V, Manor E, Buriakovsky S, Hadad Y, Goding J, Parvari R. Autosomal-recessive hypophosphatemic rickets is associated with an inactivation mutation in the ENPP1 gene. Am J Hum Genet. 2010;86(2):273–8.
10. Li Q, Guo H, Chou DW, Berndt A, Sundberg JP, Uitto J. Mutant Enpp1asj mice as a model for generalized arterial calcification of infancy. Dis Model Mech. 2013;6(5):1227–35.
11. Watanabe R, Fujita N, Sato Y, Kobayashi T, Morita M, Oike T, Miyamoto K, Kuro-O M, Michigami T, Fukumoto S, Tsuji T, Toyama Y, Nakamura M, Matsumoto M, Miyamoto T. Enpp1 is an anti-aging factor that regulates Klotho under phosphate overload conditions. Sci Rep. 2017;7(1):7786.
12. Kawaguchi Y, Nakano M, Yasuda T, Seki S, Suzuki K, Yahara Y, Makino H, Kitajima I, Kimura T. Serum biomarkers in patients with ossification of the posterior longitudinal ligament (OPLL): inflammation in OPLL. PLoS One. 2017;12(5):e0174881.
13. Koshizuka Y, Ikegawa S, Sano M, Nakamura K, Nakamura Y. Isolation of novel mouse genes associated with ectopic ossification by differential display method using ttw, a mouse model for ectopic ossification. Cytogenet Cell Genet. 2001;94(3–4):163–8.
14. Kuro-o M, Matsumura Y, Aizawa H, Kawaguchi H, Suga T, Utsugi T, Ohyama Y, Kurabayashi M, Kaname T, Kume E, Iwasaki H, Iida A, Shiraki-Iida T, Nishikawa S, Nagai R, Nabeshima YI. Mutation of the mouse klotho gene leads to a syndrome resembling ageing. Nature. 1997;390(6655):45–51.
15. Shimada T, Kakitani M, Yamazaki Y, Hasegawa H, Takeuchi Y, Fujita T, Fukumoto S, Tomizuka K, Yamashita T. Targeted ablation of Fgf23 demonstrates an essential physiological role of FGF23 in phosphate and vitamin D metabolism. J Clin Invest. 2004;113(4):561–8.
16. Ichikawa S, Imel EA, Kreiter ML, Yu X, Mackenzie DS, Sorenson AH, Goetz R, Mohammadi M, White KE, Econs MJ. A homozygous missense mutation in

human KLOTHO causes severe tumoral calcinosis. J Clin Invest. 2007;117(9):2684–91.
17. Araya K, Fukumoto S, Backenroth R, Takeuchi Y, Nakayama K, Ito N, Yoshii N, Yamazaki Y, Yamashita T, Silver J, Igarashi T, Fujita T. A novel mutation in fibroblast growth factor 23 gene as a cause of tumoral calcinosis. J Clin Endocrinol Metab. 2005;90(10):5523–7.
18. Hesse M, Fröhlich LF, Zeitz U, Lanske B, Erben RG. Ablation of vitamin D signaling rescues bone, mineral, and glucose homeostasis in Fgf-23 deficient mice. Matrix Biol. 2007;26(2):75–84.
19. Anour R, Andrukhova O, Ritter E, Zeitz U, Erben RG. Klotho lacks a vitamin D independent physiological role in glucose homeostasis, bone turnover, and steady-state PTH secretion in vivo. PLoS One. 2012;7(2):e31376.
20. Streicher C, Zeitz U, Andrukhova O, Rupprecht A, Pohl E, Larsson TE, Windisch W, Lanske B, Erben RG. Long-term Fgf23 deficiency does not influence aging, glucose homeostasis, or fat metabolism in mice with a nonfunctioning vitamin D receptor. Endocrinology. 2012;153(4):1795–805.
21. Sakuma M, Endo N, Oinuma T, Hayami T, Endo E, Yazawa T, Watanabe K, Watanabe S. Vitamin D and intact PTH status in patients with hip fracture. Osteoporos Int. 2006;17(11):1608–14.
22. Sakuma M, Endo N, Oinuma T. Serum 25-OHD insufficiency as a risk factor for hip fracture. J Bone Miner Metab. 2007;25(3):147–50.
23. Sakuma M, Endo N, Hagino H, Harada A, Matsui Y, Nakano T, Nakamura K. Serum 25-hydroxyvitamin D status in hip and spine-fracture patients in Japan. J Orthop Sci. 2011;16(4):418–23.
24. LeBoff MS, Kohlmeier L, Hurwitz S, Franklin J, Wright J, Glowacki J. Occult vitamin D deficiency in postmenopausal US women with acute hip fracture. JAMA. 1999;281(16):1505–11.

12 In Vivo Tracing of Neural Tracts in Tip-Toe Walking Yoshimura Mice by Diffusion Tensor Tractography

Tsunehiko Konomi, Morito Takano, Yuji Komaki, Keigo Hikishima, Kanehiro Fujiyoshi, Osahiko Tsuji, Hideyuki Okano, Morio Matsumoto, and Masaya Nakamura

Abstract

In ossification of the posterior longitudinal ligaments (OPLL), axonal disruption results in motor and sensory function impairment. *Twy* (tip-toe walking Yoshimura) mice develop spontaneous calcification in the cervical ligaments, thereby causing chronic compression of the spinal cords. To determine whether in vivo DTT can evaluate the axonal disruption of the chronic compressive spinal cords in *twy* mice, 6-, 15-, and 20-week-old *twy* mice were chronologically subjected to DTT. MRI was performed using a 7.0-T magnet (Biospec 70/16) with CryoProbe (Bruker biospin GmbH, Ettlingen, Germany). Diffusion tensor images were analyzed using TrackVis (Massachusetts General Hospital, MA, USA). We succeeded in depicting in vivo high-resolution DTT of the *twy* mice. The progress of the ligamentous calcification was observed at C2–3 level in each *twy* mouse, and the number of RT-97- or SMI-31-positive fibers was decreased depending on the severity of the compression of the spinal cord. We demonstrated that quantitative analysis of sequential DTT enabled to detect subtle damage of the compressed spinal cord prior to the deterioration of neurological function in *twy* mice. Thus, in a clinical setting, DTT could be a new effective imaging modality in patients with cervical OPLL.

Keywords

Diffusion tensor tractography · *twy* mouse Ossification of the posterior longitudinal ligament · Tract fiber · Cervical myelopathy Spinal cord compression · Stejskal-Tanner diffusion preparation · RT-97 · SMI-31 Rotarod treadmill · Digigait analysis

T. Konomi (✉)
Department of Orthopaedic Surgery, Keio University, Tokyo, Japan

National Hospital Organization Murayama Medical Center, Tokyo, Japan

M. Takano · O. Tsuji · M. Matsumoto · M. Nakamura
Department of Orthopaedic Surgery, Keio University, Tokyo, Japan
e-mail: masa@a8.keio.jp

Y. Komaki
Department of Physiology, Keio University, Tokyo, Japan

Central Institute for Experimental Animals, Kawasaki, Japan

K. Hikishima
Okinawa Institute of Science and Technology Graduate University, Okinawa, Japan

K. Fujiyoshi
National Hospital Organization Murayama Medical Center, Tokyo, Japan

H. Okano
Department of Physiology, Keio University, Tokyo, Japan

A. Okawa et al. (eds.), *OPLL*, https://doi.org/10.1007/978-981-15-3855-1_12

12.1 Introduction

Ossification of the posterior longitudinal ligament (OPLL) of the cervical spine compresses the spinal cord and causes deterioration of sensory and motor function. Surgical treatment for OPLL is clearly indicated when the patient shows severe myelopathy, and the surgery should be performed before progression of symptoms. However, for patients without any symptoms or with only mild myelopathy in spite of evident OPLL on plain radiography of the cervical spine, the indication for and timing of surgical treatment remain controversial. Although conventional magnetic resonance imaging (MRI) provides useful information about the compressed spinal cord [1], a discrepancy is sometimes seen between the degree of spinal cord compression and the clinical symptoms.

Diffusion tensor imaging (DTI) is an MRI technique that evaluates the diffusion of extracellular water molecules within white matter fibers. The DTI parameters are described as disclosing subtle pathological changes in white matter integrity, and they have been useful for analyzing various central nervous system disorders [2, 3]. Diffusion tensor tractography (DTT) refers to the analysis and reconstruction of the DTI data, by which the orientation of nerve fibers can be followed to trace specific neural pathways [4]. The applications of DTT were recently reported to include cases of spinal cord compression in humans [5–7]. DTT is useful for grading the neurological severity in cervical spondylotic myelopathy, because it provides objective measures in terms of microstructural changes. However, to the best of our knowledge, there are no reports on the chronological changes in this disease, including comparisons between DTT findings and histological/functional analyses in animal models.

Tip-toe walking Yoshimura (*twy*) mice are reported to be a good in vivo model for the pathological changes underlying spinal cord dysfunction related to chronic compression [8, 9]. This mouse develops spontaneous spinal cord compression, so it is suitable for investigating the effects of chronic mechanical compression of the spinal cord without any artificial manipulation. In this chapter, we describe the relevance of DTT for evaluating the tract fibers of the compressed spinal cord by comparing the chronological in vivo DTT findings with histological findings and motor performance in *twy* mice.

12.2 Comparisons of MR Images with Histology

In *twy* mice, the conventional MRI was chronologically performed at 6, 15, and 20 weeks of age using a 7.0-T magnet (BioSpec 70/16; Bruker BioSpin, Ettlingen, Germany) with a cryogenic quadrature RF surface probe (CryoProbe; Bruker BioSpin AG, Fällanden, Switzerland) to improve the sensitivity [10]. Conventional and diffusion tensor MRI was performed under general anesthesia induced by intramuscular injection of ketamine (50 mg/kg; Sankyo, Tokyo, Japan) and xylazine (5 mg/kg; Bayer, Leverkusen, Germany) and maintained by isoflurane (Foren; Abbott, Tokyo, Japan). In 20-week-old *twy* mice, severe spinal cord compression was observed at the C2–3 level due to calcification of the atlantoaxial membrane. Consistent with the histological findings, the MR images precisely depicted severe spinal cord compression. To examine the effect of ectopic calcification on the spinal cord in 20-week-old *twy* mice, we measured the transverse area of the spinal cord histologically and compared it with the canal stenosis ratio. There was a significant negative correlation between the transverse area of the spinal cord and the canal stenosis ratio ($r = -0.7840$, $p = 0.0457$).

12.3 Sequential Changes in Diffusion Tensor Tractography

Chronological T2-weighted images (T2WI) of the upper cervical spinal cord enabled the progression of spinal cord compression due to ectopic calcification to be depicted in the same *twy* mouse (Fig. 12.1a). DTI data sets were acquired with a spin-echo sequence based on the Stejskal-Tanner diffusion preparation. Mild and moderate spinal cord compression caused the tract fibers in DTI to detour around the ectopic calcification at

6 and 15 weeks of age, whereas the tract fibers were interrupted by severe spinal cord compression at 20 weeks of age (Fig. 12.1b).

Diffusion tensor tractographic images were computed using the Diffusion Toolkit and TrackVis software (Massachusetts General Hospital, MA, USA). The diffusion tensor can be represented as an ellipsoid, where a proton at the center of the voxel has an equal probability of diffusing to any point in that ellipsoid. Fiber tracking was initiated from a manually selected region of interest (ROI), from which tracking lines were propagated bidirectionally according to the principal eigenvector in each voxel. For the tractography, an ROI was placed at the C2–3 level as the epicenter ROI and at the C0–1 level as the control ROI. We determined the number of tract fibers in each specimen at the C2–3 level (epicenter site) and the C0–1 level (control/rostral site). To analyze the sequential changes in the tract fibers of the compressed spinal cords quantitatively, we determined the canal stenosis ratios and configured tract fiber (TF) ratios (Fig. 12.2a) in 6-, 15-, and 20-week-old *twy*

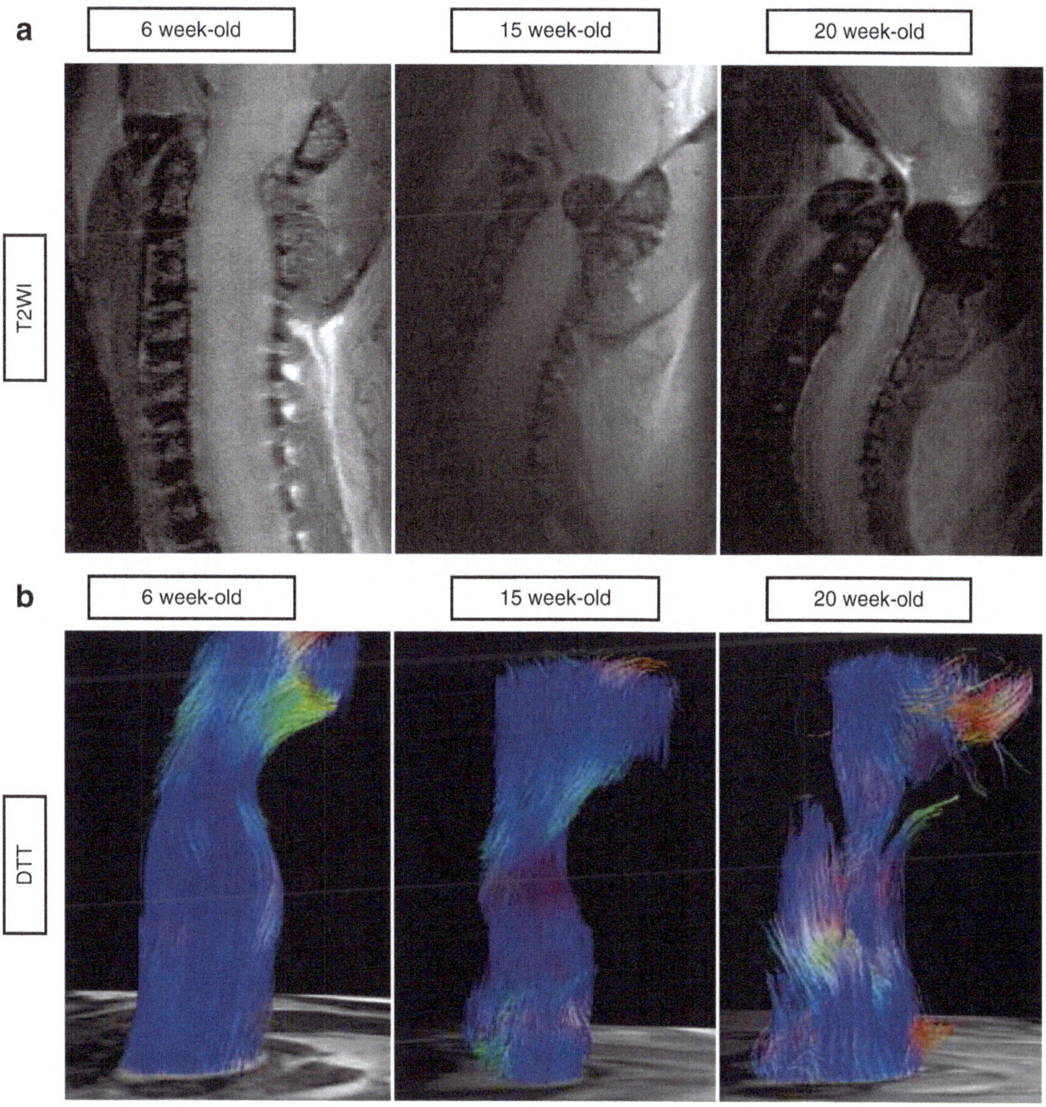

Fig. 12.1 Sagittal T2-weighted image (**a**) and diffusion tensor tractography (**b**) of the *twy* mice observed chronologically (at 6, 15, and 20 weeks of age). The results showed that calcification in the atlanto-axial membrane gradually progressed, while the number of tract fibers gradually decreased

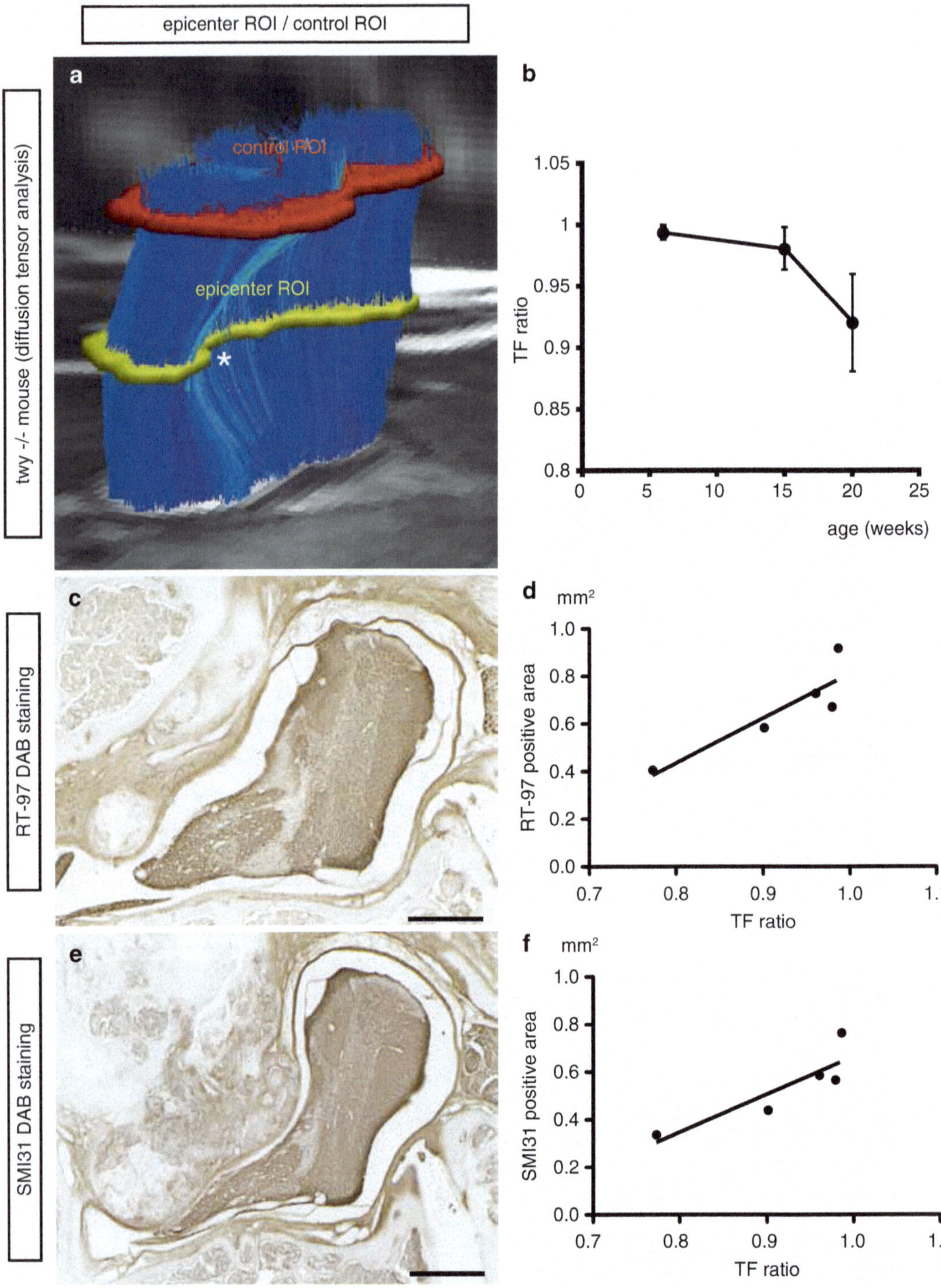

Fig. 12.2 The tract fibers were generated by placing the ROIs at the C0/1 and C2/3 levels (**a**). The TF ratio tended to decrease with the animal's age (**b**). Correlations between the TF ratio and the area of neurofilament staining for RT-97 (**c**) and SMI-31 (**e**). Scale bar: 500 μm (**d**, $r = 0.7865$: **f**, $r = 0.7746$)

mice. The canal stenosis rate is defined as 100 – (spinal cord area/spinal canal area) × 100, whereas the TF ratio is defined as the number of tract fibers at the C2–C3 level/the number of tract fibers at the C0–C1 level. The TF ratio did not significantly change in the 15-week-olds, but decreased sharply in the 20-week-olds (Fig. 12.2b). To examine the significance of the depicted tract fibers, we compared the tract fibers depicted by DTT with the RT-97- and SMI-31-positive fibers in the 20-week-old *twy* mice (Fig. 12.2c, e). The tissue sections were stained with the following primary antibodies: anti-RT-97 (mouse IgG_1, 1:200, Millipore, MA, USA) for normal neurofilaments, and anti-SMI-31 (mouse IgG_1, 1:200, Covance) for hyperphosphorylated normal axons. There was a positive correlation between the TF ratio and the RT-97-positive area ($r = 0.7865$, $p = 0.0449$, Fig. 12.2d) and SMI-31-positive area ($r = 0.7746$, $p = 0.0489$, Fig. 12.2f).

12.4 Correlations among the TF Ratio, Canal Stenosis Rate, and Motor Performance

The canal stenosis progressed with the age of the *twy* mice. To examine the chronological relationship between the TF ratio and canal stenosis ratio, we analyzed their correlation in five *twy* mice at 6, 15, and 20 weeks of age (Fig. 12.3a). As the *twy* mice became older, the canal stenosis became more prominent, causing a decrease in the TF ratio. Interestingly, two-part linear regression analysis [11] revealed that canal stenosis over 50% caused a sharp decrease in the TF ratio (intersection point: 52%, Fig. 12.3b).

Since *twy* mice show progressive paralysis due to the chronic spinal cord compression, we examined the motor function in the mice by the Rotarod treadmill test (Muromachi Kikai Co., Ltd., Tokyo, Japan) and Digigait analysis (Mouse Specifics, Quincy, MA, USA), and compared the results with the TF ratio and canal stenosis ratio in the 20-week-old *twy* mice. Both the Rotarod treadmill latency and stride length sharply decreased when the TF ratio was below 0.9 and canal stenosis ratio was over 60%. Consistent with the Rotarod treadmill analysis, the Digigait analysis revealed that two *twy* mice with severe spinal cord compression (canal stenosis ratio >60%) could not walk on the treadmill, whereas the other *twy* mice with mild or moderate spinal cord compression (canal stenosis ratio <50%) could walk on the treadmill at a speed of 8 cm/s.

12.5 Discussion

In the present study, we demonstrate that in vivo DTT could depict the chronological changes in the tract fibers of the chronic progressive spinal cord compression in *twy* mice. The number of tract fibers depicted by DTT was significantly correlated with the areas of RT-97- and SMI-31-positive neurofilaments and the results of motor function analyses. In addition, our results suggest that, in particular, over 50% spinal canal stenosis cause a sharp decrease in the tract fibers even before a prominent neurological deficit is seen.

Previous studies demonstrated that all patients with more than 60% spinal canal stenosis by OPLL exhibited myelopathy, whereas in patients with less than 60% spinal canal stenosis, the range of motion of the cervical spine was significantly larger in patients with myelopathy than in those without it [12]. Furthermore, the surgical outcomes of OPLL patients demonstrated that the postoperative recovery is poor in those with a greater than 50–60% compromise of the spinal canal by the ossified lesion [13, 14] and in those with a cervical mobility [15]. Recent reports examining the surgical option for treating patients with cervical myelopathy caused by OPLL suggested that the surgical results depend on the severity of the preoperative neurological deficit, age at the time of surgery, and duration between the onset of initial symptoms and surgery and, therefore, the cervical myelopathy must be diagnosed as early as possible [16–18].

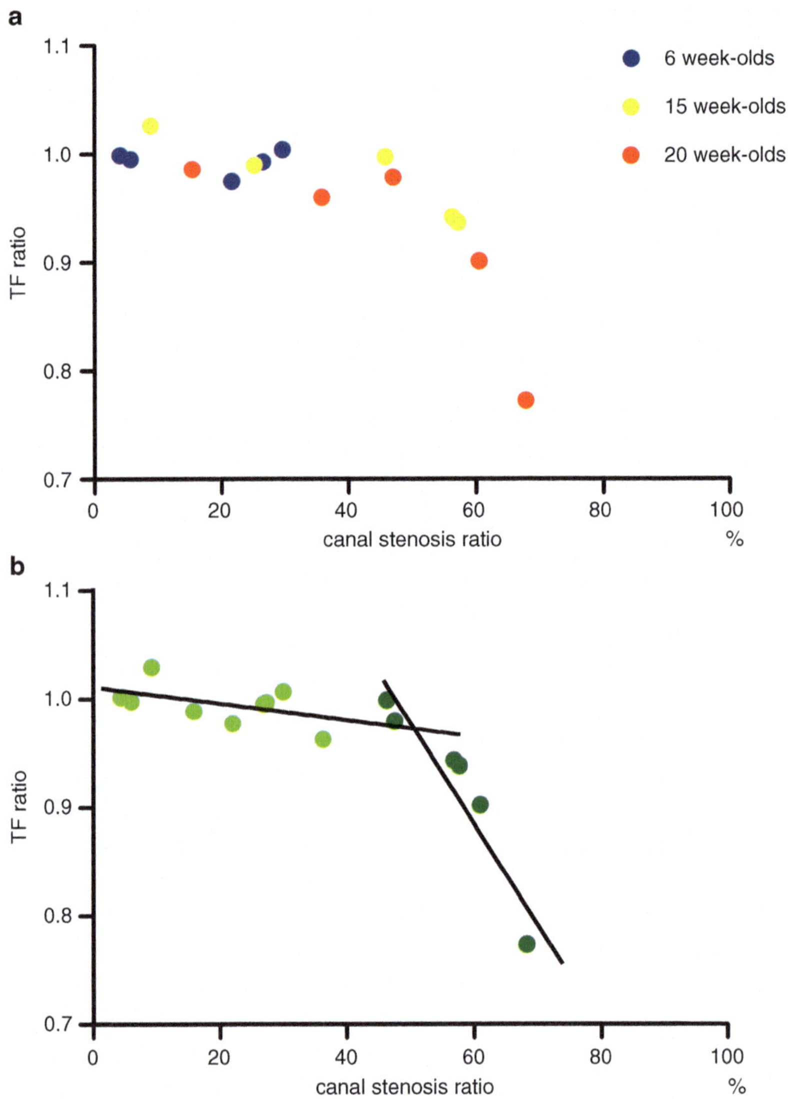

Fig. 12.3 Correlations between the TF ratio and canal stenosis ratio (**a**, blue dots: 6-week-olds, yellow dots: 15-week-olds, red dots: 20-week-olds). Two-part linear regression analysis showed that canal stenosis over 50% caused a sharp decrease in the TF ratio (**b**, light green: $r = -0.2827$, dark green: $r = -0.8705$)

However, there are no reports describing a useful and objective tool for determining the surgical indication for cervical myelopathy. Conventional MRI undoubtedly provides useful information about the compressed spinal cord. However, sometimes there is a discrepancy between the degree of spinal cord compression and the clinical symptoms.

We previously demonstrated that DTT is very useful for examining spinal cord injuries, cervical compressive myelopathy and peripheral nerve injuries in both experimental animal models and clinical situations [7, 19–21]. In the clinic, Kara et al. suggested that DTT can show abnormalities in the compressive spinal cord before the development of T2 hyperintensity on conventional MRI sequences in patients with cervical spondylotic myelopathy (CSM) [22]. Furthermore, Wang et al demonstrated DTT grading is more valuable than MRI grading for diagnosis and prognostic prediction in CSM patients [23]. Although DTT is thought to have great potential for detecting cervical myelopathy, it is unclear how DTT would show the pathological changes of the compressed spinal cord. Accordingly, we focused on *twy* mice, which develop spontaneous cervical myelopathy due to ectopic ossified ligaments.

Baba et al. previously reported that the chronic compression of the cervical spinal cord of *twy* mice causes the loss of motorneurons at the injury epicenter [24]. Yato et al. also reported that spinal motorneuron atrophy and loss in the gray matter of *twy* mice were observed when the severity of spinal canal stenosis was 30% or more [25]. Given the variation in the severity of spinal cord compression due to ligamentous calcification in these mice, it is important to observe the chronological changes in the spinal cord of live *twy* mice, which has never been reported previously.

In the present study, we performed in vivo imaging of *twy* mice with a 7 T MRI and CryoProbe, and examined the chronological changes in their compressed spinal cords. To the best of our knowledge, this is the first study to show the chronological changes of DTT parameters in *twy* mice using high-resolution MRI. We demonstrated that the TF ratio decreased sharply at around 50% spinal canal stenosis. Our results resemble clinical evidence and suggest that irreversible changes in neurofilaments increase dramatically at over 50% spinal canal stenosis. It is noteworthy that the decrease in TF ratio preceded the functional deterioration, which occurred at around 60% spinal canal stenosis.

12.6 Conclusion

In conclusion, DTT could be a new effective imaging modality in patients with cervical myelopathy due to ligamentous calcifications. In this study, subtle damage visible in the neurofilaments could be quantitatively analyzed at each stage of disease by measuring the tract fibers. Thus, in a clinical setting, the TF ratio could be a useful parameter for making decisions about the indications and timing of surgical treatment for cervical myelopathy due to OPLL.

References

1. Vedantam A, Jonathan A, Rajshekhar V. Association of magnetic resonance imaging signal changes and outcome prediction after surgery for cervical spondylotic myelopathy. J Neurosurg Spine. 2011;15(6):660–6.
2. Assaf Y, Pasternak O. Diffusion tensor imaging (DTI)-based white matter mapping in brain research: a review. J Mol Neurosci. 2008;34(1):51–61.
3. Chang Y, Jung TD, Yoo DS, Hyun JK. Diffusion tensor imaging and fiber tractography of patients with cervical spinal cord injury. J Neurotrauma. 2010;27(11):2033–40.
4. Mori S, Zhang J. Principles of diffusion tensor imaging and its applications to basic neuroscience research. Neuron. 2006;51(5):527–39.
5. Demir A, Ries M, Moonen CT, Vital JM, Dehais J, Arne P, et al. Diffusion-weighted MR imaging with apparent diffusion coefficient and apparent diffusion tensor maps in cervical spondylotic myelopathy. Radiology. 2003;229(1):37–43.
6. Facon D, Ozanne A, Fillard P, Lepeintre JF, Tournoux-Facon C, Ducreux D. MR diffusion tensor imaging and fiber tracking in spinal cord compression. AJNR Am J Neuroradiol. 2005;26(6):1587–94.
7. Nakamura M, Fujiyoshi K, Tsuji O, Konomi T, Hosogane N, Watanabe K, et al. Clinical significance of diffusion tensor tractography as a predictor of functional recovery after laminoplasty in patients with cervical compressive myelopathy. J Neurosurg Spine. 2012;17(2):147–52.
8. Okawa A, Nakamura I, Goto S, Moriya H, Nakamura Y, Ikegawa S. Mutation in Npps in a mouse model of ossification of the posterior longitudinal ligament of the spine. Nat Genet. 1998;19(3):271–3.
9. Uchida K, Baba H, Maezawa Y, Kubota C. Progressive changes in neurofilament proteins and growth-associated protein-43 immunoreactivities at the site of cervical spinal cord compression in spinal hyperostotic mice. Spine. 2002;27(5):480–6.
10. Baltes C, Radzwill N, Bosshard S, Marek D, Rudin M. Micro MRI of the mouse brain using a novel 400 MHz cryogenic quadrature RF probe. NMR Biomed. 2009;22(8):834–42.
11. Kouda K, Iki M, Fujita Y, Tamaki J, Yura A, Kadowaki E, et al. Alcohol intake and bone status in elderly Japanese men: baseline data from the Fujiwara-kyo osteoporosis risk in men (FORMEN) study. Bone. 2011;49(2):275–80.
12. Matsunaga S, Nakamura K, Seichi A, Yokoyama T, Toh S, Ichimura S, et al. Radiographic predictors for the development of myelopathy in patients with ossification of the posterior longitudinal ligament: a multicenter cohort study. Spine (Phila Pa 1976). 2008;33(24):2648–50.
13. Baba H, Imura S, Kawahara N, Nagata S, Tomita K. Osteoplastic laminoplasty for cervi-

cal myeloradiculopathy secondary to ossification of the posterior longitudinal ligament. Int Orthop. 1995;19(1):40–5.
14. Iwasaki M, Okuda S, Miyauchi A, Sakaura H, Mukai Y, Yonenobu K, et al. Surgical strategy for cervical myelopathy due to ossification of the posterior longitudinal ligament: part 1: clinical results and limitations of laminoplasty. Spine (Phila Pa 1976). 2007;32(6):647–53.
15. Ogawa Y, Chiba K, Matsumoto M, Nakamura M, Takaishi H, Hirabayashi H, et al. Long-term results after expansive open-door laminoplasty for the segmental-type of ossification of the posterior longitudinal ligament of the cervical spine: a comparison with nonsegmental-type lesions. J Neurosurg Spine. 2005;3(3):198–204.
16. Sakai K, Okawa A, Takahashi M, Arai Y, Kawabata S, Enomoto M, et al. Five-year follow-up evaluation of surgical treatment for cervical myelopathy caused by ossification of the posterior longitudinal ligament: a prospective comparative study of anterior decompression and fusion with floating method versus laminoplasty. Spine. 2012;37:367–76.
17. Tani T, Ushida T, Ishida K, Iai H, Noguchi T, Yamamoto H. Relative safety of anterior microsurgical decompression versus laminoplasty for cervical myelopathy with a massive ossified posterior longitudinal ligament. Spine. 2002;27(22):2491–8.
18. Ogawa Y, Toyama Y, Chiba K, Matsumoto M, Nakamura M, Takaishi H, et al. Long-term results of expansive open-door laminoplasty for ossification of the posterior longitudinal ligament of the cervical spine. J Neurosurg Spine. 2004;1(2):168–74.
19. Fujiyoshi K, Yamada M, Nakamura M, Yamane J, Katoh H, Kitamura K, et al. In vivo tracing of neural tracts in the intact and injured spinal cord of marmosets by diffusion tensor tractography. J Neurosci. 2007;27(44):11991–8.
20. Takagi T, Nakamura M, Yamada M, Hikishima K, Momoshima S, Fujiyoshi K, et al. Visualization of peripheral nerve degeneration and regeneration: monitoring with diffusion tensor tractography. NeuroImage. 2009;44(3):884–92.
21. Konomi T, Fujiyoshi K, Hikishima K, Komaki Y, Tsuji O, Okano HJ, et al. Conditions for quantitative evaluation of injured spinal cord by in vivo diffusion tensor imaging and tractography: preclinical longitudinal study in common marmosets. NeuroImage. 2012;63(4):1841–53.
22. Kara B, Celik A, Karadereler S, Ulusoy L, Ganiyusufoglu K, Onat L, et al. The role of DTI in early detection of cervical spondylotic myelopathy: a preliminary study with 3-T MRI. Neuroradiology. 2011;53(8):609–16.
23. Wang K, Chen Z, Zhang F, Song Q, Hou C, Tang Y, et al. Evaluation of DTI parameter ratios and diffusion tensor tractography grading in the diagnosis and prognosis prediction of cervical spondylotic myelopathy. Spine (Phila Pa 1976). 2017;42(4):E202–E10.
24. Baba H, Maezawa Y, Imura S, Kawahara N, Nakahashi K, Tomita K. Quantitative analysis of the spinal cord motoneuron under chronic compression: an experimental observation in the mouse. J Neurol. 1996;243(2):109–16.
25. Yato Y, Fujimura Y, Nakamura M, Watanabe M, Yabe Y. Decreased choline acetyltransferase activity in the murine spinal cord motoneurons under chronic mechanical compression. Spinal Cord. 1997;35(11):729–34.

Metabolomics Analysis of OPLL Patients

13

Takashi Tsuji and Morio Matsumoto

Abstract

Metabolomics is one of the "omics" technologies and is a comprehensive analysis of small molecule metabolites. The metabolomics is located at the downstream end of "omics" research; therefore, this research platform is most closely related to phenotype among other "omics" research. Recently, we compared the differences of metabolite profiling between patients with ossification of the posterior longitudinal ligament (OPLL) and control subjects for the first time and detected 259 metabolites. Among the 259 metabolites, some metabolites were significantly larger in OPLL group, even in analyses excluding patients with diabetes mellitus and hyperlipidemia. Although this research field is still in development, these results of the present study could lead to new insights into clarifying the molecular pathomechanisms of OPLL.

Keywords

Metabolomics · Metabolite · Comprehensive analysis · Ossification of the posterior longitudinal ligament · Genomics Transcriptomics · Proteomics

13.1 Metabolomics and OPLL

Ossification of the posterior longitudinal ligament (OPLL) is an abnormal ossification of the posterior longitudinal ligament in the spinal canal and is often associated with concurrent ossification of other spinal ligaments, such as the anterior longitudinal ligament, ligamentum flavum, and supraspinatus ligaments. Consequently, it has been regarded as one of the manifestations of diffuse idiopathic skeletal hyperostosis [1], and thus, the systemic factors as well as local factors have been considered to play an important role in the pathogenesis of OPLL. The relationship between underlying etiology and systemic factors of OPLL have been investigated from various standpoints including genetic factors [2], metabolic abnormalities [3], and dietary habits [4]; however, its mechanism has not been clarified.

Metabolomics is the latest of the "omics" technologies [5] that is situated downstream of genomics, transcriptomics, and proteomics and is a comprehensive analysis of small molecule metabolites (<1000 Da) which include amino

T. Tsuji (✉)
Department of Orthopaedic Surgery, Keio University School of Medicine, Tokyo, Japan

Department of Orthopaedic Surgery, Tokyo Medical Center, Tokyo, Japan

M. Matsumoto
Department of Orthopaedic Surgery, Keio University School of Medicine, Tokyo, Japan

A. Okawa et al. (eds.), *OPLL*, https://doi.org/10.1007/978-981-15-3855-1_13

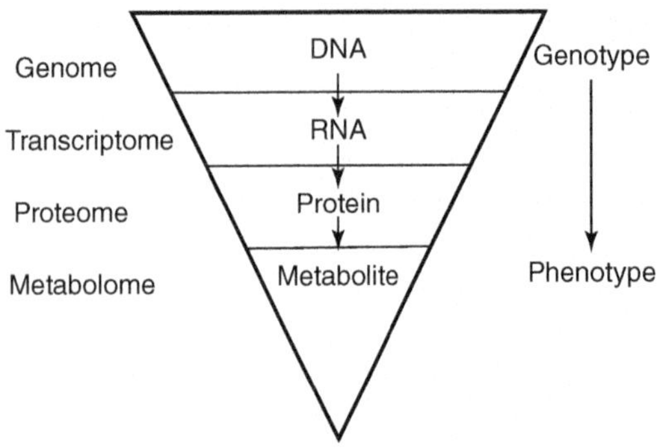

Fig. 13.1 The relationship of "omics" research

acid, nucleotides, carbohydrates, and fatty acids (Fig. 13.1). The advantages on this study are (1) the number of metabolites in human is relatively small in comparison to the number of deoxyribonucleic acid (DNA), ribonucleic acid (RNA), or proteins and (2) if the metabolites are functional, they might be related to disease pathology. Because the metabolite status reflects the pathophysiological status of a subject, the principle of metabolomics approach is that disease can be reflected by changes in metabolite concentration. Although the metabolomics approach has become widely used in the field of medical science [6], no study to date has been conducted to elucidate the metabolite profiling of patients with OPLL. Therefore, we conducted this study to compare the differences of metabolites between patients with OPLL and control subjects.

13.2 Protocol of Metabolomics

13.2.1 Materials

A total of 20 individuals (10 male patients with cervical OPLL, mean age; 61.3 ± 5.1 years, 10 male control subjects, mean age; 61.6 ± 11.8 years) participated in this study. Inclusion criteria of patients with OPLL were (1) male, (2) ossified lesion >3 levels of vertebral body and more, and (3) continuous or mixed type of OPLL. Ossified lesions were observed at 4.1 ± 0.6 (range 3–5) levels of vertebral bodies in OPLL patients. The presence of comorbidities was evaluated by medical history or laboratory examination at the time of enrollment to this study. Subjects with HbA1c ≥6.5% were diagnosed to have diabetes mellitus (DM). Those with low-density lipoprotein (LDL) ≥140 mg/dL and/or triglycerides (TG) ≥150 mg/dL were diagnosed to have hyperlipidemia (HL). In the OPLL group, two had DM and two had HL. In the control group, three had DM and two had HL.

Peripheral blood samples were drawn by experienced physicians from a peripheral vein. After blood collection, plasma samples were isolated via centrifugation at 800 × *g* for 5 min and then stored at −80 °C until use. We analyzed ionic metabolites using capillary electrophoresis time-of-flight mass spectrometry (CE-TOFMS) and lipophilic metabolites using liquid chromatography time-of-flight mass spectrometry (LC-TOFMS) (Fig. 13.2).

13.2.2 CE-TOFMS Measurement

50 μL of plasma were added to 450 μL of methanol containing internal standards (Solution ID: H3304-1002, Human Metabolome Technologies; HMT, Inc., Tsuruoka, Japan) at 0 °C in order to inactivate enzymes. The extract solution was thoroughly mixed with 500 μL of chloroform and 200 μL of Milli-Q water and centrifuged at 2300 × *g* and 4 °C for 5 min. The 350 μL of upper aqueous layer was centrifugally filtered through a Millipore 5000 Da cutoff filter to remove proteins. The filtrate was centrifugally concentrated and re-suspended in 50 μL of Milli-Q water for CE-TOFMS analysis [7].

13.2.3 LC-TOFMS Measurement

500 μL of plasma was added to 1500 μL of 1% formic acid/acetonitrile containing internal standard solution (Solution ID: H3304-1002, HMT, Inc., Tsuruoka, Japan) at 0 °C in order to inactivate enzymes. The solution was thoroughly mixed and centrifuged at 2300 × *g* and 4 °C for 5 min. The supernatant was filtrated by using Hybrid SPE phospholipid (55261-U, Supelco, Bellefonte,

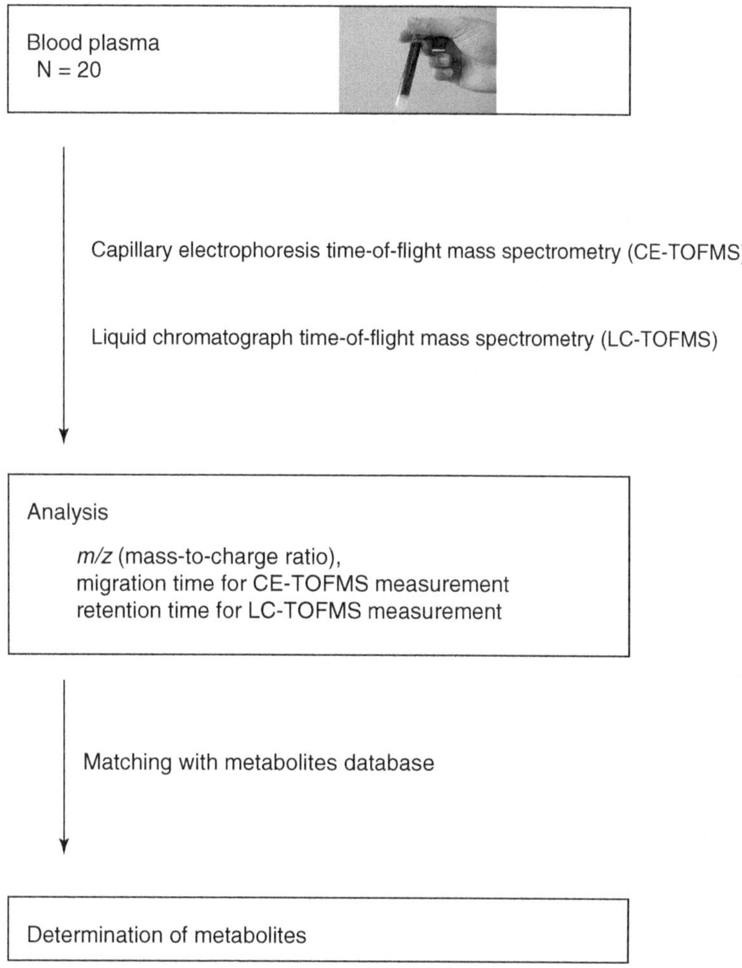

Fig. 13.2 Details of metabolome analysis

PA, USA) to remove phospholipids. The filtrate was desiccated and then dissolved with 100 μL of isopropanol/Milli-Q for LC-TOFMS analysis [8].

13.2.4 Semiquantitative Analysis of Metabolites

Peaks were extracted using automatic integration software MasterHands (Keio University, Tsuruoka, Japan) in order to obtain peak information including *m/z* (mass-to-charge ratio), migration time for CE-TOFMS measurement (MT) or retention time for LC-TOFMS measurement (RT), and peak area [9]. Signal peaks corresponding to isotopomers, adduct ions, and other product ions of known metabolites were excluded, and remaining peaks were annotated with putative metabolites from the HMT metabolite database based on their MTs/RTs and *m/z* values determined by TOFMS. The tolerance range for the peak annotation was configured at ±0.5 min for MT and ±10 ppm for *m/z*. In addition, peak areas were normalized against those of the internal standards and then the resultant relative area values were further normalized by sample amount.

13.2.5 Statistical Analysis

For each metabolite, the relative area was defined as the relative concentration of that metabolite. First, principal component analysis (PCA) was performed by using a software, SampleStat ver. 3.14. Next, the concentration of each metabolite was compared between patients with OPLL and control subjects. Finally, except for individuals with comorbidities (DM or HL), comparison of each metabolite concentration between patients with OPLL and control subjects was performed. These values were compared by using the Welch t-test. Differences with p values less than 0.05 were considered significant.

13.3 Semiquantitative Comparison of Metabolites Between OPLL and Control Subjects

A total of 259 metabolites (144 metabolites in CE-TOFMS and 115 metabolites in LC-TOFMS) were detected. The results of scatter plots in PCA comparing OPLL and control group were overlapping, and thus, no obvious differences in terms of profiling were detected between the two groups. Consequently, we compared individual metabolites between OPLL and control groups. Among the 259 metabolites, 26 metabolites were significantly different between the two groups. Of the 26 metabolites, 23 metabolites showed significantly larger and 3 metabolites showed significantly smaller in OPLL group (Table 13.1). A group of fatty acids (FA) showed large values in OPLL group as compared with the control group, and parts thereof were statistically significant (Fig. 13.3, Table 13.1).

In the analysis excluding DM patients (OPLL: n = 8, control: n = 7), 23 metabolites were significantly different between the two groups

Table 13.1 Relative concentrations of candidate metabolites comparing OPLL and control subjects

	OPLL group, n = 10		Control group, n = 10		OPLL vs. control	
Candidate metabolite	Mean	SD	Mean	SD	Ratio[a]	p-Value[b]
AC(12:1)	5.18×10^{-5}	2.33×10^{-5}	2.05×10^{-5}	1.19×10^{-5}	2.5	0.002
AC(14:3)	1.16×10^{-5}	5.69×10^{-6}	4.78×10^{-6}	3.06×10^{-6}	2.4	0.005
Glycocholic acid	2.13×10^{-5}	1.47×10^{-5}	9.26×10^{-6}	6.12×10^{-6}	2.3	0.038
AC(14:2)	6.46×10^{-5}	2.66×10^{-5}	2.87×10^{-5}	2.09×10^{-5}	2.2	0.004
AC(12:0)	8.44×10^{-5}	2.19×10^{-5}	3.85×10^{-5}	2.79×10^{-5}	2.2	<0.001
Thyroxine	6.69×10^{-6}	2.19×10^{-6}	3.24×10^{-6}	2.02×10^{-6}	2.1	0.005
AC(14:1)	1.40×10^{-4}	5.76×10^{-5}	7.01×10^{-5}	4.93×10^{-5}	2.0	0.009
FA(20:2)	3.61×10^{-5}	2.25×10^{-5}	1.87×10^{-5}	9.28×10^{-6}	1.9	0.043
AC(14:0)	5.51×10^{-5}	1.62×10^{-5}	3.00×10^{-5}	1.66×10^{-5}	1.8	0.003
AC(16:2)	1.58×10^{-5}	5.28×10^{-6}	8.76×10^{-6}	5.83×10^{-6}	1.8	0.011
FA(20:3)	3.38×10^{-5}	1.83×10^{-5}	1.91×10^{-5}	8.06×10^{-6}	1.8	0.038
AC(18:2)	2.34×10^{-4}	4.63×10^{-5}	1.34×10^{-4}	5.58×10^{-5}	1.8	<0.001
AC(16:1)	6.04×10^{-5}	2.04×10^{-5}	3.52×10^{-5}	1.84×10^{-5}	1.7	0.010
Palmitoylcarnitine, AC(16:0)	3.11×10^{-4}	9.13×10^{-5}	1.83×10^{-4}	7.76×10^{-5}	1.7	0.004
FA(24:2)	1.09×10^{-6}	2.83×10^{-7}	6.48×10^{-7}	2.24×10^{-7}	1.7	0.001
AC(18:1)	4.78×10^{-4}	1.19×10^{-4}	3.03×10^{-4}	1.27×10^{-4}	1.6	0.005
Thiaproline	6.51×10^{-4}	1.13×10^{-4}	4.33×10^{-4}	6.83×10^{-5}	1.5	0.001
AC(18:0)	1.17×10^{-4}	3.22×10^{-5}	7.86×10^{-5}	3.13×10^{-5}	1.5	0.015
22-Hydroxycholesterol	7.27×10^{-6}	2.06×10^{-6}	5.14×10^{-6}	1.39×10^{-6}	1.4	0.016
AC(20:1)	2.47×10^{-5}	5.93×10^{-6}	1.77×10^{-5}	6.43×10^{-6}	1.4	0.020
Sarsasapogenin	1.64×10^{-5}	3.69×10^{-6}	1.27×10^{-5}	3.80×10^{-6}	1.3	0.040
Hydroxyproline	2.66×10^{-3}	6.95×10^{-4}	2.09×10^{-3}	4.39×10^{-4}	1.3	0.042
3-Aminobutyric acid	1.79×10^{-4}	3.03×10^{-5}	1.47×10^{-4}	3.60×10^{-5}	1.2	0.043
Glutamine	1.36×10^{-1}	2.03×10^{-2}	1.57×10^{-1}	1.93×10^{-2}	0.9	0.033
Stigmasterol	2.97×10^{-6}	5.28×10^{-7}	4.12×10^{-6}	1.07×10^{-6}	0.7	0.009
Flavanone	2.60×10^{-6}	5.76×10^{-7}	3.66×10^{-6}	1.37×10^{-6}	0.7	0.043

OPLL ossification of the posterior longitudinal ligament, *SD* standard deviation, *AC* acylcarnitine, *FA* fatty acid
[a]Ratio shows OPLL/control
[b]Results from the Welch's t-test

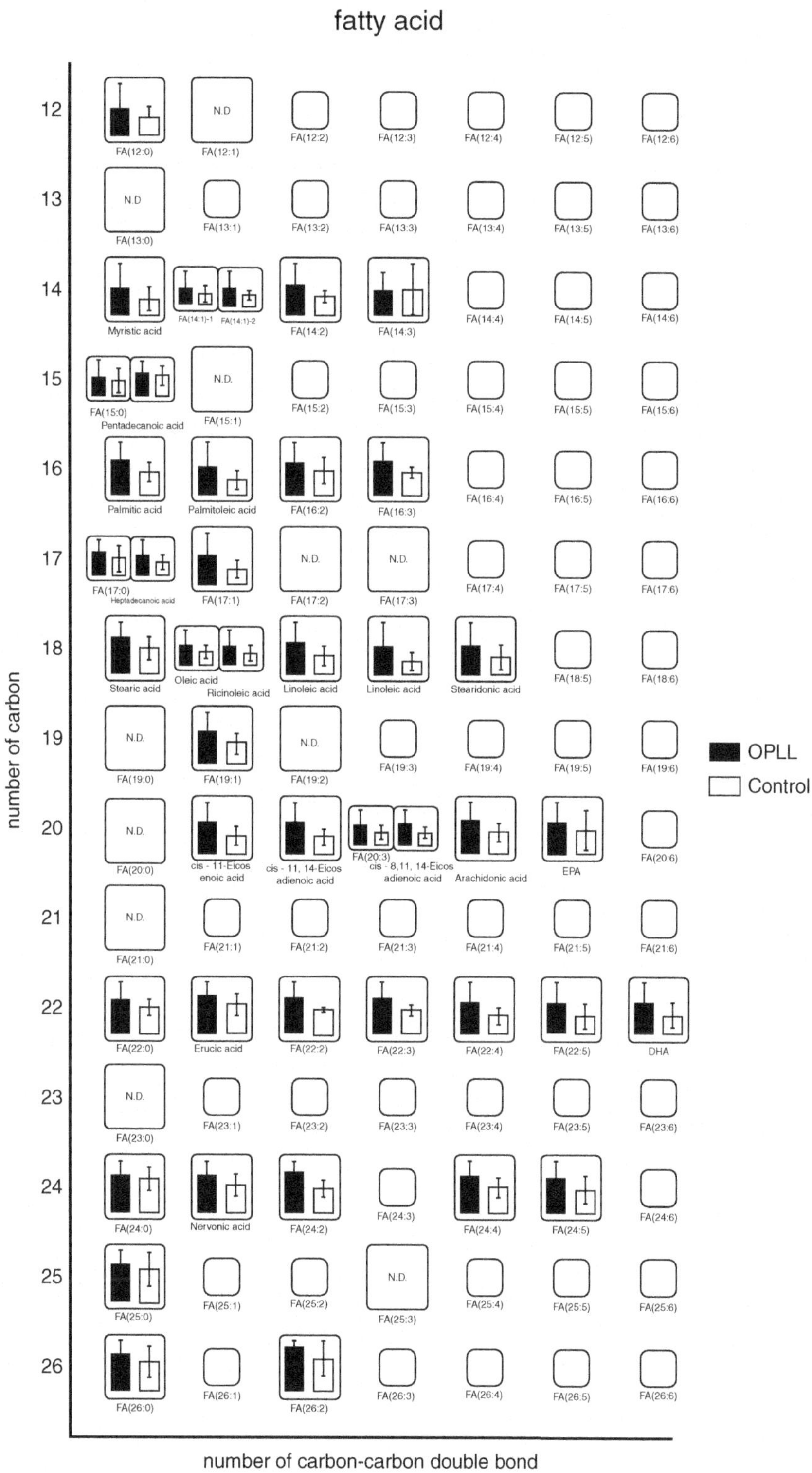

Fig. 13.3 Relative concentration of each fatty acid (FA). Most of these values are larger in OPLL patients compared with control subjects. N.D. indicates not detected

Table 13.2 Relative concentrations of candidate metabolites excluding DM patients

Candidate metabolite	OPLL group, $n = 8$		Control group, $n = 7$		OPLL vs. control	
	Mean	SD	Mean	SD	Ratio[a]	p-Value[b]
Glycocholic acid	1.88×10^{-5}	1.39×10^{-5}	6.55×10^{-6}	4.45×10^{-6}	2.9	0.046
Thyroxine	6.83×10^{-6}	2.46×10^{-6}	2.63×10^{-6}	2.05×10^{-6}	2.6	0.008
AC(12:1)	5.06×10^{-5}	2.61×10^{-5}	1.99×10^{-5}	1.25×10^{-5}	2.5	0.014
AC(12:0)	8.28×10^{-5}	2.43×10^{-5}	3.48×10^{-5}	2.84×10^{-5}	2.4	0.004
AC(14:3)	1.02×10^{-5}	5.49×10^{-6}	4.64×10^{-6}	3.22×10^{-6}	2.2	0.033
FA(24:2)	1.11×10^{-6}	2.72×10^{-7}	5.53×10^{-7}	7.20×10^{-8}	2.0	<0.001
AC(14:0)	5.33×10^{-5}	1.78×10^{-5}	2.61×10^{-5}	1.20×10^{-5}	2.0	0.004
AC(14:2)	6.01×10^{-5}	2.76×10^{-5}	2.98×10^{-5}	2.26×10^{-5}	2.0	0.036
FA(17:0)	1.41×10^{-5}	7.30×10^{-6}	7.39×10^{-5}	2.47×10^{-6}	1.9	0.037
AC(16:1)	6.03×10^{-5}	2.31×10^{-5}	3.29×10^{-5}	1.56×10^{-5}	1.8	0.018
Palmitoylcarnitine, AC(16:0)	3.13×10^{-4}	1.03×10^{-4}	1.72×10^{-4}	6.43×10^{-5}	1.8	0.008
FA(24:5)	5.66×10^{-6}	2.82×10^{-6}	3.14×10^{-6}	1.33×10^{-6}	1.8	0.047
11β-Hydroxyandrost-4-ene-3,17-dione	1.55×10^{-5}	6.63×10^{-6}	8.64×10^{-6}	2.53×10^{-6}	1.8	0.024
AC(18:2)	2.29×10^{-4}	5.13×10^{-5}	1.30×10^{-4}	5.31×10^{-5}	1.8	0.003
Nervonic acid	6.09×10^{-6}	2.31×10^{-6}	3.59×10^{-6}	6.29×10^{-7}	1.7	0.018
AC(18:1)	4.70×10^{-4}	1.34×10^{-4}	2.90×10^{-4}	1.13×10^{-4}	1.6	0.014
Thiaproline	6.51×10^{-4}	1.13×10^{-4}	4.10×10^{-4}	5.94×10^{-5}	1.6	<0.001
Decanoic acid	8.49×10^{-4}	3.12×10^{-4}	5.50×10^{-4}	1.51×10^{-4}	1.5	0.036
FA(26:2)	2.73×10^{-6}	3.29×10^{-7}	1.85×10^{-6}	7.67×10^{-7}	1.5	0.023
Hydroxyproline	2.74×10^{-3}	7.67×10^{-4}	1.98×10^{-3}	4.57×10^{-4}	1.4	0.037
3-Aminobutyric acid	1.79×10^{-4}	2.95×10^{-5}	1.34×10^{-4}	3.61×10^{-5}	1.3	0.022
Flavanone	2.58×10^{-6}	6.41×10^{-7}	3.21×10^{-6}	4.36×10^{-7}	0.8	0.043
Stigmasterol	3.03×10^{-6}	5.73×10^{-7}	4.43×10^{-6}	9.31×10^{-7}	0.7	0.007

DM diabetes mellitus, *OPLL* ossification of the posterior longitudinal ligament, *SD* standard deviation, *AC* acylcarnitine, *FA* fatty acid
[a]Ratio shows OPLL/control
[b]Results from the Welch's t-test

(Table 13.2). In the analysis excluding HL patients (OPLL: $n = 8$, control: $n = 8$), 17 metabolites were significantly different between the two groups (Table 13.3). In the analysis excluding DM and HL patients (OPLL: $n = 7$, control: $n = 5$), 25 metabolites were significantly different between the two groups (Table 13.4).

Consistently in the four analyses (i.e., Tables 13.1–13.4), six metabolites, namely AC(14:0), palmitoylcarnitine, AC(18:2), FA(24:2), thyroxine, and thiaproline, were significantly larger in OPLL group.

13.4 Characteristics and Clinical Significance of Metabolomics Profiling of OPLL Patients

Metabolomics is the comprehensive analysis of small molecule metabolites of biological samples, and this research method is expected to provide a new perspective on OPLL research. The main strengths of metabolomics are that metabolite levels can be regarded as the final response of an organism to genetic and environmental factors.

Table 13.3 Relative concentrations of candidate metabolites excluding HL patients

	OPLL group, $n = 8$		Control group, $n = 8$		OPLL vs. control	
Candidate metabolite	Mean	SD	Mean	SD	Ratio[a]	p-Value[b]
Taurodeoxycholic acid	1.43×10^{-5}	1.03×10^{-5}	4.66×10^{-6}	2.63×10^{-6}	3.1	0.034
Glycodeoxycholic acid	9.35×10^{-5}	3.55×10^{-5}	3.53×10^{-5}	2.51×10^{-5}	2.6	0.002
AC(12:1)	4.72×10^{-5}	2.37×10^{-5}	2.21×10^{-5}	1.27×10^{-5}	2.1	0.023
AC(14:3)	1.09×10^{-5}	5.98×10^{-6}	5.28×10^{-6}	3.24×10^{-6}	2.1	0.040
AC(14:2)	6.33×10^{-5}	3.00×10^{-5}	3.18×10^{-5}	2.25×10^{-5}	2.0	0.034
Thyroxine	6.86×10^{-6}	2.45×10^{-6}	3.62×10^{-6}	1.93×10^{-6}	1.9	0.017
AC(12:0)	8.02×10^{-5}	2.07×10^{-5}	4.25×10^{-5}	2.99×10^{-5}	1.9	0.012
AC(14:0)	5.29×10^{-5}	1.76×10^{-5}	3.25×10^{-5}	1.79×10^{-5}	1.6	0.038
AC(18:2)	2.32×10^{-4}	5.22×10^{-5}	1.44×10^{-4}	5.47×10^{-5}	1.6	0.005
Palmitoylcarnitine, AC(16:0)	3.06×10^{-4}	1.01×10^{-4}	1.96×10^{-4}	8.05×10^{-5}	1.6	0.031
FA(24:2)	1.04×10^{-6}	2.95×10^{-7}	6.67×10^{-7}	2.47×10^{-7}	1.6	0.017
Octanoic acid	5.29×10^{-4}	1.70×10^{-4}	3.70×10^{-4}	1.12×10^{-4}	1.4	0.046
Thiaproline	6.39×10^{-4}	1.19×10^{-4}	4.47×10^{-4}	6.84×10^{-5}	1.4	0.009
2-Hydroxyglutaric acid	2.03×10^{-4}	3.93×10^{-5}	1.48×10^{-4}	1.63×10^{-5}	1.4	0.005
Glutamine	1.34×10^{-1}	2.23×10^{-2}	1.57×10^{-1}	1.47×10^{-2}	0.9	0.034
Cholesterol	1.78×10^{-3}	5.59×10^{-4}	2.37×10^{-3}	4.79×10^{-4}	0.8	0.041
7-Dehydrocholesterol	1.67×10^{-6}	3.87×10^{-7}	2.26×10^{-6}	5.30×10^{-7}	0.7	0.026

HL hyperlipidemia, *OPLL* ossification of the posterior longitudinal ligament, *SD* standard deviation, *AC* acylcarnitine, *FA* fatty acid
[a]Ratio shows OPLL/control
[b]Results from the Welch's t-test

Table 13.4 Relative concentrations of candidate metabolites excluding DM and HL patients

	OPLL group, $n = 7$		Control group, $n = 5$		OPLL vs. control	
Candidate metabolite	Mean	SD	Mean	SD	Ratio[a]	p-Value[b]
Glycocholic acid	1.98×10^{-5}	1.47×10^{-5}	5.40×10^{-6}	4.21×10^{-6}	3.7	0.044
Glycodeoxycholic acid	9.11×10^{-5}	3.76×10^{-5}	2.71×10^{-5}	1.29×10^{-5}	3.4	0.003
Glycolithocholic acid	6.22×10^{-6}	3.68×10^{-6}	2.06×10^{-6}	9.31×10^{-7}	3.0	0.024
Deoxycholic acid	1.34×10^{-4}	8.96×10^{-5}	4.78×10^{-5}	3.11×10^{-5}	2.8	0.046
Thyroxine	6.97×10^{-6}	2.63×10^{-6}	3.03×10^{-6}	2.12×10^{-6}	2.3	0.028
FA(17:0)	1.44×10^{-5}	7.84×10^{-6}	6.72×10^{-6}	2.57×10^{-6}	2.1	0.043
FA(24:2)	1.08×10^{-6}	2.87×10^{-7}	5.45×10^{-7}	6.90×10^{-8}	2.0	0.002
Decanoic acid	8.99×10^{-4}	3.00×10^{-5}	4.71×10^{-4}	8.04×10^{-5}	1.9	0.008
Creatine	1.34×10^{-2}	4.90×10^{-3}	7.21×10^{-3}	2.84×10^{-3}	1.9	0.021
AC(14:0)	5.21×10^{-5}	1.88×10^{-5}	2.85×10^{-5}	1.38×10^{-5}	1.8	0.031
Octanoic acid	5.55×10^{-4}	1.66×10^{-4}	3.22×10^{-4}	6.01×10^{-5}	1.7	0.009
Palmitoylcarnitine, AC(16:0)	3.06×10^{-4}	1.09×10^{-4}	1.89×10^{-4}	6.70×10^{-5}	1.6	0.045
AC(18:2)	2.28×10^{-4}	5.53×10^{-5}	1.46×10^{-4}	5.00×10^{-5}	1.6	0.024
FA(26:2)	2.77×10^{-6}	3.25×10^{-7}	1.82×10^{-6}	7.01×10^{-7}	1.5	0.035
Thiaproline	6.39×10^{-4}	1.19×10^{-4}	4.21×10^{-4}	6.40×10^{-5}	1.5	0.005
Glutamic acid	1.79×10^{-2}	4.90×10^{-3}	1.22×10^{-2}	3.64×10^{-3}	1.5	0.044
2-Hydroxyglutaric acid	2.08×10^{-4}	3.98×10^{-5}	1.44×10^{-4}	1.50×10^{-5}	1.4	0.004
Hydroxyproline	2.57×10^{-3}	6.46×10^{-4}	1.84×10^{-3}	4.30×10^{-4}	1.4	0.041
Gluconic acid	4.25×10^{-4}	7.35×10^{-5}	3.40×10^{-4}	5.23×10^{-5}	1.3	0.040
Symmetric dimethylarginine	2.40×10^{-4}	3.94×10^{-5}	1.97×10^{-4}	2.68×10^{-5}	1.2	0.047

(continued)

Table 13.4 (continued)

Candidate metabolite	OPLL group, $n = 7$ Mean	SD	Control group, $n = 5$ Mean	SD	OPLL vs. control Ratio[a]	p-Value[b]
Betaine	1.80×10^{-2}	2.26×10^{-3}	2.34×10^{-2}	4.37×10^{-3}	0.8	0.046
Ethanolamine	1.03×10^{-3}	1.93×10^{-4}	1.37×10^{-3}	2.03×10^{-4}	0.8	0.019
Testosterone	3.19×10^{-5}	7.09×10^{-6}	4.23×10^{-5}	6.37×10^{-6}	0.8	0.026
7-Dehydrocholesterol	1.60×10^{-6}	3.54×10^{-7}	2.34×10^{-6}	1.74×10^{-7}	0.7	0.001
Stigmasterol	3.03×10^{-6}	6.19×10^{-7}	4.05×10^{-6}	6.31×10^{-7}	0.7	0.022

DM diabetes mellitus, *HL* hyperlipidemia, *OPLL* ossification of the posterior longitudinal ligament, *SD* standard deviation, *AC* acylcarnitine, *FA* fatty acid

[a]Ratio shows OPLL/control

[b]Results from the Welch's t-test

Therefore, this new research platform is most closely related to phenotype among other "omics" technologies. Moreover, because genomics, transcriptomics, and proteomics do not fully explain the pathophysiological condition of a large number of diseases, increased interest of metabolomic research has been observed in recent years [5]. However, to date, comprehensive metabolomics analysis in OPLL patients has not been performed. Therefore, we conducted this type of study for the first time and evaluated metabolite profiling in OPLL patients [10].

Although the underlying mechanisms of OPLL remain still obscure, OPLL has heterogenous clinical characteristics according to gender difference, ossified region (i.e., cervical, thoracic, and lumbar) and types of OPLL (i.e., continuous, mixed, segmental, and circumscribed). Therefore, we evaluated metabolite profiling of patients with OPLL focusing on male (i.e., dominant) gender, cervical (i.e., the most frequent) region, and continuous or mixed (i.e., the most frequent) types of OPLL to evaluate the typical patients and thereby reducing sample complexity and confounding factors. Furthermore, it was necessary to consider the influence of comorbidities on the metabolites because the association of OPLL with impaired glucose tolerance or abnormal lipid metabolism has been pointed out [3, 11, 12]. Therefore, we analyzed metabolites except the patients with DM and HL in our study, and consequently, there were significant differences in six metabolites between OPLL and control groups.

A group of FA was significantly larger in OPLL group. The FAs have been reported to have biological effects on bone metabolism [13, 14]. Previous in vitro studies showed that FAs can promote osteoblastogenesis and bone formation [15, 16]. Other studies reported that FAs can activate free FA receptor 4 or parathyroid hormone (PTH) type 1 receptor and, consequently, provide increased osteoblastic bone formation and decreased osteoclastic bone resorption, resulting in increases in osteoblastogenesis and decreases in osteoclastogenesis [17, 18].

Thyroid hormone, thyroxine (T4), was significantly higher in OPLL group than that in the control group. Recent in vitro study demonstrated that thyroid hormones and their metabolites cause a dose-dependent increase in the expression of osteoblast differentiation markers, osterix, and osteocalcin. Moreover, that study also demonstrated that T4 treatments elevate insulin-like growth factor 1 (IGF-1) mRNA level suggesting the involvement of IGF-1 signaling in the thyroid hormone regulation on osteoblast differentiation [19]. The other in vitro study showed that T4 increases angiopoietin 1 expression and induces bone formation, differentiation, and mineralization [20].

In our study, we evaluated the metabolite profiling in patients with OPLL for the first time. However, our studies did not identify the causative agent of OPLL. Because the present study was a cross-sectional study, the causal association between the identified metabolites and OPLL could not be elucidated. The relationship between the severity of OPLL and the identified metabolite should also be evaluated. We also needed to do a longitudinal study to see if these metabolites show dose-dependent effects for the development or progression of OPLL. Therefore, future multidisciplinary studies are needed to elucidate the real pathomechanisms of OPLL.

Finally, although the results of our study do not immediately lead to new therapies, it would be expected to be useful for clarifying the pathology of OPLL, reproducing this disease in vitro, screening therapeutic agents, and evaluating the effects of therapeutic drugs in the near future.

13.5 Conclusions

We evaluated the metabolite profiling of plasma in patients with OPLL and detected some metabolites showing suggestive association with disease. These results of the present study could lead to new insights into clarifying the molecular pathomechanisms of OPLL.

References

1. Resnick D, Shaul SR, Robins JM. Diffuse idiopathic skeletal hyperostosis (DISH): Forestier's disease with extraspinal manifestations. Radiology. 1975;115(3):513–24.
2. Nakajima M, Takahashi A, Tsuji T, Karasugi T, Baba H, Uchida K, Kawabata S, Okawa A, Shindo S, Takeuchi K, Taniguchi Y, Maeda S, Kashii M, Seichi A, Nakajima H, Kawaguchi Y, Fujibayashi S, Takahata M, Tanaka T, Watanabe K, Kida K, Kanchiku T, Ito Z, Mori K, Kaito T, Kobayashi S, Yamada K, Takahashi M, Chiba K, Matsumoto M, Furukawa K, Kubo M, Toyama Y, Genetic Study Group of Investigation Committee on Ossification of the Spinal Ligaments, Ikegawa S. A genome-wide association study identifies susceptibility loci for ossification of the posterior longitudinal ligament of the spine. Nat Genet. 2014;46(9):1012–6.
3. Shingyouchi Y, Nagahama A, Niida M. Ligamentous ossification of the cervical spine in the late middle-aged Japanese men. Its relation to body mass index and glucose metabolism. Spine (Phila Pa 1976). 1996;21(21):2474–8.
4. Wang PN, Chen SS, Liu HC, Fuh JL, Kuo BI, Wang SJ. Ossification of the posterior longitudinal ligament of the spine. A case-control risk factor study. Spine (Phila Pa 1976). 1999;24(2):142–4; discussion 145.
5. Rochfort S. Metabolomics reviewed: a new "omics" platform technology for systems biology and implications for natural products research. J Nat Prod. 2005;68(12):1813–20.
6. Newgard CB. Metabolomics and metabolic diseases: where do we stand? Cell Metab. 2017;25(1):43–56.
7. Soga T, Ohashi Y, Ueno Y, Naraoka H, Tomita M, Nishioka T. Quantitative metabolome analysis using capillary electrophoresis mass spectrometry. J Proteome Res. 2003;2(5):488–94.
8. Ooga T, Sato H, Nagashima A, Sasaki K, Tomita M, Soga T, Ohashi Y. Metabolomic anatomy of an animal model revealing homeostatic imbalances in dyslipidaemia. Mol Biosyst. 2011;7(4):1217–23.
9. Sugimoto M, Wong DT, Hirayama A, Soga T, Tomita M. Capillary electrophoresis mass spectrometry-based saliva metabolomics identified oral, breast and pancreatic cancer-specific profiles. Metabolomics. 2010;6(1):78–95.
10. Tsuji T, Matsumoto M, Nakamura M, Miyamoto T, Yagi M, Fujita N, Okada E, Nagoshi N, Tsuji O, Watanabe K. Metabolite profiling of plasma in patients with ossification of the posterior longitudinal ligament. J Orthop Sci. 2018;23(6):878–83.
11. Inamasu J, Guiot BH, Sachs DC. Ossification of the posterior longitudinal ligament: an update on its biology, epidemiology, and natural history. Neurosurgery. 2006;58(6):1027–39; discussion 1027–39.
12. Ikeda Y, Nakajima A, Aiba A, Koda M, Okawa A, Takahashi K, Yamazaki M. Association between serum leptin and bone metabolic markers, and the development of heterotopic ossification of the spinal ligament in female patients with ossification of the posterior longitudinal ligament. Eur Spine J. 2011;20(9):1450–8.
13. Watkins BA, Lippman HE, Le Bouteiller L, Li Y, Seifert MF. Bioactive fatty acids: role in bone biology and bone cell function. Prog Lipid Res. 2001;40(1–2):125–48.
14. Watkins BA, Li Y, Lippman HE, Feng S. Modulatory effect of omega-3 polyunsaturated fatty acids on osteoblast function and bone metabolism. Prostaglandins Leukot Essent Fatty Acids. 2003;68(6):387–98.
15. Shen CL, Peterson J, Tatum OL, Dunn DM. Effect of long-chain n-3 polyunsaturated fatty acid on inflammation mediators during osteoblastogenesis. J Med Food. 2008;11(1):105–10.
16. Lin G, Wang H, Dai J, Li X, Guan M, Gao S, Ding Q, Wang H, Fang H. Conjugated linoleic acid prevents age-induced bone loss in mice by regulating both osteoblastogenesis and adipogenesis. Biochem Biophys Res Commun. 2017;490(3):813–20.
17. Ahn SH, Park SY, Baek JE, Lee SY, Baek WY, Lee SY, Lee YS, Yoo HJ, Kim H, Lee SH, Im DS, Lee SK, Kim BJ, Koh JM. Free fatty acid receptor 4 (GPR120) stimulates bone formation and suppresses bone resorption in the presence of elevated n-3 fatty acid levels. Endocrinology. 2016;157(7):2621–35.
18. Candelario J, Tavakoli H, Chachisvilis M. PTH1 receptor is involved in mediating cellular response to long-chain polyunsaturated fatty acids. PLoS One. 2012;7(12):e52583.
19. Cheng S, Xing W, Pourteymoor S, Mohan S. Effects of thyroxine (T4), 3,5,3′-triiodo-L-thyronine (T3) and their metabolites on osteoblast differentiation. Calcif Tissue Int. 2016;99(4):435–42.
20. Park SH, Lee J, Kang MA, Moon YJ, Wang SI, Kim KM, Park BH, Jang KY, Kim JR. Potential of l-thyroxine to differentiate osteoblast-like cells via angiopoietin1. Biochem Biophys Res Commun. 2016;478(3):1409–15.

Part IV

Diagnosis

Diagnosis of OPLL and OLF: Overview

14

Masashi Yamazaki, Tetsuya Abe, Toru Funayama, Hiroshi Takahashi, Satoshi Maki, Takeo Furuya, and Masao Koda

Abstract

Recent progress in image diagnosis technology enables us to detect numerous new findings for the diagnosis of ossification of the posterior longitudinal ligament (OPLL) and ossification of the ligamentum flavum (OLF). In most cases of cervical OPLL and thoracic OPLL/OLF, not only static compression, but also dynamic factors contribute to the development and aggravation of the myelopathy. The rationale for posterior decompression and fusion (PDF) surgery is to suppress the motion at the nonossified segment of OPLL by stabilization. The K-line is a simple and practical parameter with utility for decisions regarding the surgical approach to cervical OPLL. Sufficient posterior shift of the spinal cord and neurological improvement will not be obtained after laminoplasty in K-line (−) OPLL patients. Multicenter CT studies of ossification of the spinal ligament have been performed by the Japanese Research Group for Ossification of the Spinal Ligament to evaluate the prevalence of OPLL in the whole spine.

M. Yamazaki (✉) · T. Abe · T. Funayama · M. Koda
Department of Orthopaedic Surgery, Faculty of Medicine, University of Tsukuba, Tsukuba City, Ibaraki, Japan
e-mail: masashiy@md.tsukuba.ac.jp

H. Takahashi · S. Maki · T. Furuya
Department of Orthopaedic Surgery, Chiba University Graduate School of Medicine, Chiba, Japan

Keywords

Ossification of posterior longitudinal ligament (OPLL) · Ossification of ligamentum flavum (OLF) · K-line

14.1 Introduction

Ossification of the posterior longitudinal ligament (OPLL) of the spine was first reported in Japan in 1960 [1]. Thereafter, OPLL has been recognized as a specific spine disease that causes compression myelopathy. Since several reports demonstrated that in Japan there were many patients with OPLL who showed severe myelopathy, in 1972 the Japanese Ministry of Health, Labor and Welfare established a special research group called The Research Group for Ossification of the Spinal Ligament to study the diagnosis and treatment of severe spinal cord disorders associated with OPLL and ossification of ligamentum flavum (OLF) [1]. Thus far, many OPLL/OLF-related studies have been advanced by the research group, which have contributed to systematize the diagnosis and treatment for OPLL/OLF. Recent progress in image diagnosis technology enables us to detect numerous new findings. In this chapter, we present our instructive cases of cervical OPLL and thoracic OPLL/OLF and describe the recent progress in their diagnosis.

A. Okawa et al. (eds.), *OPLL*, https://doi.org/10.1007/978-981-15-3855-1_14

14.2 Cervical OPLL

14.2.1 Static and Dynamic Factors for the Development of Myelopathy in Patients with Cervical OPLL

In standard textbooks, morphology of cervical OPLL has been classified using conventional lateral radiographs as (1) continuous type, (2) segmental type, (3) mixed type, and (4) localized type [1]. However, recent studies have pointed out that this classification is not necessarily useful in the clinic [2]. In many patients with OPLL, whose ossification was classified as continuous type OPLL, we can detect a gap (nonossified area) in their ossified masses by using sagittally reconstructed computed tomography (CT) (Fig. 14.1). This indicates that not only static compression, but also dynamic factors contribute to the development of myelopathy in patients with OPLL. When we look at the flexion and extension radiographs, we can detect a change in the distance between adjacent spinous processes at the level of maximum spinal cord compression, which indicates the mobility of the spine [2] (Fig. 14.1).

We previously analyzed patients who had cervical OPLL but did not show clinical symptoms of myelopathy [3]. In this study, we found that patients with massive OPLL do not develop myelopathy when the mobility of their cervical spine is highly restricted, suggesting that dynamic factors such as the segmental range of motion (ROM) preferentially contribute to the development of myelopathy in patients with cervical OPLL (Fig. 14.2). This suggests that, by controlling the dynamic factors, we might be able to reduce neurological deterioration in patients with cervical OPLL [3].

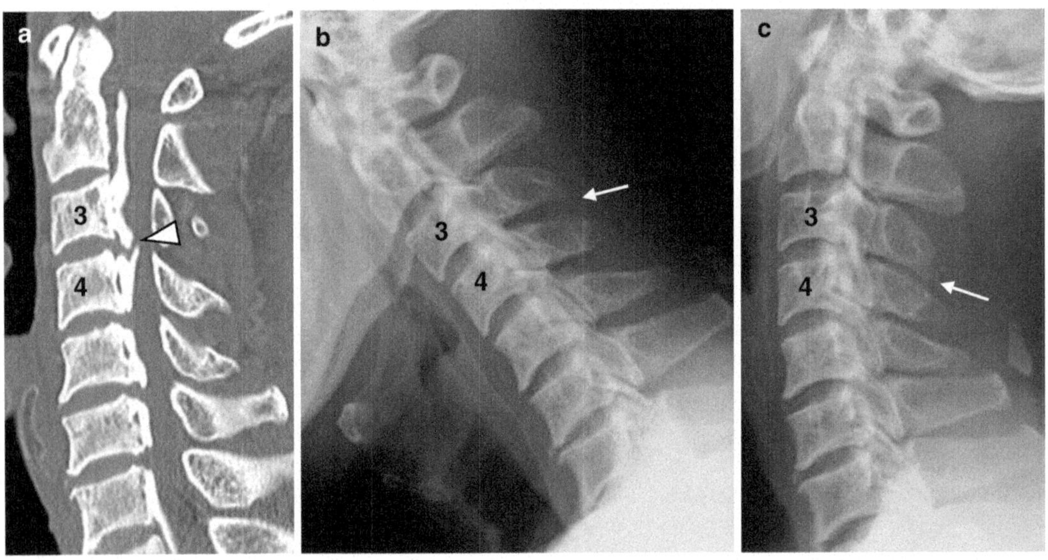

Fig. 14.1 Spinal mobility at the level of maximum cord compression in patients with cervical ossification of posterior longitudinal ligament (OPLL). In most patients with cervical OPLL who show severe myelopathy, spinal mobility remains at the level of maximum cord compression. We can detect a gap in the OPLL (noncontinuous area) by using computed tomographic (CT) sagittally reconstructed images (**a**, arrowhead) although this gap cannot usually be seen in plain radiographs. We can detect the spinal mobility at intervertebral disc levels with flexion and extension radiographs as a change in the distance between adjacent spinous processes (**b** and **c**, arrows)

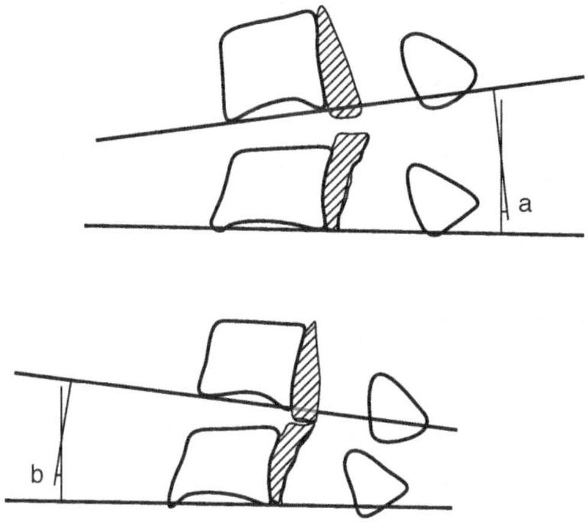

Fig. 14.2 Schematic drawings showing the segmental range of motion (ROM). The segmental ROM at the level of maximum cord compression as measured from flexion and extension radiographs. (Reproduced from Masaki et al. [2])

14.2.2 Factors Causing Poor Surgical Outcome After Laminoplasty in Patients with Cervical OPLL

In many patients with cervical OPLL, their myelopathy is relieved after laminoplasty. However, for other patients, laminoplasty alone is insufficient to improve their symptoms. We previously analyzed the factors associated with poor surgical outcome after laminoplasty [2] and found that the range of intervertebral mobility at the level of maximum cord compression before surgery was larger in the group with poor outcome than it was in the group with good outcome (Fig. 14.3). We suggest that hypermobility of vertebrae at the cord compression level is a risk factor for poor surgical outcome after laminoplasty. Based on these results, we recommend that ante-

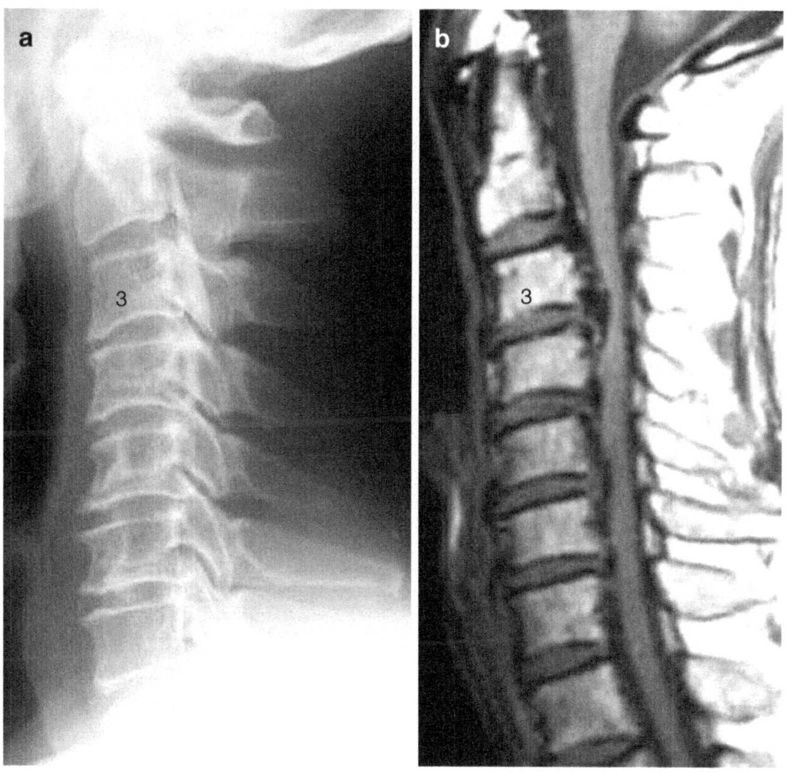

Fig. 14.3 A patient with cervical OPLL who showed poor surgical outcome after cervical laminoplasty. Preoperative radiographic image with the patient in a neutral position (**a**). T1-weighted midsagittal magnetic resonance (MR) image (**b**) of a 68-year-old man demonstrating OPLL at C2–C7 and severe compression of the spinal cord anteriorly at C3–4. Preoperative extension radiographic image (**c**) and flexion radiographic image (**d**) showing the range of motion at C3–4 was 8°. Arrows indicate the intervertebral disc mobility evident at C3–4. Postoperative radiographic image with the patient in a neutral position (**e**). T1-weighted MR midsagittal image (**f**) 1 year after C3–C7 laminoplasty, demonstrating progression of cervical kyphosis and persistent anterior impingement of the spinal cord by OPLL. The recovery rate for this case was 21.7%, representing a poor surgical outcome. (Reproduced from Masaki et al. [2])

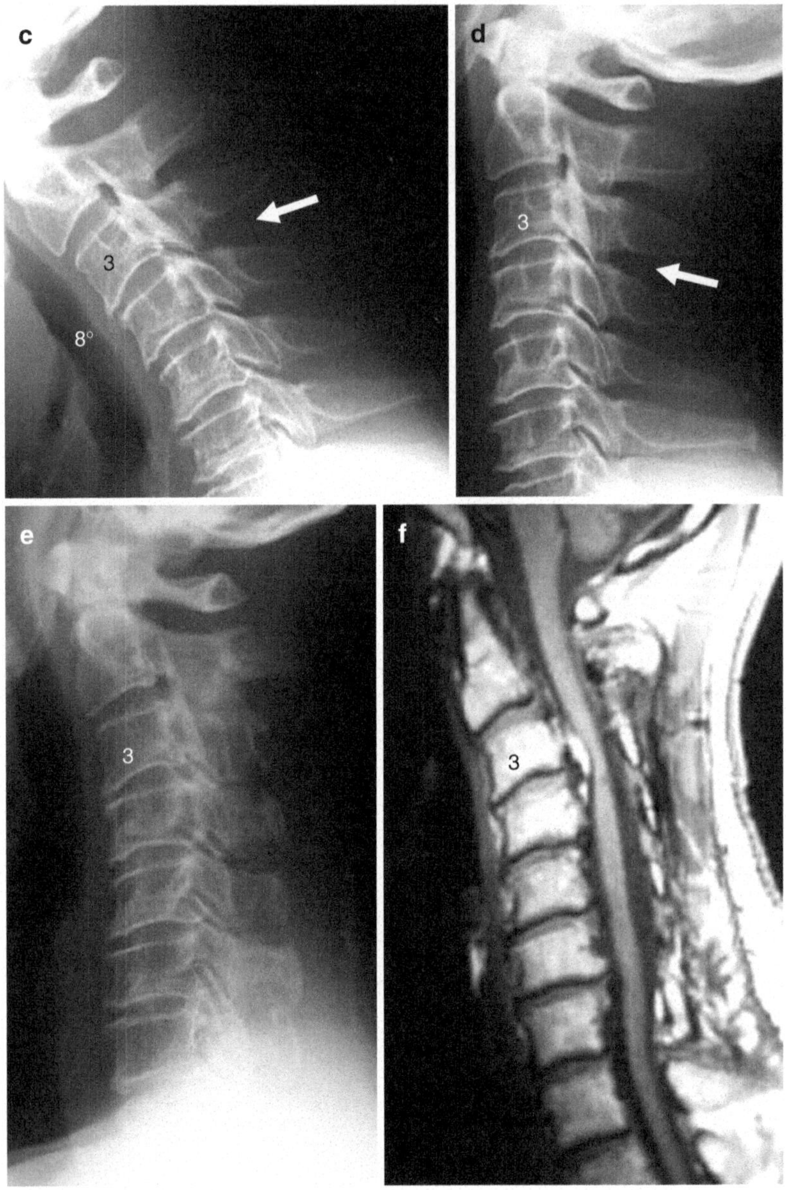

Fig. 14.3 (continued)

rior decompression with spinal fusion (ASF) should be the first choice of treatment for patients with significant OPLL and a hypermobile cervical spine. When laminoplasty is used for such cases, the addition of posterior instrumented fusion is desirable to stabilize the spine and avoid damage to the spinal cord [2].

14.2.3 The K-Line: A Concept with Utility for Decisions Regarding Surgical Approach to Cervical OPLL

Previous studies showed that kyphotic alignment of the cervical spine and a large OPLL are major factors causing poor surgical outcome after laminoplasty in patients with cervical OPLL [4, 5]. However, these parameters are complicated and not practical to use in the clinic. We were the first to report a new index, the K-line, to help decide the surgical approach to cervical OPLL. The K-line was defined as a line that connects the midpoints of the spinal canal at C2 and C7 [6] (Fig. 14.4). OPLL did not exceed the K-line in the K-line (+) group and did exceed it in the K-line (−) group. We found that the surgical outcomes of K-line (−) patients after laminoplasty were inferior to those of K-line (+) patients. We suggest that a sufficient posterior shift of the spinal cord and neurological improvement will not be obtained after posterior decompression surgery in the K-line (−) group [7, 8] (Fig. 14.5). Thus, the K-line is a simple and practical tool with utility for decisions regarding the surgical approach to cervical OPLL (Fig. 14.6).

14.2.4 The K-Line in Cervical OPLL Patients Is Different on Plain Radiographs and CT Images

Although K-line was originally measured on plain radiographs, CT reconstruction is applied for K-line measurement by several surgeons. Thus, we analyzed whether there is a difference in K-lines obtained from radiographs of standing patients and those obtained from CT sagittal images of supine patients [9] (Fig. 14.7). The results showed that the X-P-based K-line was found to be (+) in 35 patients and (−) in 30 patients. Four of 35 patients with an X-P-based K-line (11%) showed a change from K-line (+) to (−) in CT-based K-line measurements. One of 30 patients with an X-P-based K-line (3%) showed a change from (−) to (+) in CT-based measurements. Thus, we conclude that the

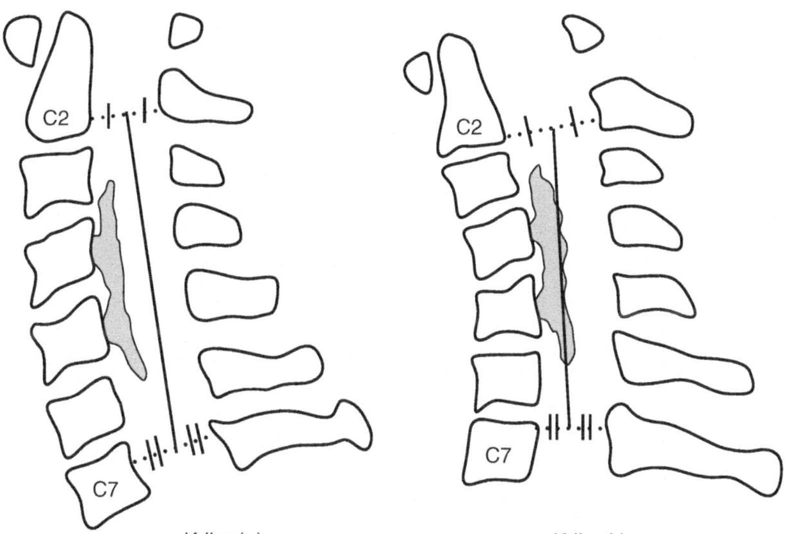

Fig. 14.4 Schematic drawings of the "K-line". The K-line is a straight line that connects the midpoints of the spinal canal at C2 and C7 on lateral cervical radiographs. Patients with cervical OPLL are divided into two groups according to the K-line. OPLL does not exceed the K-line in the K-line (+) group and does exceed it in the K-line (−) group. (Reproduced from Fujiyoshi et al. [6])

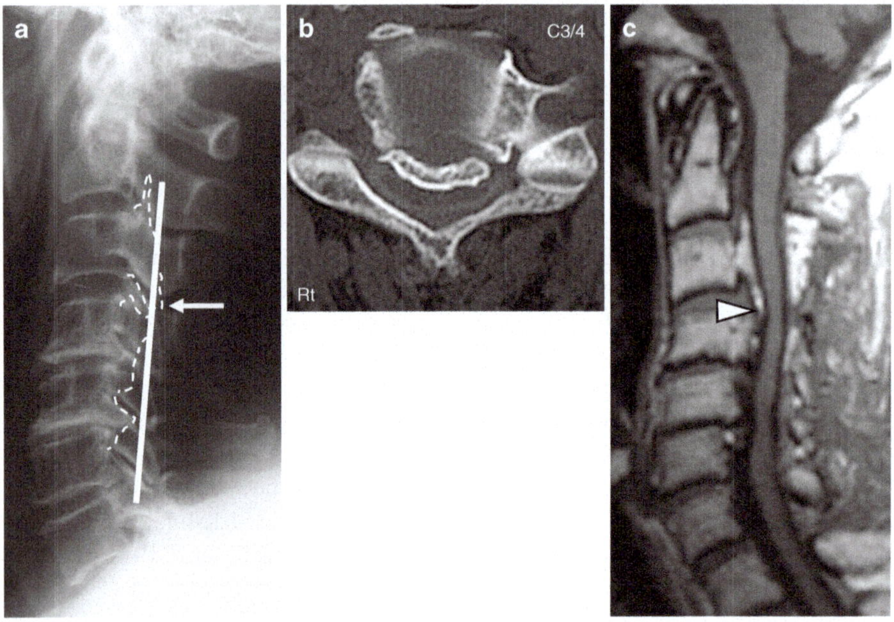

Fig. 14.5 A patient with K-line (–) OPLL who showed neurological deterioration after laminoplasty. Preoperative radiographic image of an 81-year-old woman in a neutral position (**a**) demonstrating OPLL at C2–C6 and severe anterior impingement of the spinal cord at C3–4. The OPLL exceeded the K-line (arrow). Her preoperative JOA score was 9/17. Axial CT image at C3–4 showing the OPLL occupation ratio was 70% (**b**). The segmental ROM at C3–4 was 12°. Postoperative T1-weighted MR midsagittal image (**c**) after C3–C7 laminoplasty demonstrating persistent anterior impingement of the spinal cord by OPLL at C3–4 (arrowhead). After surgery, the patient deteriorated neurologically, showing a postoperative JOA score 5/17 (recovery rate: –50%)

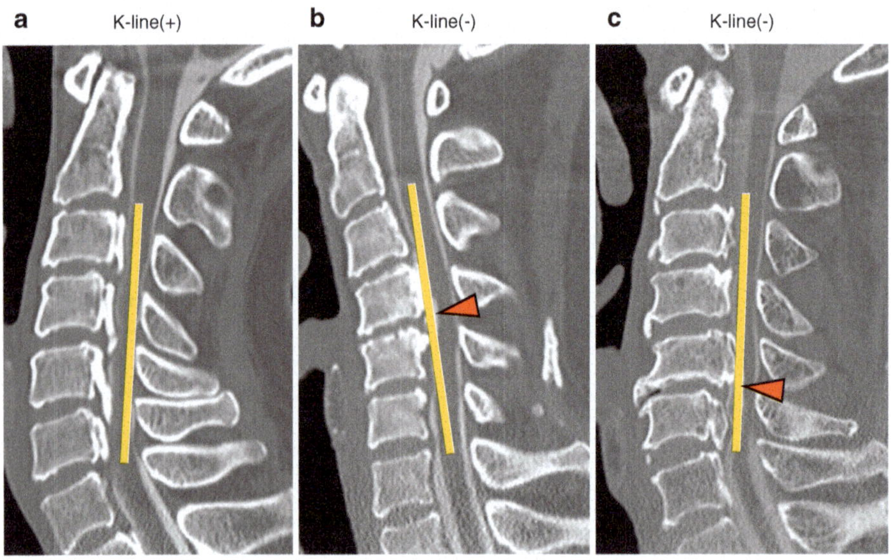

Fig. 14.6 Determination of the K-line. We classified three patients with cervical OPLL using the K-line depicted in their CT midsagittal images. K-line is defined as (+) when the peak of ossification foci does not exceed the K-line (**a**). K-line is defined as (–) when the peak of ossification foci exceeds the K-line (**b**, **c**, arrowheads). K-line can be (–) when the cervical alignment is kyphosis (**b**), ossification foci are extremely thick (**c**), and a combination of kyphosis and thick OPLL

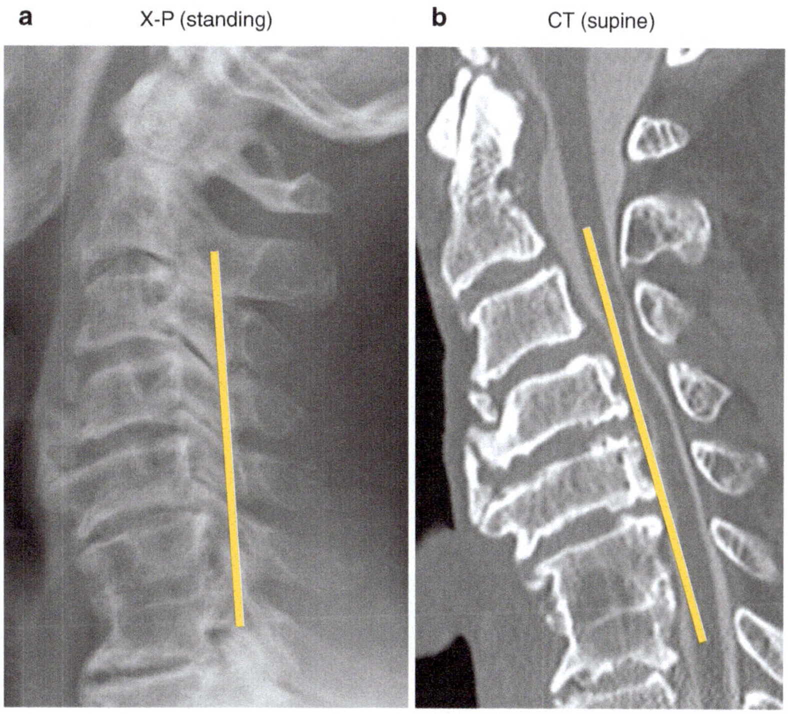

Fig. 14.7 Representative cervical radiographs and CT midsagittal images of the same patient with cervical OPLL. The X-P-based K-line was found to be (+) (**a**) whereas the CT-based K-line was found to be (−) (**b**). The K-line was different between radiographs and the CT midsagittal images. (Reproduced from Ijima et al. [9])

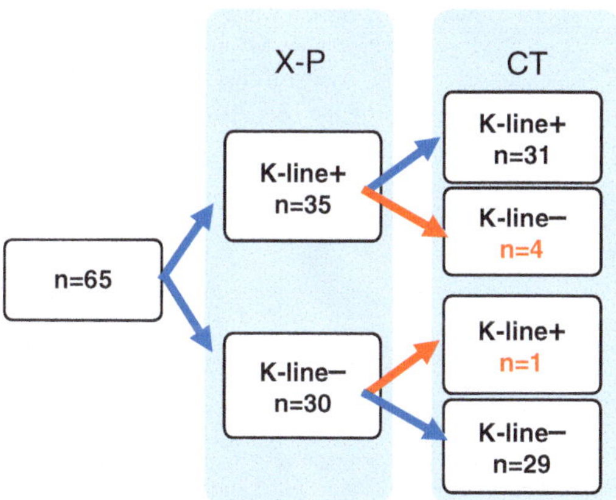

Fig. 14.8 Tree diagram showing the X-P-based K-line and the CT-based K-line of 65 patients with cervical OPLL. The X-P-based K-line was found to be (+) in 35 patients and (−) in 30 patients. Four of 35 patients with an X-P-based K-line (11%) showed a change from K-line (+) to (−) in CT-based K-line measurements. One of the 30 patients with an X-P-based K-line (3%) showed a change from (−) to (+) in CT based measurements. (Reproduced from Ijima et al. [9])

K-line should be measured using plain radiographs of standing patients because X-P-based K-line and CT-based K-line measurements can be different [9] (Fig. 14.8).

14.3 Thoracic OPLL and PLF

14.3.1 Static and Dynamic Factors for the Development of Myelopathy in Patients with Thoracic OPLL and OLF

We previously evaluated the clinical results of PDF surgery for thoracic myelopathy due to OPLL/OLF. The results demonstrate that despite persistent anterior impingement of the spinal cord by residual OPLL, PDF can result in considerable neurological recovery with a low risk of postoperative paralysis [10–12]. For these cases of PDF, we measured the kyphotic angles at instrumented fusion levels. The preoperative kyphotic angles were measured with patients supine and sitting (Fig. 14.9). The difference between the kyphotic angle when the patients were supine and the kyphotic angle measured when they were sitting ranged from 8° to 20° (mean spinal mobility per disc was 1.3°). In patients with thoracic OPLL/OLF, the spinal column still showed some mobility at the level of cord compression despite the presence of massive heterotopic vertebral ossification. Moreover, the postoperative kyphotic angle at the level of instrumented fusion was greater than the preoperative kyphotic angle while the patient was supine, but less than the preoperative kyphotic angle while the patient was sitting. We suggest that the remaining mobility of the spinal column at the level of cord compression correlates with the development and aggravation of myelopathy in patients with thoracic OPLL/OLF.

14.3.2 Bone Union and Remodeling of the Nonossified Segment in Thoracic OPLL After PDF Surgery

The motion at the nonossified segment of the OPLL/OLF is thought to be highly correlated with aggravation of symptoms of myelopathy (Fig. 14.9). The rationale for PDF surgery is to suppress the motion at the nonossified segment of

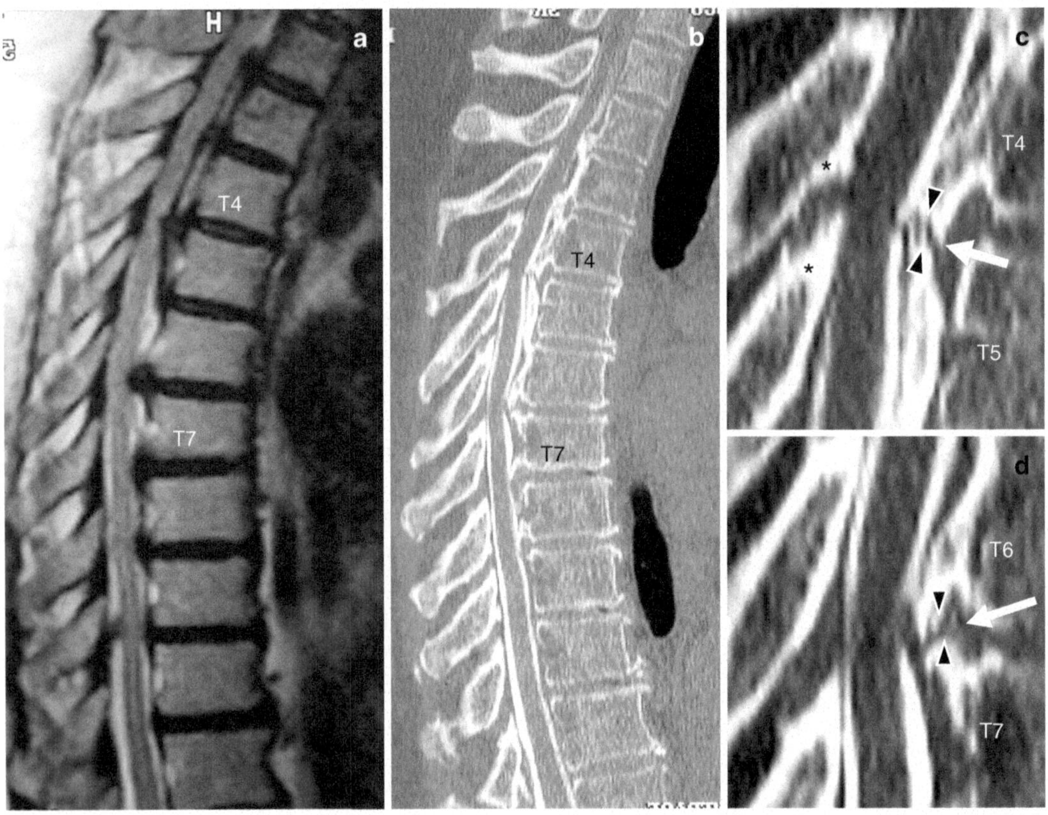

Fig. 14.9 A case of thoracic OPLL and ossification of ligamentum flavum (OLF) who underwent posterior decompression with instrumented fusion (PDF). Preoperative T2-weighted MR image at the midsagittal plane (**a**) of a 55-year-old woman, showing severe narrowing of the spinal cord at T4–5 and T6–7. CT midsagittal images after myelography (**b**–**d**) showing her spinal cord was impinged by a beak-type OPLL at T4–5 and T6–7 (**c**, **d**, arrows) and OLF (**c**, asterisks). The mid-portion of the beak-type OPLL contains a nonossified area (**c**, **d**, arrowheads). Radiographic images showing that the kyphotic angle at T1–T10 was 27° when she was supine (**e**) and 35° when sitting (**f**). A postoperative radiographic image after PDF (**g**) showing a kyphotic angle at T1–T10 of 32°. A midsagittal reconstruction CT image 2 weeks after surgery (**h**) showing a nonossified area at the mid-portion of the ossified mass at T4–5 (**h**, arrow) and T6–7 (**h**, arrowheads). The CT images 2 years and 3 months (**i**) and 6 years and 7 months (**j**) after surgery showing progression of the union at the nonossified areas (**i**, **j**, arrows and arrowheads). (Reproduced from Yamazaki et al. [11])

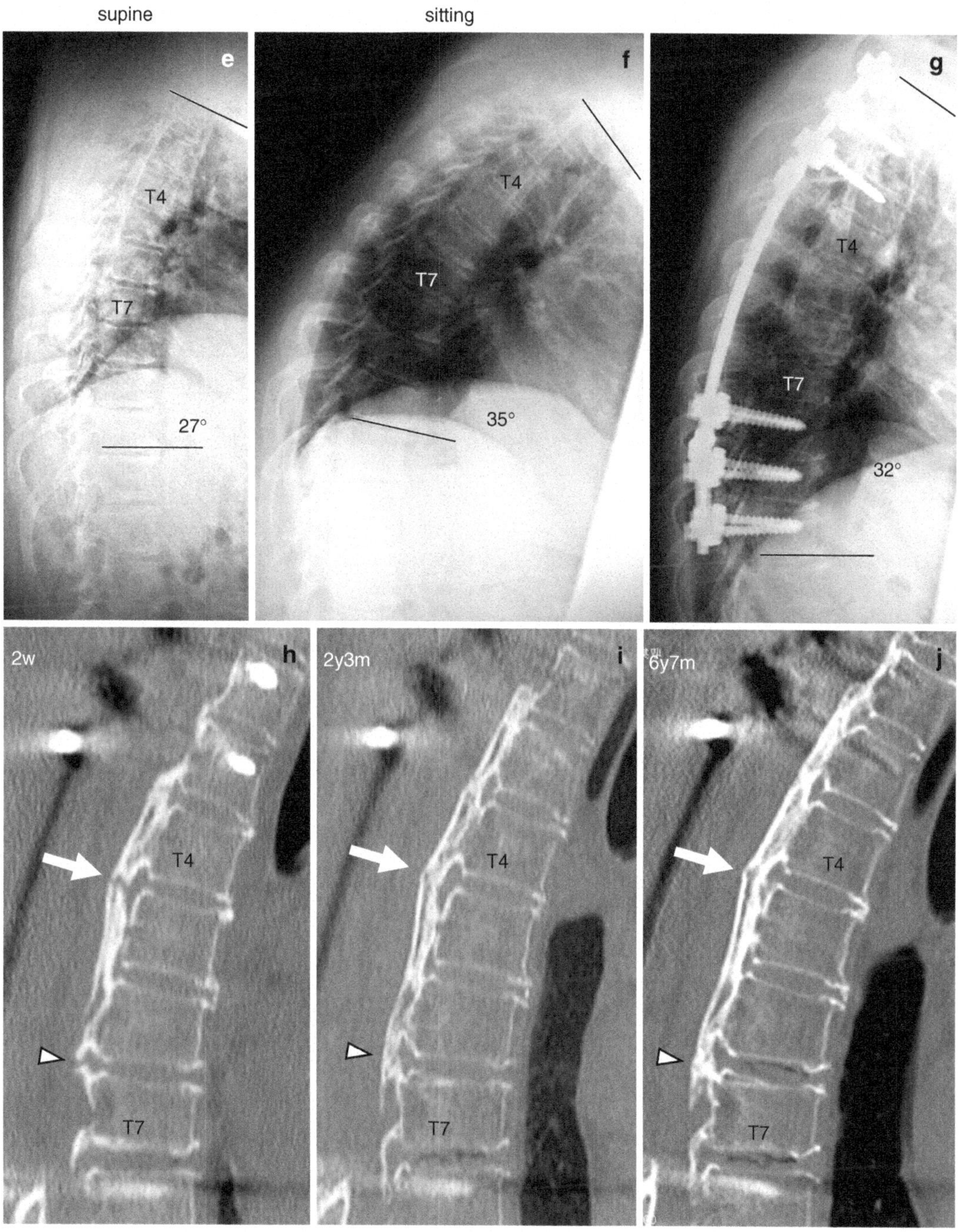

Fig. 14.9 (continued)

OPLL by stabilization. We previously investigated the course of bone union and remodeling of the nonossified segment of thoracic OPLL after PDF surgery. The results showed that nonossified segments of OPLLs fused in most thoracic OPLL patients (Fig. 14.9). The thickness of the OPLL at its thickest segment also decreased after PDF surgery. The decrease in ossification thickness was significantly greater in the patients who showed fusion of nonossified segments of OPLL compared with that in patients who did not show fusion [13]. The results showed that remodeling of the OPLLs, following fusion of nonossified segment of OPLLs, resulted in a decreased OPLL thickness, with the potential for reducing spinal cord compression.

14.3.3 Pathogenesis of Severe Myelopathy Caused by Thoracic OPLL and OLF

We experienced postoperative transient paraparesis in a patient with thoracic OPLL/OLF [14] (Fig. 14.10). The patient's spinal cord was severely impinged anteriorly by a beak-type OPLL and posteriorly by OLF at the level of maximum cord compression. The patient underwent PDF surgery. Immediately after surgery, he developed a Brown–Séquard-type paralysis, which spontaneously resolved without requiring the addition of OPLL extirpation. This example highlights that the risk of postoperative neurological deterioration cannot be eliminated even when PDF is selected as the surgical procedure for thoracic OPLL/OLF, especially in instances in which the spinal cord is severely compressed.

We suggest that pathogenesis of severe myelopathy caused by thoracic OPLL/OLF is a fragile spinal cord, which is repeatedly impinged from an anterior and posterior direction by a heterotopic ossified mass. The impingement of the spinal cord is not only static but also dynamic. We suppose that the decompression surgery itself for such fragile spinal cords carries a great risk of postoperative paralysis.

14.4 Multicenter CT Study by The Research Group for Ossification of the Spinal Ligament

We utilized the CT image data from the Japanese Research Group for Ossification of the Spinal Ligament and conducted the multicenter CT studies. We aimed to evaluate the prevalence of OPLL in the whole spine among patients with cervical OPLL. In addition, we used a multiple regression model to investigate the factors that correlate with the presence and distribution of ossified lesions in the whole spine.

14.4.1 A New CT Classification

We proposed three classification systems of cervical OPLL based on CT imaging: A, B, and axial. Classification A comprises two lesion types: bridge and nonbridge. Classification B requires examiners to describe all vertebral and interverte-

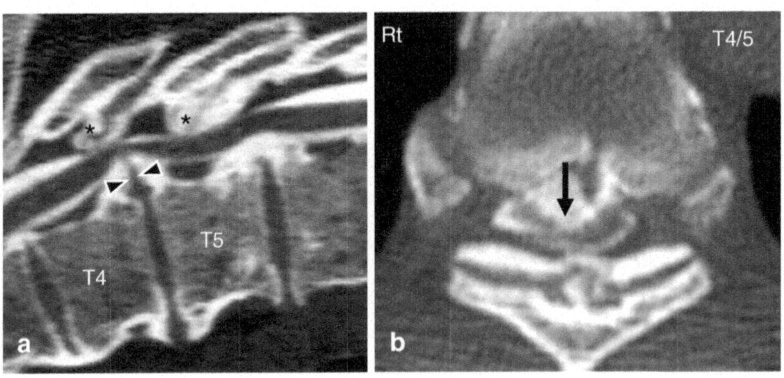

Fig. 14.10 A case of thoracic OPLL and OLF who showed transient postoperative paralysis after PDF. Preoperative midsagittal (**a**) and axial (**b**) reconstruction images from a CT myelogram showing impingement of the spinal cord anteriorly by a beak-type OPLL (**b**, arrow) and posteriorly by OLF (**a**, asterisks) at T4–5. The mid-portion of the beak-type OPLL contains a nonossified area (**a**, arrowheads). (Reproduced from Yamazaki et al. [14])

bral levels where OPLL exits in the cervical spine. Axial classification comprises central and lateral lesions identified on axial CT images [15].

14.4.2 The Extent of OPLL in the Whole Spine

We evaluated the prevalence and distribution of OPLL using CT images of the whole spine to analyze what factors predict the presence of ossified lesions in the thoracolumbar spine in patients who were diagnosed with cervical OPLL using plain X-ray images. The extent of OPLL in the whole spine is significantly associated with the extent of cervical OPLL, female sex, and obesity [16].

14.4.3 Ossification of the Supra/Interspinous Ligaments

The prevalence and distribution of ossification of the supra/interspinous ligaments (OSIL) was analyzed in symptomatic patients with cervical OPLL. We found a significant positive correlation between the sum of the levels involving OPLL (OP-index) and that by OSI (OSI-index) [17].

14.4.4 Distribution of OPLL

We evaluated the distribution of ossified spinal lesions in patients with severe OPLL and prediction of ossification at each segment based on the cervical OP index classification. Thoracolumbar OPLL occurred most often at the level of T1 in men and at T3–4 in women. In case of severe OPLL, although ossified lesions were frequently seen at the intervertebral and vertebral levels around the cervicothoracic and thoracolumbar junctions in men, OPLL was observed more diffusely in the thoracic spine in women [18].

14.4.5 Diffuse Idiopathic Skeletal Hyperostosis

The prevalence and distribution of diffuse idiopathic skeletal hyperostosis (DISH) was analyzed using whole-spine CT of patients with cervical OPLL. DISH was present in nearly half of the patients with cervical OPLL and more common in older patients. DISH developed at the thoracic level and progressed into the cervical or lumbar spine with age [19].

14.4.6 Ossification of the Nuchal Ligament

We determined the coexistence of ossification of the nuchal ligament (ONL) associated with the severity of ossification in the whole spine in patients with cervical OPLL. Coexistence of ONL in patients with cervical OPLL was associated with the severity of spinal hyperostosis, especially in those with cervical OPLL and ossification of anterior longitudinal ligament (OALL), and thoracolumbar OALL and OSIL [20].

14.5 Conclusion

In most cases of cervical OPLL and thoracic OPLL/OLF, not only static compression, but also dynamic factors contributed to the development and aggravation of the myelopathy. The rationale for PDF surgery is to suppress motion at the non-ossified segment of OPLL by stabilization. The K-line is a simple and practical parameter with utility in decisions regarding surgical approach to cervical OPLL.

References

1. Tsuyama N. Ossification of the posterior longitudinal ligament of the spine. Clin Orthop Relat Res. 1984;184:71–84.
2. Masaki Y, Yamazaki M, Okawa A, Aramomi M, Hashimoto M, et al. An analysis of factors causing poor surgical outcome in patients with cervical myelopathy due to ossification of the posterior longitudinal ligament: anterior decompression with spinal fusion versus laminoplasty. J Spinal Disord Tech. 2007;20(1):7–13.
3. Fujiyoshi T, Yamazaki M, Okawa A, Kawabe J, Hayashi K, Endo T, et al. Analysis of static versus dynamic factors for the development of myelopathy in patients with cervical ossification of the posterior longitudinal ligament. J Clin Neurosci. 2010;17:320–4.

4. Iwasaki M, Okuda S, Miyauchi A, Sakaura H, Mukai Y, Yonenobu K, et al. Surgical strategy for cervical myelopathy due to ossification of the posterior longitudinal ligament: part 1: clinical results and limitations of laminoplasty. Spine. 2007;32(6):647–53.
5. Yamazaki A, Homma T, Uchiyama S, Katsumi Y, Okumura H. Morphologic limitations of posterior decompression by midsagittal splitting method for myelopathy caused by ossification of the posterior longitudinal ligament in the cervical spine. Spine. 1999;24(1):32–3.
6. Fujiyoshi T, Yamazaki M, Kawabe J, Endo T, Furuya T, Koda M, et al. A new concept for making decisions regarding the surgical approach for cervical ossification of the posterior longitudinal ligament: the K-line. Spine. 2008;33(26):E990–3.
7. Koda M, Mochizuki M, Konishi H, Aiba A, Kadota R, Inada T, et al. Comparison of clinical outcomes between laminoplasty, posterior decompression with instrumented fusion, and anterior decompression with fusion for K-line (−) cervical ossification of the posterior longitudinal ligament. Eur Spine J. 2016;25:2294–301.
8. Saito J, Maki S, Kamiya K, Furuya T, Inada T, Ota M, et al. Outcome of posterior decompression with instrumented fusion surgery for K-line (−) cervical ossification of the longitudinal ligament. J Clin Neurosci. 2016;32:57–60.
9. Ijima Y, Furuya T, Ota M, Maki S, Saito J, Kitamura M, et al. The K-line in the cervical ossification of the posterior longitudinal ligament is different on plain radiographs and CT images. J Spine Surg. 2018;4(2):403–7.
10. Yamazaki M, Mochizuki M, Ikeda Y, Sodeyama T, Okawa A, Koda M, et al. Clinical results of surgery for thoracic myelopathy caused by ossification of the posterior longitudinal ligament: operative indication of posterior decompression with instrumented fusion. Spine. 2006;31(13):1452–60.
11. Yamazaki M, Okawa A, Fujiyoshi T, Furuya T, Koda M. Posterior decompression with instrumented fusion for thoracic myelopathy caused by ossification of the posterior longitudinal ligament. Eur Spine J. 2010;19:691–8.
12. Koda M, Furuya T, Okawa A, Inada T, Kamiya K, Ota M, et al. Mid- to long-term outcomes of posterior decompression with instrumented fusion for thoracic ossification of the posterior longitudinal ligament. J Clin Neurosci. 2016;27:87–90.
13. Koda M, Furuya T, Okawa A, Aramomi M, Inada T, Kamiya K, et al. Bone union and remodelling of the non-ossified segment in thoracic ossification of the posterior longitudinal ligament after posterior decompression and fusion surgery. Eur Spine J. 2015;24(11):2555–9.
14. Yamazaki M, Okawa A, Mannoji C, Fujiyoshi T, Furuya T, Koda M. Postoperative paralysis after posterior decompression with instrumented fusion for thoracic myelopathy due to ossification of the posterior longitudinal ligament. J Clin Neurosci. 2011;18(2):294–6.
15. Kawaguchi Y, Matsumoto M, Iwasaki M, Izumi T, Okawa A, Matsunaga S, et al. New classification system for ossification of the posterior longitudinal ligament using CT images. J Orthop Sci. 2014;19(4):530–6.
16. Hirai T, Yoshii T, Iwanami A, Takeuchi K, Mori K, Yamada T, et al. Prevalence and distribution of ossified lesions in the whole spine of patients with cervical ossification of the posterior longitudinal ligament: a multicenter study (JOSL CT study). PLoS One. 2016;11(8):e0160117.
17. Mori K, Yoshii T, Hirai T, Iwanami A, Takeuchi K, Yamada T, et al. Prevalence and distribution of ossification of the supra/interspinous ligaments in symptomatic patients with cervical ossification of the posterior longitudinal ligament of the spine: a CT-based multicenter cross-sectional study. BMC Musculoskelet Disord. 2016;17(1):492.
18. Hirai T, Yoshii T, Nagoshi N, Takeuchi K, Mori K, Ushio S, et al. Distribution of ossified spinal lesions in patients with severe ossification of the posterior longitudinal ligament and prediction of ossification at each segment based on the cervical OP index classification: a multicenter study (JOSL CT study). BMC Musculoskelet Disord. 2018;19(1):107.
19. Nishimura S, Nagoshi N, Iwanami A, Takeuchi A, Hirai T, Yoshii T, et al. Japanese organization of the study for ossification of spinal ligament (JOSL). Prevalence and distribution of diffuse idiopathic skeletal hyperostosis on whole-spine computed tomography in patients with cervical ossification of the posterior longitudinal ligament: a multicenter study. Clin Spine Surg. 2018;31(9):E460–5.
20. Yoshii T, Hirai T, Iwanami A, Nagoshi N, Takeuchi K, Mori K, et al. Co-existence of ossification of the nuchal ligament is associated with severity of ossification in the whole spine in patients with cervical ossification of the posterior longitudinal ligament—a multi-center CT study. J Orthop Sci. 2019;24(1):35–41.

Clinical Manifestation of Cervical OPLL

15

Hiroshi Ozawa

Abstract

The clinical symptoms and signs caused by cervical ossification of the posterior longitudinal ligament (OPLL) are divided into three categories: (1) cervical myelopathy or spinal cord injury with motor and sensory disturbance of the upper and lower limbs, spasticity, and bladder dysfunction; (2) cervical radiculopathy with pain and motor and sensory disturbance of the upper limb; and (3) axial discomfort with pain and stiffness around the neck. Occasionally, an acute spinal cord injury occurs after a minor trauma due to the narrow spinal canal caused by massive OPLL.

Keywords

Ossification of the posterior longitudinal ligament · Cervical spine · Myelopathy Radiculopathy · Neck pain · Spinal cord injury

15.1 Introduction

Ossification of the posterior longitudinal ligament (OPLL) of the spine can be radiographically identified at any level of the whole spine, including the cervical, thoracic, and lumbar regions; the cervical region has the most frequent occurrences. In cases wherein cervical OPLL is identified by radiography, the syndrome may range from asymptomatic to severe paralysis. The clinical entity of cervical OPLL is defined as patients with neurological complaints or deficits or with annoying discomfort around the neck originating from compressed or entrapped neural tissues due to OPLL of the cervical spine.

OPLL is one of the essential factors associated with stenosis of the cervical spinal canal, which causes the spinal cord and nerve roots to be entrapped or compressed. On the basis of the varied shape and volume of OPLL, the clinical symptoms differ among individuals. The clinical symptoms and syndromes caused by cervical OPLL are divided into (1) cervical myelopathy or spinal cord injury with motor and sensory disturbance of the upper and lower limbs, spasticity, and bladder dysfunction; (2) cervical radiculopathy with pain and motor and sensory disturbance of the upper limb; and (3) discomfort with pain and stiffness around the neck. Usually, a combination of these symptoms in varying degrees is observed.

15.1.1 Age and Gender

On the basis of a large cohort study for age groups [1], the occurrence of cervical OPLL evaluated by lateral radiograms was 2.2% in the age group

H. Ozawa (✉)
Department of Orthopaedic Surgery, Tohoku Medical and Pharmaceutical University, Sendai, Japan
e-mail: hozawa@tohoku-mpu.ac.jp

A. Okawa et al. (eds.), *OPLL*, https://doi.org/10.1007/978-981-15-3855-1_15

of 50s, 1.9% in the 60s, 2.1% in the 70s, and 1.3% in the 80s. There was no significant difference in the occurrence of OPLL between the age groups. The occurrence of OPLL was significantly higher in males (3.2%) than in females (1.3%, $p < 0.05$).

15.1.2 Lifestyle and OPLL

No specific occupation has been reported to result in more prevalent OPLL. Regarding sleep, 6–8 h of moderate sleep was found to be correlated with a reduced incidence of OPLL compared with <5 or >9 h of sleep. There was no clear correlation between the incidence of OPLL and exercise, smoking, and alcohol consumption [2]. Patients with OPLL tended to be taller and heavier than those without OPLL ($p < 0.05$). Furthermore, the plasma pentosidine levels and bone mineral density values for both the lumbar spine (L2–4) and the femoral neck ($p < 0.05$) were higher in patients with OPLL than in those without OPLL [1].

15.1.3 Clinical Features

The clinical presentation depends on the size of OPLL, diameter of the spinal canal, and range of motion of the spine. Some patients have no symptoms although radiography indicates massive OPLL.

In general, the clinical symptoms and syndromes caused by cervical OPLL are divided into (1) cervical myelopathy or spinal cord injury with motor and sensory disturbance of the upper and lower limbs, spasticity, and bladder dysfunction; (2) cervical radiculopathy with pain and motor and sensory disturbance of the upper limb; and (3) discomfort with pain and stiffness around the neck. The most common complaint at the onset is paresthesia or numbness in the upper limb, followed by neck and nuchal pain or discomfort [3] (Table 15.1). Myelopathy is a common syndrome [4] (Table 15.2), and its onset is usually gradual; however, some studies have reported trauma-induced myelopathy.

Table 15.1 Initial symptoms at the onset of OPLL and their frequency

Symptom	Frequency (%)
Pain/numbness of the upper limb	48
Neck and nuchal pain/stiffness	42
Pain/numbness of the lower limb	19

Table 15.2 Frequency of syndromes caused by cervical OPLL

Syndrome	Frequency (%)
Myelopathy	45
Neck and nuchal pain/stiffness	25
Radiculopathy	7
Combined	43

15.1.4 Myelopathy

Cervical myelopathy is an essential syndrome associated with OPLL because OPLL compresses the spinal cord under the narrow spinal canal, and the compressed spinal cord produces severe disturbance in the activities of daily living. In general, myelopathy due to OPLL follows this course. Over a period of months, patients may notice a peculiar sensation in the hands that is associated with clumsiness and weakness. The lower limbs may precede or follow the arms in terms of development of these symptoms. Patients typically have difficulty in walking with fairly symmetrical leg weakness. Wasting and atrophy of the upper extremities (mostly to a slight degree) according to the severity of OPLL also occur. At the time of the first visit to the hospital, a clinical examination usually indicates a lack of dexterity in the hands and spastic involvement of the lower extremities.

A precise neurological diagnosis of myelopathy due to OPLL is critical. To determine the symptoms of OPLL, the spinal level of initiation and maximum symptoms should be evaluated. The segmental sign caused by the disturbance of gray matter needs must also be examined. The long tract sign, with an increase in deep tendon reflexes, the frequent presence of Hoffmann's sign, and sensory changes in the limbs caused by disturbance of the pyramidal, anterior spinothalamic, and posterior column are also examined. Myelopathy can be diagnosed by the presence of both the segmental and long tract signs. Finally, the functional motor, sensory, and bladder status are evaluated using the Japanese Orthopaedic Association scoring system for cervical myelopathy. Neurological findings are occasionally complicated because patients with cervical OPLL often have associated thoracic OPLL or ossification of the ligamentum flavum at the level of the thoracic or lumbar spine.

Myelopathy is frequently induced by an accident such as a fall. Presence of spinal stenosis due to OPLL can easily induce damage to the fragile spinal cord. The occurrence and increase of symptoms are largely based on spinal canal stenosis caused by OPLL acting as a static compressive force. Intervertebral motion also contributes to dynamic stress to the spinal cord although the intervertebral motion is limited. The cause of deterioration varies among individuals, and the progression is often slow. Occasionally, the progression is rapid or acute, similar to that of acute spinal cord injury (SCI) after a minor accident such as a fall or a forceful extension injury of the cervical spine. It has been reported that 23% of patients experience a previous mild trauma to the neck, which in most cases produces symptoms directly after the trauma [5].

15.1.5 Radiculopathy

Discomfort and pain in the affected side of the scapular area, arm, and hand with or without associated motor weakness may be a symptom of cervical radiculopathy due to OPLL. Similar to that in cases of cervical spondylotic radiculopathy, radicular pain and numbness caused by OPLL are sometimes severe and are correlated with the level of cervical nerve root involvement.

15.1.6 Pain and Stiffness

Patients with OPLL often complain about dull neck pain and stiff neck. This discomfort is experienced in the middle of the neck and subsequently spreads to the suboccipital region or across the shoulders where the suffering sensation may appear to emanate from the levator scapulae muscles. This type of discomfort is mostly vague. The pain, whose source remains unclear, might be stimulated by the formation and growth of ossification either to the sinuvertebral nerve spreading in the longitudinal ligament or to the constricted nerve root in the spinal canal. Although annoying pain usually does not occur according to neck motion, the neck motion is often limited or severely stiff, especially in lateral bending, depending on the longitudinal volume of OPLL, which restricts intervertebral motion.

Takeshita et al. [6] have investigated the occurrence and severity of pain in 184 patients with OPLL in comparison with 122 patients with cervical spondylotic myelopathy (CSM) and 44 healthy volunteers. Approximately 10% of patients with OPLL and CSM reported pain with severe disabilities. Additionally, patients with OPLL had relatively lower cervical function and higher psychological stress. The duration of symptoms, severity of spinal cord damage, and stiffness of the trunk were correlated with pain or numbness in patients with OPLL as well as in patients with CSM.

Regarding the relationship between OPLL and neuropathic pain [7], the numerical rating scale (NRS) showed that patients with cervical OPLL had an average pain NRS score of 4.3 ± 2.7 and a numbness NRS score of 4.6 ± 2.8. A pain NRS score of ≥ 5 was reported in 48.8% of the patients, and a numbness NRS score of ≥ 5 was reported in 52.3% of the patients. According to the pain DETECT test (i.e., a neuropathic pain screening questionnaire), approximately 60% of the patients presented with neuropathic pain or suspected pain.

15.1.7 Natural Course

The formation and growth of OPLL are considered to be slow; therefore, OPLL is not always symptomatic. OPLL is occasionally identified with the absence of any symptoms during routine medical checkups. When asymptomatic OPLL is identified by radiography, the ossification is considered to be a radiological finding of the spine similar to a degenerative spinal change. In patients without myelopathy at the initial examination who frequently complained neck stiffness and limited neck motion, the life prognosis and ability to manage activities of daily living without an attendant were satisfactory in 91% of the patients at 13 years of follow-up [8].

A long-term follow-up of 109 asymptomatic patients with OPLL was reported by Matsunaga et al. [9]. All the patients were followed up for at least 5 years with a mean follow-up period of 11.3 years. Only 24.8% of the patients without myelopathy at the first examination developed myelopathy during the follow-up period. In 22% of the patients with myelopathy onset, myelopathy was induced after a minor accident such as a fall from the stairs or a whiplash injury of the cervical spine. In trauma-induced myelopathy, the types of OPLL include mixed and segmental types in the plain radiograph classification. The myelopathy-free rate was shown by the Kaplan–Meier method (Fig. 15.1). All the patients with >60% spinal canal stenosis in the plain radiograph developed myelopathy within 15 years of follow-up, whereas the myelopathy-free rate of patients with <60% spinal canal stenosis was 66% at the maximum follow-up period of 26 years.

15.1.8 SCI and OPLL

The clinical syndrome of cervical OPLL mostly develops insidiously, and the time of onset is usually unclear. However, an acute SCI occasionally occurs in cases of accidental falls or a hyperextension force to the neck in patients with cervical OPLL.

The prevalence of OPLL among cervical SCI was relatively high, especially in those without bone injury. Most cervical SCIs associated with OPLL were incomplete and predominantly caused by low-energy trauma. Therefore, bone injuries such as fracture and dislocation were rarely observed. The majority of patients were unaware of OPLL (Fig. 15.2).

OPLL and the subsequent cervical stenosis can predispose to SCI following minor trauma. Chikuda et al. [10] have reported that among 453 patients with acute traumatic cervical SCI, OPLL was found in 106 (23%) patients. In a series of 106 patients with SCI accompanied by OPLL, 88.7% (94/106) had a central cord syndrome and did not have a concurrent fracture. The average age was 66 years, and the most common cause was a fall (74%). Only 25% of the patients were previously aware that they had OPLL. Koyanagi

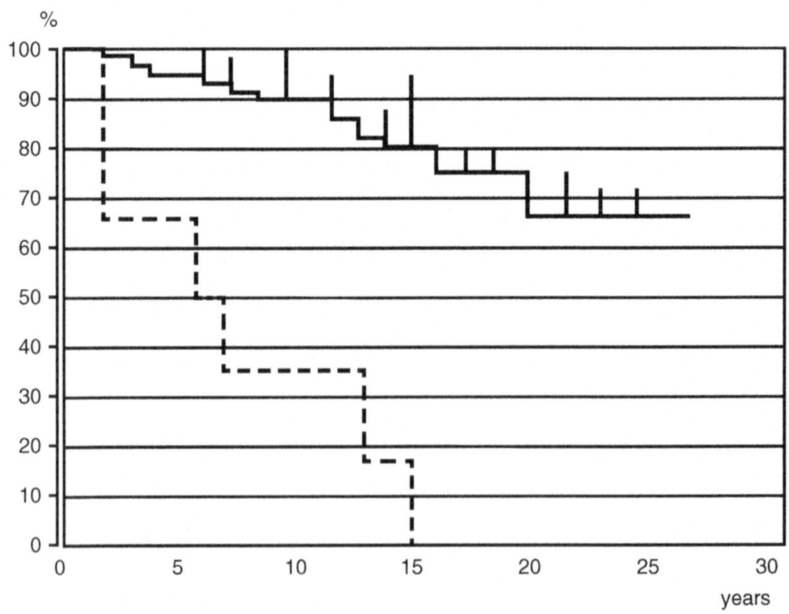

Fig. 15.1 Myelopathy-free rate of asymptomatic subjects with OPLL by the Kaplan–Meier method. The bold line indicates the data of subjects with <60% spinal canal stenosis. The dotted line indicates the data of subjects with >60% spinal canal stenosis

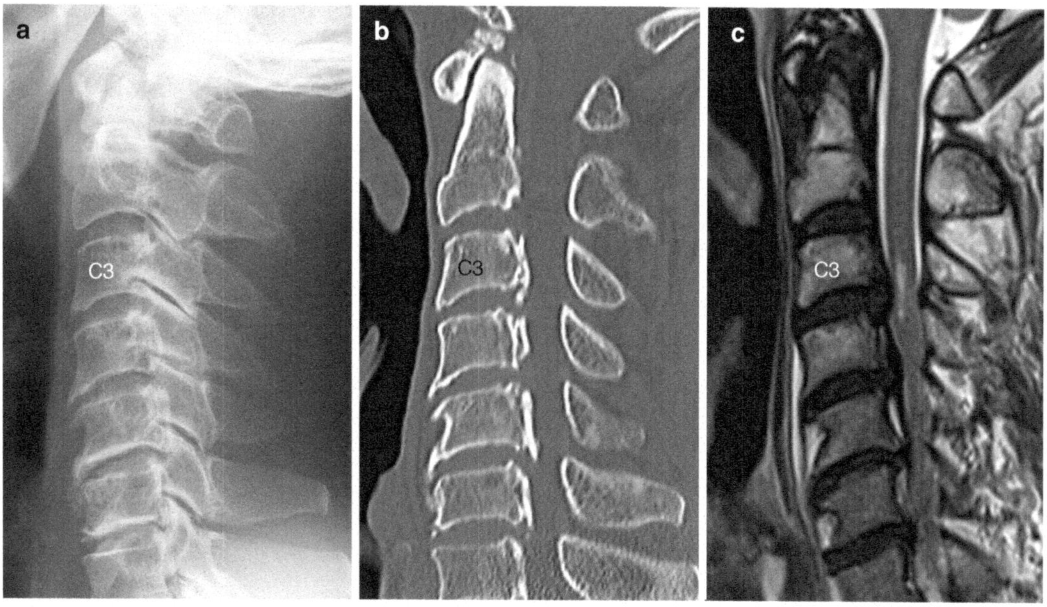

Fig. 15.2 Lateral plain radiograph (**a**) and sagittal reconstruction CT image (**b**) showing segmental type OPLL between C2 and C7. Sagittal T2WI MRI image (**c**) showing intramedullary high signal area indicating cervical cord injury at C3/4 intervertebral disc level

et al. [11] have reported that in 28 patients with OPLL and cervical SCI, the average age was 63 years and 61% of OPLL and cervical SCI were caused due to a ground-level fall. Overall, 8 patients had a continuous type of OPLL, 6 had a mixed type, and 14 had a segmental type. The authors noted that in the group with continuous OPLL, SCI occurred at the caudal end of the OPLL analogous to an ankylosed spine. In the segmental type OPLL group, SCI occurred most commonly at the intervertebral disc level. With segmental OPLL, a hyperextension mechanism can cause compression of the spinal cord and subsequent SCI.

15.2 Conclusions

The radiological findings of OPLL at the cervical spine are not rare and are not always correlated with clinical severity. The clinical entity of cervical OPLL is defined as patients with neurological complaints or deficits originating from compressed or entrapped neural tissues caused by OPLL of the cervical spine. Furthermore, patients with OPLL often complain of discomfort with pain and stiffness around the neck. The onset of symptoms is insidious, and myelopathy mostly progresses slowly. Occasionally, an acute spinal cord lesion occurs after a minor trauma due to the narrow spinal canal caused by massive OPLL.

References

1. Yoshimura N, Nagata K, Muraki S, Oka H, Yoshida M, Enyo Y, Kagotani R, Hashizume H, Yamada H, Ishimoto Y, Teraguchi M, Tanaka S, Kawaguchi H, Toyama Y, Nakamura K, Akune T. Prevalence and progression of radiographic ossification of the posterior longitudinal ligament and associated factors in the Japanese population: a 3-year follow-up of the ROAD study. Osteoporos Int. 2014;25:1089–98.
2. Washio M, Kobashi G, Okamoto K, Sasaki S, Yokoyama T, Miyake Y, Sakamoto N, Ohta K, Inaba Y, Tanaka H. Sleeping habit and other life styles in the prime of life and risk for ossification of the posterior longitudinal ligament of the spine (OPLL): a case-control study in Japan. J Epidemiol. 2004;14:168–73.
3. Terayama K, Kurokawa K, Seki H. Report on the ossification of the spinal ligaments. In: Terayama K, editor. Investigation Committee report on the ossification of the spinal ligaments of Japanese Ministry of Public

Health and Welfare, Tokyo; 1976. p. 8–33 [article in Japanese].
4. Kawai S. Clinical manifestation of cervical ossification of the posterior longitudinal ligaments. In: Yonenobu K, Sakou T, Ono K, editors. OPLL: ossification of posterior longitudinal ligament. Tokyo: Springer; 1997. p. 81–4.
5. Matsunaga S, Sakou T. Ossification of the posterior longitudinal ligament of the cervical spine: etiology and natural history. Spine. 2012;37:E309–14.
6. Takeshita K, Fujiwara N, Nakamura K. Pain and numbness in patients with ossification of the posterior longitudinal ligament of the spine. J Musculoskelet Pain Res. 2010;2:48–53 [article in Japanese].
7. Takeshita K. The ossification of the posterior longitudinal ligament and neuropathic pain. Spine Spinal Cord. 2013;26:175–80 [article in Japanese].
8. Matsunaga S, Sakou T, Arishima Y, Koga H, Hayashi K, Komiya S. Quality of life in elderly patients with ossification of the posterior longitudinal ligament. Spine. 2001;26:494–8.
9. Matsunaga S, Tsuji T, Toyama Y, Ijiri K, Komiya S, Numasawa T, Toh S, Ichimura S, Satomi K, Seichi A, Hoshino Y, Takeshita K, Nakamura K, Endo K, Yamamoto K, Kato Y, Kato T, Shinomiya K, Tokuhashi Y, Kawaguchi Y, Kimura T, Matsuyama Y, Ishiguro N, Neo M, Nakamura T, Fujimori T, Iwasaki M, Yoshikawa H, Taniguchi S, Tani T, Kato Y, Taguchi T, Sato K, Nagata K. Risk factors for development of myelopathy in patients with asymptomatic ossification of the posterior longitudinal ligament. J Spine Res. 2013;4:116–22.
10. Chikuda H, Seichi A, Takeshita K, Matsunaga S, Watanabe M, Nakagawa Y, Oshima K, Sasao Y, Tokuhashi Y, Nakahara S, Endo K, Uchida K, Takahata M, Yokoyama T, Yamada K, Nohara Y, Imagama S, Hosoe H, Ohtsu H, Kawaguchi H, Toyama Y, Nakamura K. Acute cervical spinal cord injury complicated by preexisting ossification of the posterior longitudinal ligament: a multicenter study. Spine. 2011;36:1453–8.
11. Koyanagi I, Iwasaki Y, Hida K, Imamura H, Fujimoto S, Akino M. Acute cervical cord injury associated with ossification of the posterior longitudinal ligament. Neurosurgery. 2003;53:887–91; discussion 891–2.

Three-Dimensional Imaging of Cervical Ossification of the Posterior Longitudinal Ligament

16

Keiichi Katsumi, Toru Hirano, Kei Watanabe, Tomohiro Izumi, Masayuki Ohashi, Tatsuki Mizouchi, and Naoto Endo

Abstract

On the basis of a three-dimensional (3D) image analysis method for cervical ossification of the posterior longitudinal ligament (OPLL) and analysis of the progression of ossified lesions with this method, the mean annual rate of lesion increase in non-surgically treated patients ($n = 41$) was 4.1%/year. Risk factors for OPLL progression are younger age and obesity; younger age is the most important predictor. These findings reflect the natural course of OPLL, which is important in the clinical management of patients with the aforementioned risk factors.

Furthermore, we evaluated whether laminoplasty with instrumented fusion further suppresses the progression of OPLL compared with stand-alone laminoplasty using novel 3D analysis. A comparison of patients treated with posterior decompression and fusion (PDF) (the PDF group, $n = 19$) and laminoplasty (LP) alone (the LP group, $n = 22$) showed that the mean annual rate of lesion increase was 2.0%/year in the PDF group, which was significantly lower than the rate of 7.5%/year in the LP group. Notably, the mean annual rate of increase was gradually decreasing over time in the PDF group. This is the first study to prove a possible suppressant effect of posterior instrumented fusion on OPLL progression.

Keywords

Ossification of the posterior longitudinal ligament · Progression · Three-dimensional analysis · Volume · Risk factors

K. Katsumi (✉)
Department of Orthopedic Surgery, Niigata University Medical and Dental General Hospital, Niigata, Japan

Spine Center, Department of Orthopedic Surgery, Niigata Central Hospital, Niigata, Japan

T. Hirano
Department of Orthopedic Surgery, Uonuma Institute of Community Medicine, Niigata University Medical and Dental Hospital, Minami-uonuma City, Niigata, Japan
e-mail: thirano@med.niigata-u.ac.jp

K. Watanabe · M. Ohashi · T. Mizouchi · N. Endo
Department of Orthopedic Surgery, Niigata University Medical and Dental General Hospital, Niigata, Japan
e-mail: keiwatanabe_39jp@live.jp; masayuki-ohashi@ksh.biglobe.ne.jp; endless@med.niigata-u.ac.jp

T. Izumi
Department of Orthopedic Surgery, Niigata Minami Hospital, Niigata, Japan
e-mail: t_izm@pop01.odn.ne.jp

A. Okawa et al. (eds.), *OPLL*, https://doi.org/10.1007/978-981-15-3855-1_16

16.1 Introduction

Cervical ossification of the posterior longitudinal ligament (OPLL) is a progressive disease resulting in a narrowed spinal canal. Knowledge on the natural course of OPLL and especially the risk factors of OPLL progression is important for the careful observation of this disease or for an indication for surgical treatment. Several studies demonstrated that approximately more than 60% of patients showed radiographic evidence of OPLL progression [1–6], and the rate of progression was significantly greater in patients undergoing surgery than those treated conservatively [3, 5, 7, 8]. The risk factors of OPLL progression are younger age at surgery, continuous or mixed type of OPLL, higher Japanese Orthopedic Association score [9] at the last follow-up, and wide anteroposterior width of the space available for the spinal cord (SAC) [1–6]. In particular, several studies indicated that younger age was the most significant risk factor for OPLL progression [1–4]; however, some reports have found no correlation between age and OPLL progression [8, 10]. Thus, consensus has not been reached on many proposed risk factors for progression. One of the reasons for this is that several previous reports measured ossified lesions using manual or computerized measurement systems based on lateral X-ray images [1–5, 8, 9]. These measurements mainly evaluated the progression in the craniocaudal direction (length), making it difficult to evaluate the caudal progression (due to the interference of the shoulders) and to evaluate the progression in the anteroposterior direction (width). Although there are recent reports that measure the length and width of the ossified lesions using bone computed tomography (CT) [11, 12], these are based on two-dimensional analyses such as length and width, which cannot evaluate three-dimensional (3D) images and the volume of the ossified lesion. Therefore, to date, the 3D structure of the ossified lesions has not been accurately evaluated.

16.2 Three-Dimensional Image Analysis

Our coauthors Izumi et al. [13] developed a 3D image analysis method for cervical OPLL using the Mimics® software (Materialise Japan Co., Ltd., Yokohama, Japan), which observes the detailed morphology of the ossified lesions and the quantitative evaluation of their volume. The following were the detailed steps in this method: The first step was to identify the affected vertebra and ossification based on the DICOM data for CT images using the Mimics® software. In the second step, the ossification was detached from the posterior aspect of the vertebral body using both axial and sagittal slice images. In the third step, the region of ossification was isolated, and a 3D model was created. In the last step, the ossification volume was calculated, based on the 3D model (Fig. 16.1) [13]. The novel method described here appears to be useful for the quantitative evaluation of OPLL with only minimal measurement error (Fig. 16.2). The results of our study using 3D image analysis are shown below.

16.2.1 Natural Course of Ossified Volume Progression Using 3D Analysis in Non-Surgically Treated Patients with Cervical OPLL: Risk Factors for the Progression of Ossification Are Younger Age and Obesity [14]

There have been no reports regarding the risk factors for OPLL volume progression in non-surgically treated patients based on 3D image analysis. We investigated the natural course of OPLL and the risk factors for volume progression using 3D image analysis.

A total of 41 OPLL patients (22 males, 19 females; mean age, 61.8 years; range, 35–80 years) who had been followed conservatively at the affiliated hospitals between 2006 and 2015

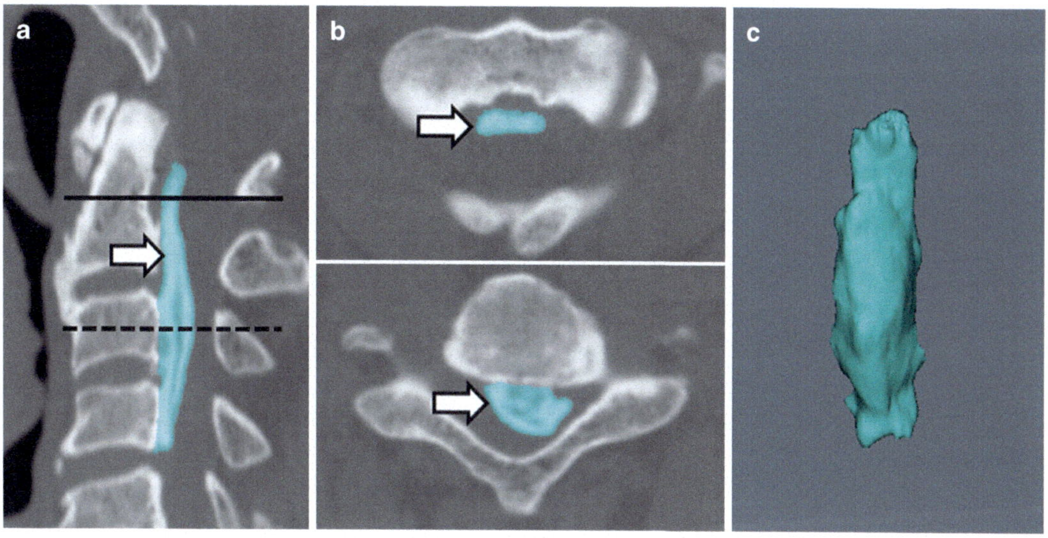

Fig. 16.1 (**a**, **b**) Ossification was detached from the affected vertebral body semi-automatically using computed tomography (CT) axial and sagittal planes (so-called segmentation). (**b**) Axial planes of CT at C2 (straight line) and C3 (dotted line). (**c**) The region of ossification was isolated, and a three-dimensional model was created (3854 mm^3)

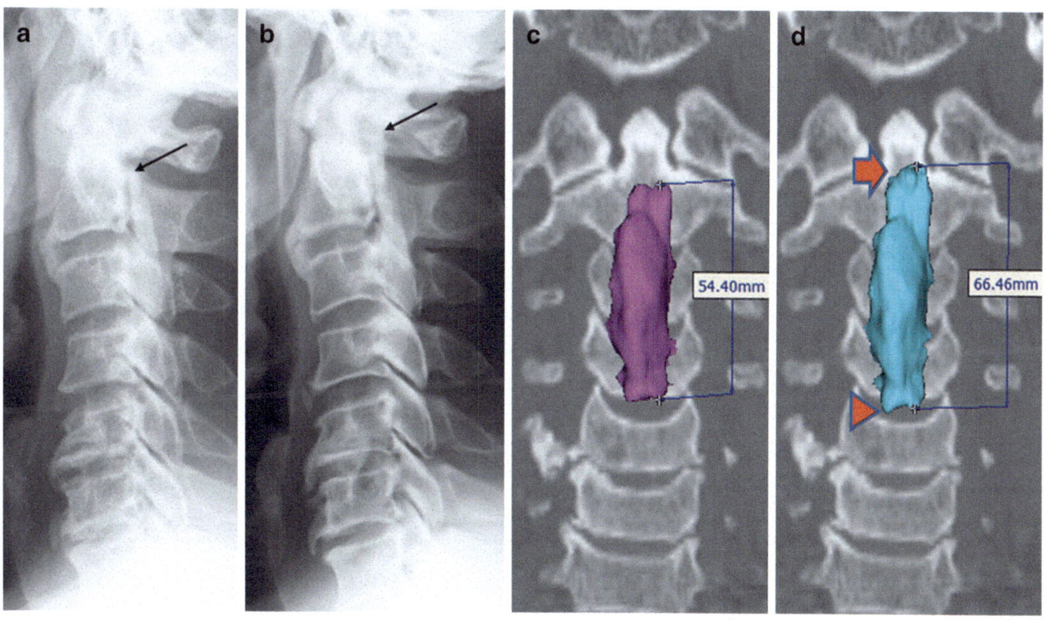

Fig. 16.2 (**a**) Plain radiography of a 62-year-old male with continuous ossification of the posterior longitudinal ligament (OPLL) at C2–C4. (**b**) Plain radiography at 3 years after initial examination revealed OPLL progression in the craniocaudal direction. The arrows indicate the edge of OPLL. (**c**) The length and volume of the ossified lesion were 54.4 mm and 3654.1 mm^3 according to the three-dimensional (3D) imaging analysis in the initial examination. (**d**) Three years later, OPLL had grown 12 mm in the craniocaudal direction, and the volume of the ossified lesion increased to 4092.7 mm^3. The annual rate of lesion increase was 4.0%. 3D imaging analysis revealed growth of not only the cranial part (arrow) but also the caudal part (arrowhead)

Table 16.1 Patient demographic data at initial measurement

Age at operation (years)	62 ± 9 (35–85)
Sex (male:female)	22:19
Follow-up period (months)	26 ± 17 (12–84)
Body height (cm)	160.7 ± 8.7 (145–180)
Body weight (kg)	63.6 ± 11.6 (43–87)
BMI (kg/m^2)	24.5 ± 3.3 (17.6–32.9)
Type of OPLL, number of patients	
Continuous	3
Segmental	5
Mixed	33
Circumscribed	
Occupation ratio of OPLL (%)	43.2 ± 12.5 (19.0–71.6)
Number of ossified vertebra	3.7 ± 1.4 (1–6)
Thickness of ossification (mm)	5.1 ± 1.6 (2.4–8.6)
Space available for the spinal cord (mm)	6.7 ± 1.7 (3.4–10.2)
C2–C7 angle (°)	11.2 ± 9.1 (-11–35)
C2–C7 ROM (°)	32.5 ± 9.9 (13–55)
JOA score (point)	15.6 ± 1.8 (11–17)

Mean ± standard deviation
JOA Japanese Orthopaedic Association

were included in the analysis (Table 16.1) [14]. We evaluated the clinical examination, radiological examination, and 3D measurements of the ossified lesion and performed risk factor analysis for OPLL progression.

16.2.1.1 Clinical Examinations

Patients' body height, body weight (BW), and body mass index (BMI) were recorded. Neurological severity was evaluated using the Japanese Orthopedic Association (JOA) score.

16.2.1.2 Radiological Examinations

The numbers of the ossified vertebrae, ossification thickness, and SAC were measured using CT. Spinal canal occupation rates were expressed as the percentage ratio of the maximum thickness of ossification to the midsagittal diameter of the canal using the CT axial view. The C2–C7 lordotic angle was measured between the lower endplates of C2 and C7 on lateral radiographs. Additionally, we evaluated the C2–C7 range of motion (ROM) based on flexion and extension radiographs.

16.2.1.3 Measurement of the Ossified Lesion

OPLL measurements were obtained twice with an interval of at least 1 year (initial examination and final examination). The ossified lesion volume was calculated twice during each examination to determine the mean volume and evaluate the intra-observer error. We evaluated the volume change of OPLL using the annual rate of lesion increase. The ossified increase rate (a) was measured from the ossified volume between the initial and final measurements. The annual rate of lesion increase (b) was calculated by dividing the increase rate by the interval from the initial to the final measurement.

(a) Increase rate (%) = (increased volume/initial volume) × 100
(b) Annual rate of lesion increase (%/year) = (increase rate/interval (months)) × 12

16.2.1.4 Statistical Analyses

Stepwise regression analysis was performed to identify variables independently associated with the annual rate of lesion increase as a dependent variable. First, the significance of the variable was evaluated using a univariate analysis. Next, variables with $p < 0.1$ were subjected to a multivariate analysis; $p < 0.05$ was considered statistically significant.

16.2.1.5 Results

The results demonstrated that the mean C2–C7 angle, C2–C7 ROM, and JOA score were 11.5 ± 10.5° (range, −6° to 39°), 30.0 ± 8.8° (range, 13–51°), and 15.5 ± 1.8 (range, 10–17) in the final examination, respectively. The C2–C7 ROM was significantly decreased from the initial to final examinations ($p < 0.05$). The mean ossification volume was 2047.4 ± 1437 mm^3 (range, 26–5704 mm^3) in the initial examination and 2201.0 ± 1524 mm^3 (range, 35–5935 mm^3) in the final examination, indicating a significant increase in ossification volume (153.6 mm^3, $p < 0.001$) over the course of 25 months. The mean increase rate of ossified lesion between the initial and final examinations was 8.8 ± 8.5% (range, 0.1–36.5%). The mean annual rate of lesion increase was 4.1 ± 2.7%/year (range, 0.1–10.8%/year).

The univariate regression analysis demonstrated significant relationships between the annual rate of lesion increase and age ($\beta = -0.48$, $p = 0.001$) (Fig. 16.3), BW ($\beta = 0.36$, $p = 0.02$), and BMI ($\beta = 0.35$, $p = 0.03$). Furthermore, age

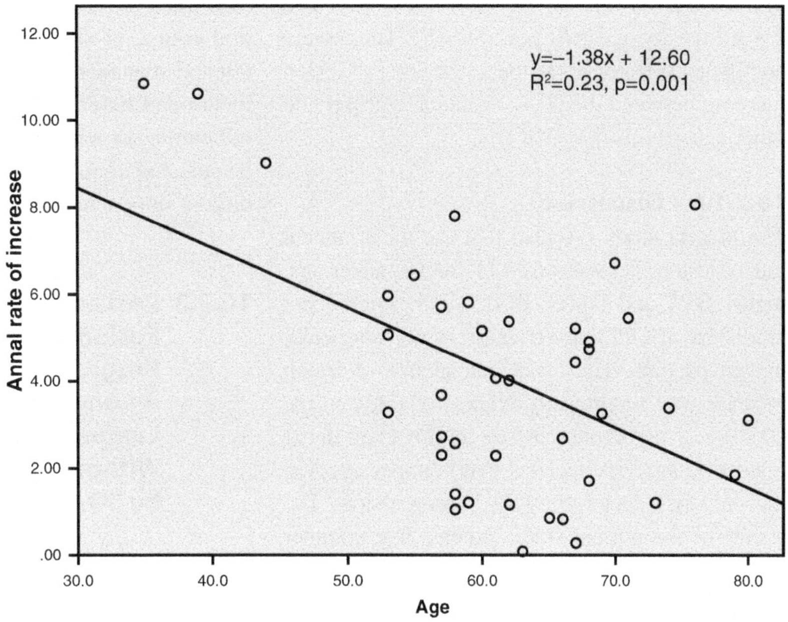

Fig. 16.3 Relationship between the annual rate of lesion increase and age. A significant negative correlation was found between the annual rate of lesion increase and age ($y = -1.38 \times +12.60$, $R^2 = 0.23$, $p = 0.001$)

Table 16.2 Linear regression analysis of risk factors for ossification of the posterior longitudinal ligament progression

	Annual rate of lesion increase				
	Univariate linear regression		Multivariate linear regression		
Characteristics	β	p Value	β	p Value	$R^2 = 0.23$
Age	−0.48	0.001**	−0.48	0.001**	
Body height	0.11	0.48			
Body weight	0.36	0.02*	0.21	0.17	
Body mass index	0.35	0.03*	0.21	0.17	
Spinal canal occupation rate	−0.07	0.66			
Thickness of ossification	−0.03	0.85			
Space available for the spinal cord	0.10	0.52			
JOA score (initial)	0.07	0.68			
JOA score (final)	0.04	0.82			
C2–C7 angle (initial)	−0.30	0.05	−0.25	0.08	
C2–C7 angle (final)	−0.31	0.05	−0.18	0.24	
C2–C7 ROM (initial)	0.27	0.09	0.14	0.35	
C2–C7 ROM (final)	0.18	0.27			
Ossification volume (initial)	−0.12	0.45			

The multivariate model includes variables with $p < 0.1$ according to univariate analysis

β standardized partial regression coefficient, R^2 coefficient of determination, *JOA* Japanese Orthopaedic Association

*$p < 0.05$

**$p < 0.01$

was the only significant predictor of OPLL progression ($R^2 = 0.23$; $p = 0.001$) in the multivariate liner regression analysis (Table 16.2).

The mean annual rate of lesion increase was 10.2 ± 1.0% by age 30–49 years ($n = 3$), 3.9 ± 2.2% by age 50–59 years ($n = 14$), 3.0 ± 1.9% by age 60–69 years ($n = 17$), and 4.3 ± 2.6% by age ≥70 years ($n = 7$). There were significant differences in the annual rate of lesion increase between the 30–49 years age group and other age groups ($p < 0.05$).

16.2.1.6 Discussion

The present study revealed that the mean annual rate of lesion increase was 4.1% and younger age, higher BW, and higher BMI are the significant predictors of OPLL progression in non-surgically treated patients. The mean annual rate of lesion increase was significantly higher for those in the 30–49-year age group, and the multivariate linear regression analysis revealed that younger age was the only risk factor for OPLL progression. The results of the present study indicate that younger age is the best predictor of OPLL progression and reflect the natural course of OPLL. Therefore, we consider the natural course of non-surgically treated OPLL as follows: (1) The volume of OPLL increases rapidly in ages 30–49 years and (2) OPLL progression decelerates after the age of 50 years, and the aging process tends to slow the OPLL progression throughout the lifetime. The following are some of the reasons why younger patients have an increased risk of OPLL progression: high bioactivity, large biomechanical stress such as wider ROM, and increased load of the cervical spine [11].

In this study, obesity (BW and BMI) is the significant predictor of OPLL progression in a univariate linear regression analysis. Previous reports revealed a significant relationship between obesity, glucose intolerance, and presence of OPLL [6, 15, 16]. It is well known that obesity causes insulin resistance and glucose intolerance, and insulin is thought to be an osteogenic factor of bone anabolism [17]. Akune et al. [15] reported that the upregulation of insulin production due to the impairment of insulin action may stimulate osteoprogenitor cells to induce ossification. These metabolism-related factors could affect the presence and volume progression of OPLL.

The present study revealed that younger age, higher BW, and higher BMI are the significant predictors of OPLL progression in non-surgically treated patients; younger age is the most important predictor. Moreover, the annual rate of OPLL progression tends to gradually decrease in patients older than 50 years. These findings reflect the natural course of OPLL, which is important in the clinical management of patients with the aforementioned risk factors. Furthermore, in terms of indication for surgery, proper procedures should be selected considering the natural course of the disease in patients with these risk factors.

16.2.2 Posterior Instrumented Fusion Suppresses the Progression of Cervical OPLL: A Comparison of Laminoplasty with and Without Instrumented Fusion by 3D Analysis [18]

The hypothesis that spinal fusion suppresses the progression of OPLL was based on previous reports [3, 6]; however, there have been no reports that describe any definitive evidence on the matter. This study aimed to evaluate whether laminoplasty with instrumented fusion suppresses the progression of OPLL compared to stand-alone laminoplasty using novel 3D analysis.

The present study comprised a group of 19 patients (14 males, 5 females) with OPLL treated with posterior decompression and fusion (PDF) (the PDF group) and a group of 22 patients (14 males, 8 females) treated with laminoplasty (LP) alone (the LP group) (Table 16.3) [18]. There were no significant differences except the preoperative C2–C7 angle between the two groups (Table 16.3). The volume change of OPLL was compared between the two groups.

16.2.2.1 Measurement of the Ossified Lesion

OPLL measurements were obtained three times with an interval of at least 1 year (1st measurement, 2nd measurement, and 3rd measurement). The 1st measurement was performed before surgery, and both the 2nd and 3rd measurements

Table 16.3 Demographic characteristics of the PDF and LP groups before surgery

	PDF group (n = 19)	LP group (n = 22)
Age at operation (years)	61 ± 9 (49–85)	59 ± 12 (39–77)
Sex (male:female)	14:5	14:8
Follow-up period (months)	51 ± 21 (17–103)	52 ± 19 (24–103)
Type of OPLL, number of patients		
Continuous	1	
Segmental	3	6
Mixed	15	16
Circumscribed		
Occupation ratio of OPLL (%)	51.5 ± 10.5 (34.3–77.8)	45.7 ± 13.3 (20.6–65.6)
Number of ossified vertebra	3.6 ± 1.4 (1–6)	3.8 ± 1.4 (1–6)
Number of opened lamina	4.1 ± 1.0 (2–6)	4.2 ± 1.1 (2–6)
C2–C7 lordotic angle (°)	−1.8 ± 16.9 (−45 to 30)	10.5 ± 8.7 (−3 to 26)
JOA score (point)	10.8 ± 3.8 (2–17)	10.5 ± 2.7 (5–15)

PDF posterior decompression and fusion, *LP* laminoplasty, *OPLL* ossification of the posterior longitudinal ligament, *JOA* Japanese Orthopaedic Association

were performed after surgery. Both the mean intervals from the 1st to the 2nd measurement and the 2nd to the 3rd measurement were not significantly different between the two groups.

16.2.2.2 Surgical Procedure

We have referred to the K-line to make decisions on the indication of additional instrumented fusion [19]. We have commonly performed laminoplasty for patients with K-line (+) OPLL and performed laminoplasty concomitant with posterior instrumented fusion for patients with K-line (−). As a basic principle, laminoplasty with instrumented fusion was performed using pedicle screws at the uppermost and lowermost instrumented levels, and lateral mass screws were used at the other levels, and the mean number of fixation levels was 4.5 ± 0.9 vertebrae (range, 2–5).

16.2.2.3 Results

The results demonstrated that the mean ossified volume in the PDF group was 2363 ± 1823 mm^3 (range, 292–6684 mm^3) at the 1st measurement, 2471 ± 1926 mm^3 (range, 300–7112 mm^3) at the 2nd measurement, and 2596 ± 2219 mm^3 (range, 306–7853 mm^3) at the 3rd measurement. The mean ossified volume in the LP group was 2361 ± 1962 mm^3 (range, 123–6250 mm^3) at the 1st measurement, 2553 ± 2053 mm^3 (range, 128–6378 mm^3) at the 2nd measurement, and 2889 ± 2196 mm^3 (range, 144–7197 mm^3) at the 3rd measurement. The volume of the ossified lesion significantly increased at the final follow-up in both groups (all, $p < 0.05$), whereas that from the 2nd to the 3rd measurement did not change in the PDF group.

The mean annual rate of lesion increase was 2.0 ± 1.7%/year (range, −3.0% to 5.3%/year) in the PDF group and 7.5 ± 5.6%/year (range, 1.0–19.2%/year) in the LP group, and there were significant differences in the annual rate of increase between the two groups ($p < 0.001$) (Fig. 16.4). Notably, the annual rate of increase from the 2nd to the 3rd measurement (2.5%/year) significantly decreased more compared to that from the 1st to the 2nd measurement (1.3%/year) in the PDF group ($p < 0.05$).

16.2.2.4 Illustrative Case

The patient was 57 years old with mixed-type OPLL. K-line (−)-type OPLL was found at the C3–C6 level on CT at the initial visit with a volume of 1909 mm^3 (Fig. 16.5a). Three years and 9 months later, the patient had progressive myelopathy, the volume of the ossified lesion increased to 2172 mm^3, and the annual rate of increase in the preoperative period was 3.7%/year (Fig. 16.5b). PDF from C2–C7 was performed (Fig. 16.5c). The volume of the ossified lesion was 2199 mm^3, and the mean annual rate of increase in the postoperative period decreased to 0.4%/year (Fig. 16.5d).

16.2.2.5 Discussion

In the present study, the mean annual rate of lesion increase in the PDF group was significantly lower than that in the LP group using novel 3D analysis. Notably, the mean annual rate of increase was gradually decreasing over time in the PDF group, which might be related with the process of bony fusion after PDF. These

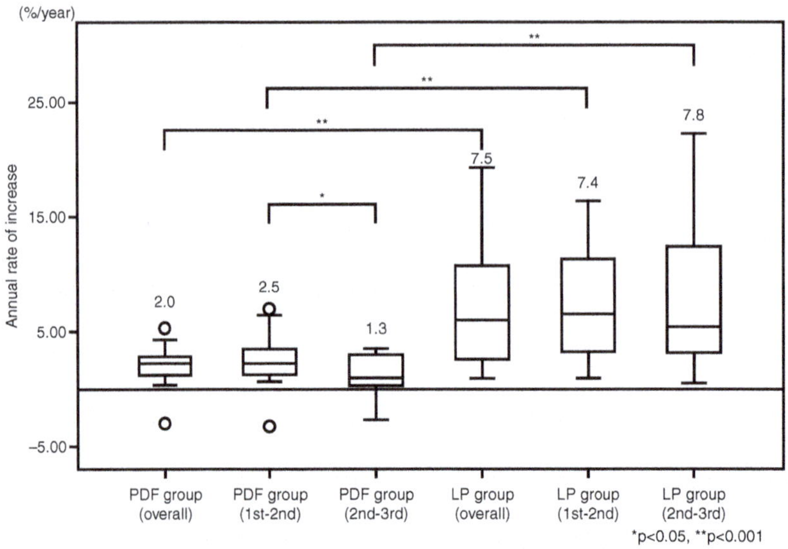

Fig. 16.4 The annual rate of lesion increase was evaluated in the PDF and LP groups. There was a significant difference in the annual rate of lesion increase between the two groups. In the PDF group, the annual rate of increase from the 1st to the 2nd measurement and from the 2nd to the 3rd measurement was significantly lower than that in the LP group. In the PDF group, the rate of increase from the 2nd to the 3rd measurement was significantly lower than that from the 1st to the 2nd measurement. *LP* laminoplasty, *PDF* posterior decompression and fusion

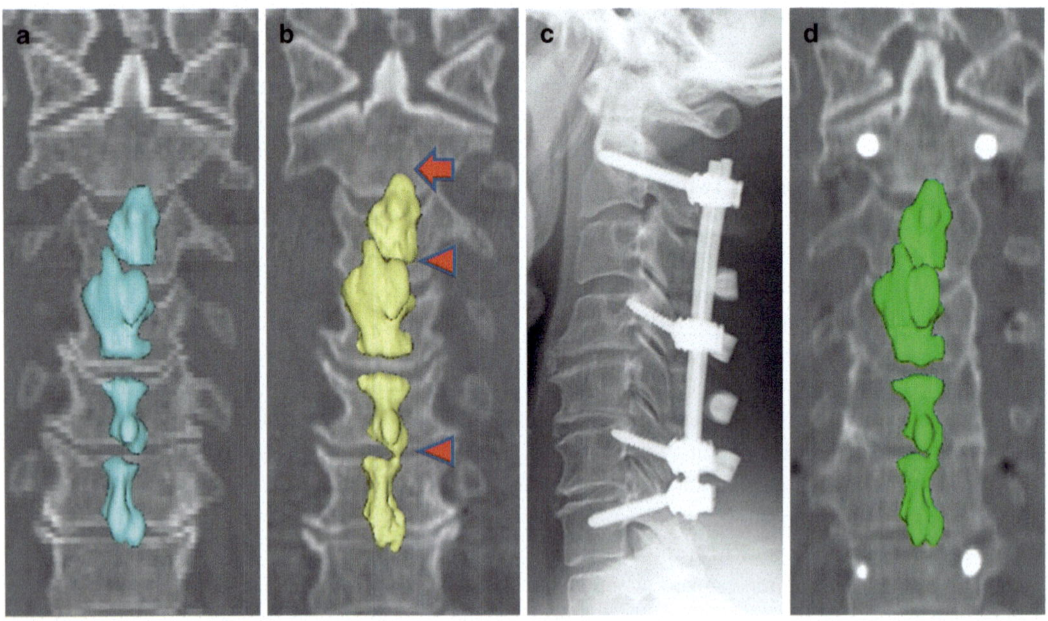

Fig. 16.5 (**a**) A 3D model of mixed-type OPLL showing the C3–C6 level at the initial visit. (**b**) A preoperative 3D model of OPLL showing progression at both the cranial portion of the OPLL (arrow) and C3/C4 and C5/C6 intervertebral area (arrowhead). (**c**) A plain radiography revealing the C2–C7 PDF. (**d**) A 3D model of OPLL at 3 years after the operation showing a lower progression of the OPLL. *OPLL* ossification of the posterior longitudinal ligament, *PDF* posterior decompression and fusion, *3D* three-dimensional

findings suggested that additional posterior instrumented fusion following laminoplasty suppresses the progression of OPLL. In an in vitro study, Tanno et al. [20] provided evidence that mechanical stress plays a key role in the progression of OPLL through the induction of osteogenic differentiation in spinal ligament cells and the promotion of the mechanism of bone morphogenetic proteins. These results supported the hypotheses that dynamic factors stimulate the progression of OPLL and stabilization may lead to the decreased progression of OPLL [3, 6, 20]. There are previous reports that confirm that the posterior fusion for thoracic OPLL reduced the size of the ossified lesions [21, 22]. Moreover, recently, a number of similar reports have been published indicating that additional fusion surgery for cervical OPLL suppresses the progression of ossification [23, 24].

This is the first study that validates the possible suppressant effect of posterior instrumented fusion on OPLL progression. Posterior decompression surgery is difficult to resect the ossified lesion itself and may not avoid OPLL progression or kyphotic change of cervical alignment, which are risk factors for late neurological deterioration. However, additional posterior instrumented fusion is useful to maintain both the cervical alignment and positive clinical outcomes, that is, suppression of OPLL progression. Our results suggest that posterior instrumented fusion has a beneficial effect on the long-term outcomes of OPLL patients with K-line (−) group. The novel CT-based 3D analysis method described here can measure the volume of OPLL accurately and thus can be useful for the examination of OPLL progression.

References

1. Iwasaki M, Kawaguchi Y, Kimura T, et al. Long-term results of expansive laminoplasty for ossification of the posterior longitudinal ligament of the cervical spine: more than 10 years follow up. J Neurosurg. 2002;96:180–9.
2. Kawaguchi Y, Kanamori M, Ishihara H, et al. Progression of ossification of the posterior longitudinal ligament following en bloc cervical laminoplasty. J Bone Joint Surg Am. 2001;83:1798–802.
3. Chiba K, Yamamoto I, Hirabayashi H, et al. Multicenter study investigating the postoperative progression of ossification of the posterior longitudinal ligament in the cervical spine: a new computer-assisted measurement. J Neurosurg Spine. 2005;3:17–23.
4. Hori T, Kawaguchi Y, Kimura T. How does the ossification area of the posterior longitudinal ligament thicken following cervical laminoplasty? Spine. 2007;32:E551–6.
5. Matsunaga S, Sakou T, Taketomi E, et al. Clinical course of patients with ossification of the posterior longitudinal ligament in the cervical spine: a new computer assisted measurement. J Neurosurg Spine. 2005;3:17–23.
6. Fragen KM, Cox JB, Hoh DJ. Does ossification of the posterior longitudinal ligament progress after laminoplasty? Radiographic and clinical evidence of ossification of the posterior longitudinal ligament lesion growth and the risk factors for late neurologic deterioration. J Neurosurg Spine. 2012;17:512–24.
7. Takatsu T, Ishida Y, Suzuki K, et al. Radiological study of cervical ossification of the posterior longitudinal ligament. J Spinal Disord. 1998;12:271–3.
8. Taketomi E. Progression of ossification of the posterior longitudinal ligament in the cervical spine. J Neurospinal Soc Jpn. 1997;8:359–66.
9. Hirabayashi K. Japanese Orthopaedic Association scoring system for cervical myelopathy. J Jpn Orthop Assoc. 1994;68:134–47 (in Japanese).
10. Kajiura K, Ikata T, Kato S, et al. Progression of ossification of the posterior longitudinal ligament of the cervical spine observed for 10 or more years. Ministry of Health, Labour and Welfare Specific Disease Report. Bone and Joint Disease Research Team; 1998. p. 146–8.
11. Matsunaga S, Nakamura K, Seichi A, et al. Radiographic predictors for the development of myelopathy in patients with ossification of the posterior longitudinal ligament: a multicenter cohort study. Spine. 2008;33:2648–50.
12. Chang H, Kong CG, Won HY, et al. Inter-and intra-observer variability of a cervical OPLL classification using reconstructed CT images. Clin Orthop Surg. 2010;2:8–12.
13. Izumi T, Hirano T, Watanabe K, et al. Three-dimensional evaluation of volume change in ossification of the posterior longitudinal ligament of the cervical spine using computed tomography. Eur Spine J. 2013;22:2569–74.
14. Katsumi K, Watanabe K, Izumi T, et al. Natural history of the ossification of cervical posterior longitudinal ligament: a three-dimensional analysis. Int Orthop. 2018;42:835–42.

15. Akune T, Ogata N, Seichi A, et al. Insulin secretory response is positively associated with the extent of ossification of the posterior longitudinal ligament of the spine. J Bone Joint Surg Am. 2001;83:1537–44.
16. Shingyouchi Y, Nagahama A, Niida M. Ligamentous ossification of the cervical spine in the late middle-aged Japanese men. Its relation to body mass index and glucose metabolism. Spine. 1996;21:2474–8.
17. Thomas DM, Hards DK, Rogers SD, et al. Insulin and bone, clinical and scientific view. Endocrinol Metab North Am. 1997;4:5–17.
18. Katsumi K, Izumi T, Ito T, et al. Posterior instrumented fusion suppresses the progression of ossification of the posterior longitudinal ligament: a comparison of laminoplasty with and without instrumented fusion by three-dimensional analysis. Eur Spine J. 2016;25:1634–40.
19. Fujiyoshi T, Yamazaki M, Kawabe J, et al. A new concept for making decisions regarding the surgical approach for cervical ossification of the posterior longitudinal ligament: the K-line. Spine. 2008;33:990–3.
20. Tanno M, Furukawa K, Ueyama K, et al. Uniaxial cyclic stretch induces osteogenic differentiation and synthesis of bone morphogenetic proteins of spinal ligament cells derived from patients with ossification of the posterior longitudinal ligaments. Bone. 2003;33:475–84.
21. Kimura H, Fujibayashi S, Takemoto M, et al. Spontaneous reduction in ossification of the posterior longitudinal ligament of the thoracic spine after posterior spinal fusion without decompression: a case report. Spine. 2014;39:E417–9.
22. Koda M, Furuya T, Okawa A, et al. Bone union and remodelling of the nonossified segment in thoracic ossification of the posterior longitudinal ligament after posterior decompression and fusion surgery. Eur Spine J. 2015;24:2555–9.
23. Lee CH, Sohn MJ, Lee CH, et al. Are there differences in the progression of ossification of the posterior longitudinal ligament following laminoplasty versus fusion? A meta-analysis. Spine. 2017;42:887–94.
24. Mehdi SK, Alentado VJ, Lee BS, et al. Comparison of clinical outcomes in decompression and fusion versus decompression only in patients with ossification of the posterior longitudinal ligament: a meta-analysis. Neurosurg Focus. 2016;40:E9.

17 Clinical Manifestations of Thoracic Ossification of the Posterior Longitudinal Ligament (OPLL) and Ossification of the Ligament Flavum (OLF)

Yukihiro Matsuyama, Go Yoshida, and Tomohiro Banno

Abstract

Thoracic OPLL (T-OPLL) is rarer than cervical OPLL and an ossified ligament compresses the spinal cord and nerve root, causing serious neurological dysfunction. T-OPLL often causes severe myelopathy that requires surgical intervention. However, the rate of occurrence, natural history, and optimal treatment for T-OPLL have not yet been investigated. Ossification of the ligament flavum (OLF) is also found in the thoracic spine and causes myelopathy. In this chapter, we review the clinical and neurological manifestations of T-OPLL and OLF.

Keywords

OPLL · Thoracic OPLL · Thoracic OLF

17.1 Introduction

Ossification of the posterior longitudinal ligament (OPLL) in the spinal canal affects 0.8–3.0% of Asians and 0.1–1.7% of European Caucasians [1]. Thoracic OPLL (T-OPLL) is rarer than cervical OPLL and has several unique characteristics. The ossified ligament compresses the spinal cord and nerve root, causing serious neurological dysfunction. T-OPLL often causes severe myelopathy that requires surgical intervention. However, the rate of occurrence, natural history, and optimal treatment for T-OPLL have not yet been investigated. Ossification of the ligament flavum (OLF) is mostly found in the thoracic spine and causes myelopathy. In this chapter, we review the clinical and neurological manifestations of T-OPLL and OLF.

17.2 Etiology and Pathogenesis of OPLL

Previous studies found that genetic background was strongly related to OPLL; sibling-pair linkage studies and candidate gene association studies identified a number of genes or loci that were linked to OPLL [2–5]. Recently, Nakajima et al. reported a replication study on the Japanese population, which identified six new susceptibility loci for OPLL. Analyses of gene expression in and around the OPLL-associated loci suggested that *RSPH9* and *STK38L* might be involved in OPLL etiology through the process of membranous ossification while *HAO1*, *RSPO2*, and *CCDC91* might be involved through the process of endochondral ossification [6].

Y. Matsuyama (✉) · G. Yoshida · T. Banno
Department of Orthopaedic Surgery, Hamamatsu University School of Medicine, Hamamatsu, Shizuoka, Japan

A. Okawa et al. (eds.), *OPLL*, https://doi.org/10.1007/978-981-15-3855-1_17

17.3 Prevalence of OPLL and OLF

Generally, OPLL is found in the cervical spine, and OLF in the lower thoracic spine. Ehara et al. reported that the prevalence of OPLL was 93%, 5.5%, and 4.5% in the cervical spine, thoracic spine, and lumbar spine, respectively, while that of OLF was 67%, 6%, 17%, and 11% in the lower thoracic spine, upper thoracic spine, cervical spine, and lumbar spine, respectively [7]. Ono et al. found that the prevalence of thoracic OPLL was 0.6%, and three times as many women as men were affected. In addition, they found that thoracic OPLL can be associated with OLF (14/39, 36% among women; 4/7, 57% among men) [8]. The prevalence of OLF has been estimated as 3.8–26% [9, 10]. Fujimori et al. reported data from computed tomographic images of 1500 healthy Japanese subjects. Thoracic and lumbar OLF were detected in 12% and 0.3% subjects, respectively [11]. OLF is predominantly observed in the upper or lower third of the thoracic spine, which can be attributed to increased mechanical stress where the thoracic vertebrae form the junction between the rigid rib cage and elastic cervical or lumbar spine [12].

17.4 Clinical Characteristics of T-OPLL and OLF

17.4.1 OPLL

T-OPLL causes specific thoracic myelopathy of its pathological feature. T-OPLL shows physiological kyphosis and poor vascular supply, which are not seen in the cervical or lumbar spine. Therefore, the symptoms and course might be dramatic. Isolated T-OPLL is rare, accounting for only 10% of the cases. In the remaining 90%, T-OPLL is associated with OPLL in the cervical spine. Because the movement of the thoracic spine is limited by the rib cage, dynamic factors may not play an important role in the development of myelopathic symptoms in cases of T-OPLL, unlike in cases with OPLL of the cervical or lumbar spine [13]. However, physiologic kyphosis of the thoracic spine renders the spinal cord the capacity to hold against the ventrally located OPLL. Moreover, thoracic OPLL occurs frequently in the mid-thoracic spine, where the spinal cord receives scarce blood supply under physiological conditions; this intramedullary hypocirculation may also render the spinal cord more vulnerable to compression by OPLL [13, 14].

17.4.2 Classification of Thoracic OPLL

The most common classification of cervical OPLL is by the Investigation Committee on OPLL of the Japanese Ministry of Health and Welfare. A lateral radiograph is used to classify OPLL into four subtypes: continuous, segmental, mixed, and localized or other. The continuous type is an ossified mass that spans several vertebral bodies and intervening disk spaces. The segmental type involves ossification behind each vertebral body. The mixed type is a mixture of both continuous and segmental types. The localized or other type has been described as a variant in which the ossification is localized to the intervertebral disk space without involvement of the vertebral body. The mixed and continuous types are most frequently associated with progression to myelopathy (Fig. 17.1).

17.4.3 OLF

OLF develops in the thoracic spine, either alone or in combination with OPLL. The lower thoracic spine is most often affected. Unlike OPLL, OLF occurs more frequently among men. Asymptomatic OLF may not be rare. The lower thoracic spine has more mobility than the upper or middle thoracic spine; thus, it is considered that mechanical stress on the ligamentous flavum may contribute to the development and progression of the ossification of the ligamentous flavum. In most cases, OLF arises from the capsular portion of the ligamentous flavum and extends medially. There is often a difference in the thickness of the ossification between the right and left sides, causing asymmetry of the neurological symptoms.

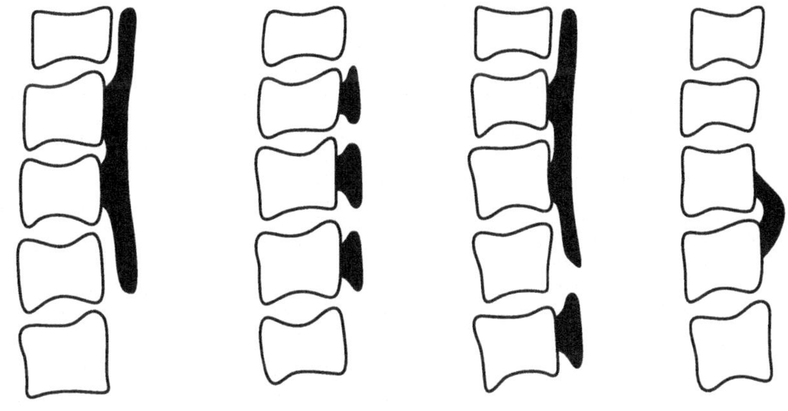

Fig. 17.1 Classification of thoracic ossification of the posterior longitudinal ligament (OPLL) by the investigation committee on the Ossification of the Spinal Ligaments of the Japanese Ministry of Public Health and Welfare

17.5 Neurological Symptoms

Spinal cord compression owing to the thoracic lesion may manifest as various neurological symptoms depending on the level of the lesion. Additionally, owing to the rarity of thoracic myelopathy, its diagnosis is often delayed [15, 16], or it is misdiagnosed as cervical or lumbar disorders. OPLL is mainly distributed in the upper to middle thoracic segment, whereas OLF is mainly distributed at the lower thoracic segment. However, in some cases, multiple cord compression by multi-segmental OPLL and/or OLF makes it difficult to identify the most affected lesion.

17.5.1 OPLL

Patients with OPLL may be asymptomatic or present with severe clinical symptoms, such as back pain, muscle motor weakness, sensory disturbance, bowel bladder dysfunction, and gait disturbance. Some patients have slight pain or discomfort on their back despite severe cord compression owing to ossification. In most cases, the neurological symptoms gradually progress over time. Some patients showed rapid progression of the symptoms causing an inability to walk within a short time (Fig. 17.2). Especially after myelopathy occurs, neurological symptoms steadily deteriorate. Ando et al. [17] revealed that age, weight, BMI, discontinuity between rostral and caudal OPLL lesions, and occurrence of high intensity area on MRI are likely to be associated with development of myelopathy.

The initial neurological manifestations of myelopathy are pain or numbness of the lower extremity followed by muscle motor weakness of the lower extremity and unsteady gait [18]. Patients also complain of tightness and stiffness of the trunk and lower extremities.

On neurological examination, they demonstrate hyperreflexia in their lower extremities. Pathological reflexes and clonus are also observed. In cases with peripheral neuropathy, such as diabetes or when accompanied with lumbar canal stenosis, these findings may disappear. Sensory disturbances, including impaired sense of light touch, pinprick, temperature, vibration, and position, are observed below the dermatome corresponding to the level of OPLL. Spasticity, ataxia, and severe muscle motor weakness of the lower extremities lead to gait disturbances and, occasionally, inability to walk. In cases of severe myelopathy, bladder bowel dysfunction could be observed.

17.5.2 OLF

OLF is commonly seen in the lower thoracic spine (T9–12); thus, the clinical manifestations differ depending on the level of the spinal cord

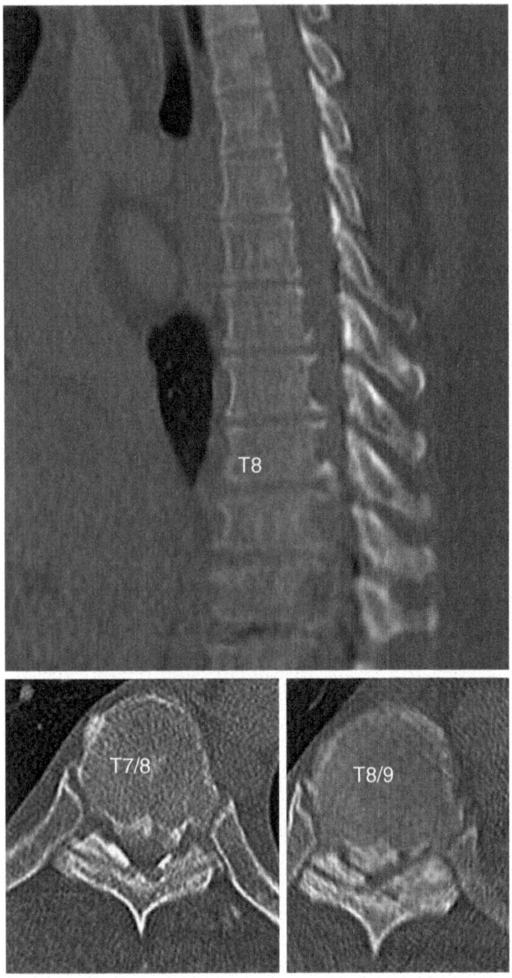

Fig. 17.2 A 52-year-old female patient with beak-type OPLL at T7/T8 and T8/T9. She had severe myelopathy, including spastic gait and bladder dysfunction. Axial view of computed tomography at T8/T9 shows the spinal cord severely compressed by OPLL and OLF

compression [18]. Various neurological manifestations arise from the OLF of the lower thoracic spine because this area is composed of epiconus, conus medullaris, and cauda equina; furthermore, although the localization depends on the individual (Fig. 17.3) [19], the termination level of the conus medullaris is mostly located from the middle third of L1 vertebra to the L1/2 intervertebral disc [18]. Epiconus and conus medullaris are located approximately at the T12 and L1 vertebrae, respectively (Fig. 17.4) [19].

When epiconus, which consists of spinal cord segment L4-S2, is compressed, muscle motor weakness and atrophy of the lower extremity are observed, referred to as the "epiconus syndrome." Sensory disturbances are often observed below the knee. Deep tendon reflex abnormalities differ among patients and depend on the affected level. Babinski reflex is sometimes positive. Some patients of epiconus syndrome represent only segmental signs, such as flaccid paralysis with muscle atrophy and stocking-type sensory disturbances, without deep tendon abnormalities. In such cases, motor neuron disease or peripheral neuropathy should be distinguished [14]. When conus medullaris, which consists of spinal cord segment below S2, is compressed sensory disturbance around the anus along with urinary dysfunction were typically observed called "conus medullaris syndrome." The deep tendon reflex is usually normal, and Babinski's reflex is negative. Patients with OLF above T11 usually present with typical thoracic myelopathy with hyperreflexia of the deep tendon reflex and muscle motor weakness and sensory disturbance below the affected level. On the other hand, patients with OLF below L1 represent the cauda equine syndrome. Intermittent claudication and pain and numbness of lower extremities are typical symptoms. The deep tendon reflex is diminished, and no Babinski's reflex is observed. Sensory disturbance is observed below the knee and around the genital area.

The clinical characteristics of epiconus, conus medullaris, and cauda equina syndromes are different. However, these symptoms often coexist, and in such cases, it may be difficult to identify the affected lesion.

17.5.3 Combined

Simultaneous OPLL and OLF was observed in the mid-thoracic spine in two-thirds of the patients [20]. Moreover, Kawaguchi et al. [21] revealed that approximately 10% of the patients had OPLL and OLF at the same level of the thoracic spine. In patients with combined OPLL and OLF at multiple levels, the neurological symp-

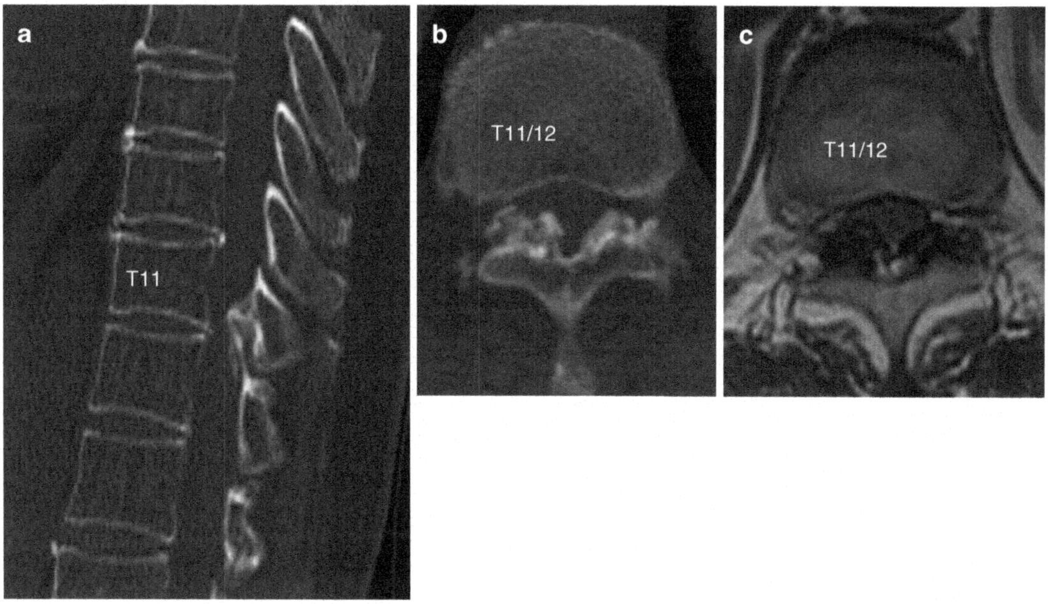

Fig. 17.3 A 62-year-old female patient with OLF at T11/12. She had severe myelopathy including spastic gait and numbness in bilateral lower extremities. (**a**) Sagittal view of computed tomography (CT). (**b**) Axial view of CT. (**c**) Axial view of magnetic resonance imaging. Spinal cord severely compressed by OLF at the T11/12 level

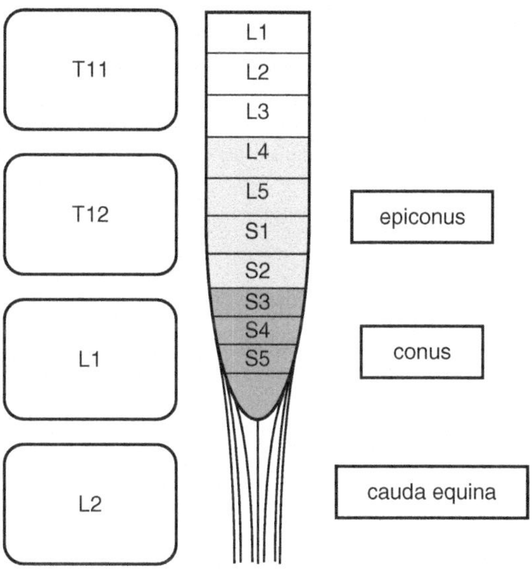

Fig. 17.4 Anatomical distribution of spinal cord segments at thoracolumbar spine. Epiconus, which consists of L4 to S2 spinal cord segments, is located at the T12 vertebra. Conus medullaris, which consists of spinal cord segments below L2, is located at the L1 vertebra

toms may be complex. Therefore, accurate diagnosis should be made with reference to imaging findings not only at the whole thoracic but also at the cervical and lumbar levels.

References

1. Matsunaga S, Sakou T. In: Yonenobu K, Nakamura K, Toyama Y, editors. Disease entity, incidence, literature search and prognosis. OPLL: ossification of the posterior longitudinal ligament. 2nd ed. Tokyo: Springer; 2006. p. 11–7.
2. Matsunaga S, Sakou T. Overview of epidemiology and genetics. In: Yanenobu K, Nakamura K, Toyone Y, editors. Ossification of the posterior longitudinal ligament. Tokyo: Springer; 2006. p. 7–9.
3. Sakou T, Matsunaga S, Koga H. Recent progress in the study of pathogenesis of ossification of the posterior longitudinal ligament. J Orthop Sci. 2000;5:310–5.
4. Taketomi E, Sakou T, Matsunaga S, Yamaguchi M. Family study of a twin with ossification of the posterior longitudinal ligament in the cervical spine. Spine. 1992;17:S55–6.

5. Okawa A, et al. Mutation in *Npps* in a mouse model of ossification of the posterior longitudinal ligament of the spine. Nat Genet. 1998;19:271–3.
6. Nakajima M, Takahashi A, Tsuji T, et al. Genetic study group of investigation committee on ossification of the spinal ligaments. A genome-wide association study identifies susceptibility loci for ossification of the posterior longitudinal ligament of the spine. Nat Genet. 2014;46(9):1012–6.
7. Ehara S, Shimamura T, Nakamura R, Yamazaki K. Paravertebral ligamentous ossification: DISH, OPLL and OLF. Eur J Radiol. 1998;27:196–205.
8. Ono M, Russell WJ, Kudo S, Kuroiwa Y, Takamori M, Motomura S, Murakami J. Ossification of the thoracic posterior longitudinal ligament in a fixed population. Radiological and neurological manifestations. Radiology. 1982;143:469–74.
9. Guo JJ, Luk KD, Karppinen J, et al. Prevalence, distribution, and morphology of ossification of the ligamentum flavum: a population study of one thousand seven hundred thirty-six magnetic resonance imaging scans. Spine. 2010;35:52–6.
10. Kudo S, Ono M, Russell WJ. Ossification of thoracic ligamenta flava. AJR Am J Roentgenol. 1983;141:117–21.
11. Fujimori T, Watabe T, Iwamoto Y, et al. Prevalence, concomitance, and distribution of ossification of the spinal ligaments. Result of whole spine CT scan in 1500 Japanese patients. Spine. 2016;41:1668–76.
12. Okada K, Oka S, Tohge K, et al. Thoracic myelopathy caused by ossification of the ligamentum flavum. Clinicopathologic study and surgical treatment. Spine. 1991;16:280–7.
13. Fujimura Y, Nishi Y, Nakamura M, Watanabe M, Matsumoto M. Myelopathy secondary to ossification of the posterior longitudinal ligament of the thoracic spine treated by anterior decompression and bony fusion. Spinal Cord. 1997;35(11):777–84.
14. Matsumoto M, Chiba K, Toyama Y. Clinical manifestations of thoracic OPLL and OLF. In: Yanenobu K, Nakamura K, Toyama Y, editors. Ossification of the posterior longitudinal ligament. Tokyo: Springer; 2006. p. 7–9.
15. Ohtsuka K, Terayama K, Yanagihara M, Wada K, Kasuga K, et al. A radiological population study on the ossification of the posterior longitudinal ligament in the spine. Arch Orthop Trauma Surg. 1987;106:89–93.
16. Yonenobu K, Ebara S, Fujiwara K, Yamashita K, Ono K, et al. Thoracic myelopathy secondary to ossification of the spinal ligament. J Neurosurg. 1987;66:511–8.
17. Ando K, Imagama S, Kobayashi K, Hida T, Ito K, et al. Comparative study of surgical treatment and nonsurgical follow up for thoracic ossification of the posterior longitudinal ligament: radiological and clinical evaluation. Spine. 2017;42:407–10.
18. Takenaka S, Kaito T, Hosono N, Miwa T, Oda T, et al. Neurological manifestations of thoracic myelopathy. Arch Orthop Trauma Surg. 2014;134:903–12.
19. Ando T. Epiconus syndrome and conus medullaris syndrome. Spine Spinal Cord. 2015;28(3):185–90.
20. Onishi E, Sano H, Matsushita M. Surgical treatment for thoracic myelopathy due to simultaneous ossification of the posterior longitudinal ligament and ligamentum flavum at the same level. Clin Spine Surg. 2016;29:E389–95.
21. Kawaguchi Y, Nakano M, Yasuda T, Seki S, Hori T, et al. Characteristics of ossification of the spinal ligament; incidence of ossification of the ligamentum flavum in patients with cervical ossification of the posterior longitudinal ligament—analysis of the whole spine using multidetector CT. J Orthop Sci. 2016;21:439–45.

18 Evaluation of Distribution Patterns of Spinal Ligament Ossification Using Whole-Spine Computed Tomography in Patients with Cervical Ossification of the Posterior Longitudinal Ligament

Takashi Hirai, Toshitaka Yoshii, Atsushi Okawa, and Yoshiharu Kawaguchi

Abstract

Ossification of the posterior longitudinal ligament (OPLL) and other types of spinal ligament ossification are common in Japan and are known to frequently cause neuropathy. Cervical OPLL is a common form of OPLL that often involves ossification of not only the cervical vertebrae but also ligaments in other parts of the spine, and therefore evaluation of ossification by 360° whole-spine imaging is considered important. In this study, we analyzed data from a large multicenter retrospective study to evaluate the distribution of spinal ligament ossification across the entire spine in patients with cervical OPLL with a focus on correlations between OPLL, ossification of the nuchal ligament, ossification of the supraspinous and interspinous ligaments, and diffuse idiopathic skeletal hyperostosis.

T. Hirai (✉) · T. Yoshii · A. Okawa
Department of Orthopedic Surgery, Tokyo Medical and Dental University, Tokyo, Japan

Y. Kawaguchi
Department of Orthopedic Surgery, Faculty of Medicine, University of Toyama, Toyama, Japan

Keywords

Ossification of the posterior longitudinal ligament · Diffuse idiopathic skeletal hyperostosis · Ossification of the anterolateral ligament · Ossification of the supraspinous and interspinous ligaments · Ossification of the nuchal ligament · Computed tomography Whole spine

18.1 Introduction

Spinal ligament ossification is heterotopic bone formation that can occur in any region of the spine. Notably, ossification of the posterior longitudinal ligament (OPLL) is the most frequent type of ossification. Compression of the spinal cord by these lesions can cause myelopathy and major functional impairment. As reported by Fujimori et al. [1], epidemiological studies have shown that the prevalence of OPLL is 0.1–1.3% in Caucasians but is higher in Asians and particularly the Japanese population (1.9–4.3%), demonstrating a strong predisposition to ossification in the spine. Ossified lesions develop at a relatively higher rate in the cervical vertebrae, but it is not uncommon to see concurrent OPLL in the thoracic vertebrae,

A. Okawa et al. (eds.), *OPLL*, https://doi.org/10.1007/978-981-15-3855-1_18

a highly vulnerable part of the spinal cord, where the lesions can cause severe paralysis. Detection of any such concurrent lesions is considered critical. Before the advent of computed tomography (CT), when it was common practice to make assessments using plain X-rays, it was found that 17.5% of patients with cervical OPLL had concurrent thoracic OPLL and 12.6% had concurrent lumbar OPLL [2]. Kawaguchi et al. [3] evaluated 178 sequential patients with cervical OPLL in a single-center study using whole-spine CT and found that more than half (53.4%) had concurrent thoracolumbar ossification. They concluded that it would be important to compile more data from patients in different regions to identify risk factors for the presence of thoracolumbar OPLL.

Ossification of the anterolateral ligament (OALL) is a type of spinal ligament ossification shown to be relatively prevalent in Japan. Diffuse idiopathic skeletal hyperostosis (DISH), a condition first described by Resnik that is characterized by bridging of at least four sequential thoracic vertebral bodies, is particularly noteworthy because it is believed to be clinically asymptomatic in the majority of cases but is known to result in fracture following even minor trauma due to morphological characteristics, occasionally leading to severe paralysis. The condition is often difficult to diagnose on plain X-rays alone and is sometimes overlooked even when images are interpreted by an orthopedic surgeon. Therefore, it is important to always pay attention to the possibility of latent DISH. However, the prevalence and precise distribution of concurrent DISH across the spinal cord in patients with cervical OPLL have never been investigated.

This is a project of the working group of the Japanese Multicenter Research Organization for Ossification of the Spinal Ligament (JOSL), funded by a Health and Labour Science Research Grant for research on measures to address rare and intractable diseases from the Ministry of Health, Labour and Welfare. We retrospectively evaluated data from consenting patients with cervical OPLL who underwent whole-spine CT at collaborating institutions. We determined the prevalence of concurrent thoracolumbar OPLL [4], DISH [5], ossification of the nuchal ligament (ONL) [6], and ossification of the supraspinous and interspinous ligaments (OSIL) [7] to identify predictive factors for thoracolumbar OPLL and analyzed DISH distribution across the spine using clustering classification.

18.2 Methods

18.2.1 Subjects

We retrospectively evaluated data for 322 patients from the 20 participating JOSL institutions with a diagnosis of cervical OPLL on plain X-ray after complaints of symptoms such as neck pain, upper or lower extremity numbness, or gait disturbance who had not undergone spinal surgery, were older than 15 years, and consented to undergoing whole-spine CT and other study assessments (mean age 64.6 years, 242 men and 80 women). All patients were Asians of Japanese heritage.

18.2.2 Assessments

Data on age, sex, diabetes, and body mass index (BMI) were evaluated as basic patient data, and the 322 patients from whom mid-sagittal images of the entire spine were successfully obtained (242 men and 80 women) were included in analysis. Images were evaluated by five board-certified spine surgeons of the Japanese Orthopaedic Association who reviewed the distribution of OPLL on paramedian sagittal oblique images. OPLL and OALL were defined as ossified lesions of at least 2 mm in thickness extending along the course of the ligament, and OSIL was defined as complete formation of a bone bridge between the superior and inferior spinous process. To evaluate the severity of ossification, the number of vertebral body and intervertebral disc levels with OPLL across the entire spine was defined as the OP-index (sum for cervical vertebrae: cervical OP-index, sum for thoracic vertebrae: thoracic OP-index, sum for lumbar vertebrae: lumbar OP-index) [3]. DISH was defined as bridging involving four or more sequential vertebral bodies. With reference to the definition of DISH, OSIL involving four sequential spinous processes was defined as diffuse OSIL [7]. The ONL level was determined as a line joining the superior endplate of the upper spine and the inferior endplate of the lower spine. Severity was further classified into three grades by cervical OP-index (≤5: grade I, 6–9: grade II, ≥10: grade 3) [4].

Analysis of DISH, OSIL, and ONL was performed in the 234 patients for whom sagittal images could be easily interpreted and evaluated fully to both the left and right edges to allow for comprehensive thoracic OALL evaluation.

18.2.3 Statistical Analysis

The student's t-test was used to compare results between male and female patients, and the chi-square test was used to analyze differences in sex and prevalence of concurrent diabetes. Multivariate analysis was performed to identify predictive factors for the spinal OP-index. In addition, cluster analysis using a correlation matrix was used for statistical classification to evaluate the distribution of DISH.

18.3 Results

18.3.1 Prevalence of Concurrent Thoracolumbar OPLL and Distribution of Ossification in Cervical OPLL Patients by Sex

Thoracolumbar OPLL was detected in 181 of 322 patients (56.2%). Prevalence was significantly higher in women than in men (71.5 vs. 51.2%) (Table 18.1). Both the prevalence of concurrent diabetes and BMI did not differ between men and women. Mean spinal OP-index was also higher in women than in men (12.1 vs. 8.2).

Evaluating the distribution of OPLL across each level showed that OPLL was most frequently detected at vertebral body C5 level and intervertebral disc C3/4 level in both men and women (Fig. 18.1). The thoracic vertebral body and intervertebral disc levels at which OPLL was most frequently detected were T1 (14.9%) and T1/2 (13.6%) in men, and T1 (27.5%) and T3/4 (33.8%) in women. For the lower thoracic vertebrae and the lumbar vertebrae, OPLL was most frequently detected at L1 (5.8%) and T12-L1 (14.5%) in men and L1 and L2 (11.3%) and T12-L1 (27.5%) in women with no difference between the sexes. OPLL was more commonly detected at L5/S disc level than any other lumbar level, at a rate of 10.7% in men and 16.3% in women. A higher cervical OP-index classification was associated with significantly higher prevalence of ossification at the upper and lower thoracic vertebrae and the upper lumbar vertebrae in men and at all thoracic vertebrae in women. Women tended to have OPLL at multiple sites as evidenced by the high percentage of female patients with a spinal OP-index of ≥20 (4.5%, n = 11 in men vs. 20%, n = 16 in women) (Table 18.1); this is indicative of extensive ossification. Among these patients with a spinal OP-index of ≥20, OPLL was most frequently detected at the cervicothoracic junction and other upper thoracic vertebrae in men and at the middle thoracic vertebrae in women (Fig. 18.2 and Table 18.2).

Table 18.1 Patient data by sex

	Men (n = 242)	Women (n = 80)	p
Age (years)	64.7 ± 11.6	64.6 ± 10.0	ND
Body mass index (kg/m^2)	25.8 ± 4.8	25.5 ± 4.7	ND
Prevalence of concurrent diabetes (%)	31.8%	31.3%	ND
Prevalence of concurrent thoracolumbar OPLL (%)	51.2%	71.3%	<0.01
Cervical OP-index	5.86 ± 2.9	5.75 ± 3.0	ND
Spinal OP-index	8.24 ± 5.5	12.1 ± 9.0	<0.01
OP-index ≥20	11 (4.5%)	16 (20%)	<0.01

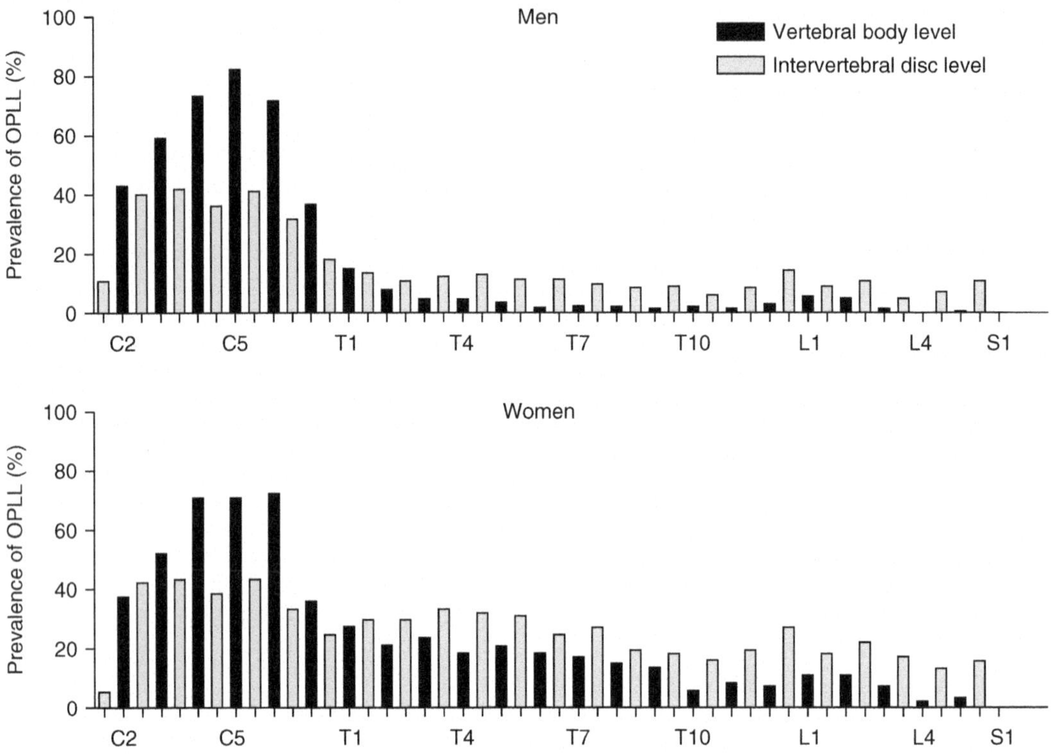

Fig. 18.1 Spinal distribution of OPLL by sex

Fig. 18.2 Distribution of OSIL

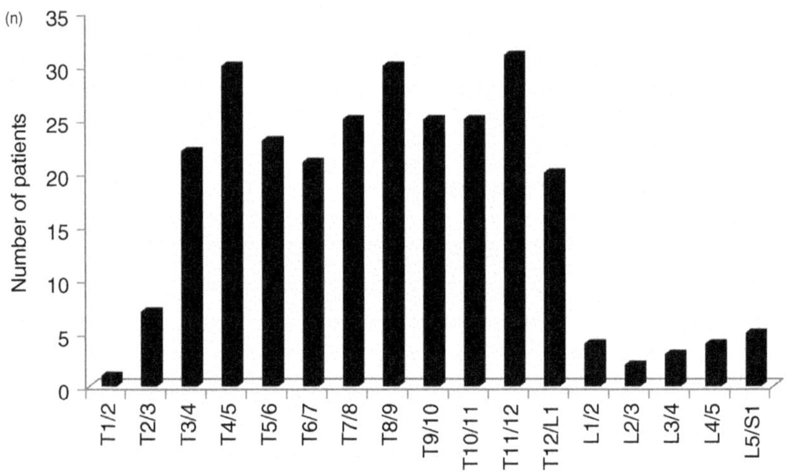

18.3.2 Predictive Factors of the Spinal OP-Index

Multiple regression analysis with age, sex, BMI, diabetes, cervical OP-index, cervical OA-index, and CNR classification as explanatory variables and spinal OP-index as the response variable was performed to determine whether spinal OP-index can be predicted. Sex, BMI, and cervical OP-index were found to have significant influence, as expressed by the equation $Y = -8.707 + 4.108X_1 + 1.558X_2 + 0.143X_3$ (Y: spinal

Table 18.2 Comparison of OPLL prevalence between all patients and patients with an OP-index of 20 or higher (Cited in [11])

OPLL prevalence	Men		Women	
Level	Total	OP >20	Total	OP >20
T1	14.9%	72.7%	27.5%	75.0%
T1–2	13.6%	81.8%	30.0%	68.8%
T2	7.9%	54.5%	21.3%	62.5%
T2–3	10.7%	81.8%	30.0%	81.3%
T3	4.5%	54.5%	23.8%	68.8%
T3–4	12.4%	81.8%	33.8%	81.3%
T4	5.0%	54.5%	18.8%	56.3%
T4–5	13.2%	72.7%	32.5%	100.0%
T5	3.7%	18.2%	21.3%	62.5%
T5–6	11.6%	45.5%	31.3%	87.5%
T6	2.1%	18.2%	18.8%	56.3%
T6–7	11.6%	36.4%	25.0%	75.0%
T7	2.5%	18.2%	17.5%	43.8%
T7–8	9.9%	54.5%	27.5%	68.8%
T8	2.1%	18.2%	15.0%	37.5%
T8–9	8.7%	36.4%	20.0%	56.3%
T9	1.7%	18.2%	13.8%	43.8%
T9–10	9.1%	36.4%	18.8%	56.3%
T10	2.1%	9.1%	6.3%	18.8%
T10–11	6.2%	18.2%	16.3%	43.8%
T11	1.7%	18.2%	8.8%	18.8%
T11–12	8.7%	54.5%	20.0%	43.8%
T12	2.9%	36.4%	7.5%	31.3%
T12–L1	14.5%	54.5%	27.5%	81.3%
L1	5.8%	45.5%	11.3%	37.5%
L1–2	9.1%	45.5%	18.8%	50.0%
L2	5.0%	45.5%	11.3%	37.5%
L2–3	10.7%	54.5%	22.5%	56.3%
L3	1.7%	18.2%	7.5%	25.0%
L3–4	5.0%	27.3%	17.5%	31.3%
L4	0.4%	9.1%	2.5%	12.5%
L4–5	7.4%	18.2%	13.8%	31.3%
L5	0.8%	9.1%	3.8%	12.5%
L5–S1	10.7%	45.5%	16.3%	50.0%
S1	0.4%	9.1%	0.0%	0.0%

OP-index, X_1: sex [male = 0, female = 1], X_2: cervical OP-index, X_3: BMI [kg/m^2]).

18.3.3 Correlation of Cervical OP-Index Classification with Thoracolumbar OPLL Lesions

On the basis of results from multivariate analysis, analysis was performed to determine whether concurrent thoracolumbar OPLL could be easily predicted from the cervical OP-index. To that end, the correlation of cervical OP-index classification with OPLL distribution was assessed. Mean thoracolumbar OP-index was 1.93 for grade I, 3.93 for grade II, and 7.37 for grade III, and prevalence of concurrent thoracolumbar OPLL was 42.3% for grade I, 70.4% for grade II, and 82.6% for grade III (Table 18.3). The percentage of patients with a spinal OP-index of 20 or higher was 1.2% for grade I, 8.3% for grade II, and 32.6% for grade III.

Table 18.3 Cervical OP-index classification and hazard ratios for thoracolumbar OPLL and spinal OP-index of 20 or higher

Cervical OP-index classification	Number of patients	Thoracolumbar OP-index	Prevalence of concurrent thoracolumbar OPLL	Percentage with spinal OP-index ≥20
Grade 1	168	1.9 ± 3.6	42.3%	1.2%
Grade 2	108	3.9 ± 5.3	70.4%	8.3%
Grade 3	46	7.4 ± 7.5	82.6%	32.6%

18.3.4 Prevalence of Concurrent OSIL and Relationship with OPLL

In total, 68 (54 men and 14 women) of the 234 patients had OSIL between 278 spinous processes (260 thoracic and 18 lumbar). Only a few lesions were detected at T1/2/3, but these were distributed evenly across other levels (Fig. 18.2). Diffuse OSIL, defined as OSIL involving four sequential spinous processes, was detected in 26 patients (21 men and 5 women, 11.1%).

Analyzing the relationship between cervical OP-index classification and OSIL revealed that the number of OSIL sites increased with grade (Fig. 18.3).

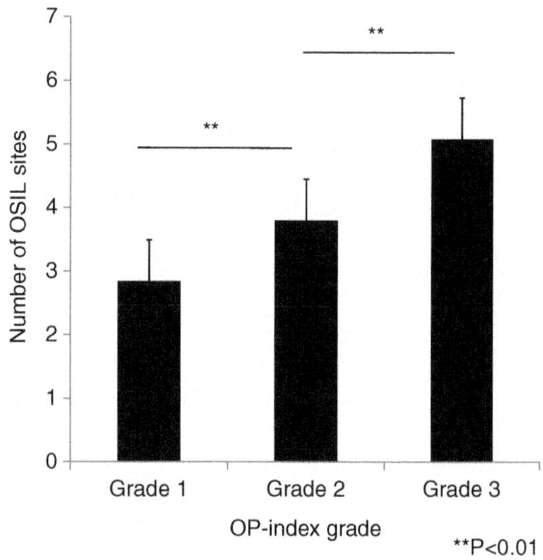

Fig. 18.3 Relationship between cervical OP-index classification and number of vertebrae with OSIL

18.3.5 Relationship Between ONL and OPLL Across the Entire Spine

ONL was detected in 130 of 234 patients (65.5%) and was particularly common at the C4/5 (64.6%) and C5/6 (59.2%) levels (Fig. 18.4). The group of patients with ONL (ONL[+]) had a higher percentage of men and was older than the group of patients without ONL (ONL[−]), but there were no differences in prevalence of concurrent diabetes or BMI (Table 18.4). Also, patients with ONL had a significantly higher cervical OP-index (5.5 vs. 3.8) and prevalence of concurrent DISH (57.7% vs. 44.7%) than patients without ONL.

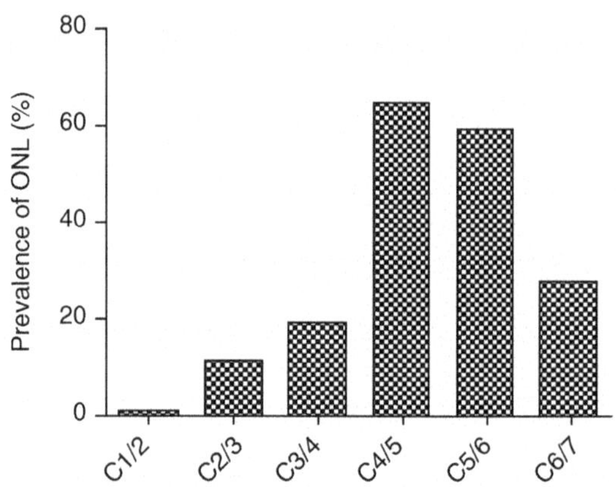

Fig. 18.4 Distribution of ONL

18.3.6 Morphological Classification of DISH in Patients with Cervical OPLL

DISH was detected in 114 of 234 patients (48.7%, 91 men and 23 women) with a mean age of 67.3 years. These patients were significantly older than those without DISH (mean age, 63.4 years, Table 18.5). On clustering analysis, DISH distribution was classified into six categories on the basis of pattern: (1) C2–5,

Table 18.4 Relationship of ONL with concurrent OPLL and DISH

	ONL+	ONL−	*p*
Sex (% male)	81.5%*	68.9%	<0.05
Age (years)	66.8 ± 10.4*	63.2 ± 10.9	<0.05
Prevalence of concurrent diabetes (%)	33.1%	26.2%	ND
Body mass index (kg/m²)	25.5 ± 4.9	25.3 ± 4.0	ND
Cervical OP-index	5.5 ± 4.5**	3.8 ± 3.8	<0.01
Prevalence of concurrent DISH	57.7%*	44.7%	<0.05

*<0.05
**<0.01

Table 18.5 Relationship between DISH and concurrent OPLL

	DISH+	DISH-	*p*
Number of patients	114*	120%	–
Sex (% male)	51.4%	40.4%	ND
Age (years)	67.3 ± 0.9	63.4 ± 1.0	ND
Prevalence of concurrent diabetes (%)	31.6	29.2	ND
Body mass index (kg/m²)	25.9 ± 0.5	25.1 ± 0.4	ND
Cervical OP-index	6.3 ± 3.0	7.0 ± 3.0	ND

(2) C3-T1, (3) C6-T5, (4) T3–10, (5) T8-L2, and (6) T12-S1. Category 4 (T3–10), the most frequent pattern, was seen in 98 patients. The next most frequent patterns were category 5 with 75 patients, category 3 with 49 patients, category 6 with 8 patients, and category 1 with 2 patients. Patients with DISH were further split into three categories by extent of spread (DISH classification). DISH only at the thoracic vertebral level was defined as grade 1, DISH extending to either the cervicothoracic junction (C6-T2) or thoracolumbar junction (T11-L2) was defined as grade 2, and DISH extending to the cervical (C1–5) or lumbar (L3-S1) levels was defined as grade 3; 34 patients were grade 1, 54 were grade 2, and 14 were grade 3. Mean age was also found to increase with grade (grade 1, 64.3 years; grade 2, 68.1 years; grade 3, 71.3 years). Analysis of the relationship between cervical OP-index classification and DISH identified a positive correlation between the number of cervical OPLL sites and the extent of OALL spread (Fig. 18.5).

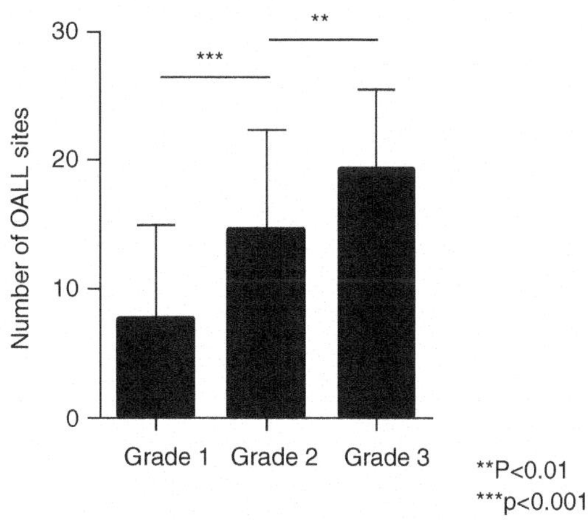

Fig. 18.5 Relationship between cervical OP-index classification and number of vertebrae with OALL

18.4 Discussion

OPLL has long been a topic of research in Japan, and several epidemiological studies have been conducted to date, but were all single-center studies. This study is thus the first large multicenter detailed evaluation of the distribution of ligament ossification across the entire spine in patients with cervical OPLL. Before the advent of multidetector CT, accurate evaluation of ossification was limited due to the difficulty in visualizing OPLL of the upper to middle thoracic vertebrae on plain X-rays. With the current availability of detailed imaging of ossified lesions using reconstructed whole-spine CT images, accurate evaluation is now possible for not only OPLL but also other spinal ligament ossification in 360°. In this study, we showed that more than half of patients with cervical OPLL (56%) had concurrent OPLL at some thoracolumbar level. Though no study has yet evaluated CT images in the general population for OPLL, Mori et al. [8] reported a prevalence of 1.9% for thoracic OPLL in 3013 patients who underwent chest CT for lung disease, and Fujimori et al. [9] reported a 1.6% rate of thoracic OPLL on CT images in 1500 patients who underwent positron-emission tomography/CT. These findings, along with the high prevalence of ossification in this study, suggest that OPLL across the entire spine is likely to occur in people who have a strong tendency toward ligament ossification.

We also discovered that sex, BMI, and cervical OP-index strongly influenced spinal OP-index. Cervical OP-index showed a particularly strong correlation with the number of ossified lesions across the spine, and so we proposed a new cervical OP-index classification [4]. Quite interestingly, the cervical OP-index influenced not only the number of thoracolumbar OPLL sites but also the prevalence of concurrent OSIL and DISH. DISH has long been recognized as a disease entity, and studies show that even the minor trauma it results in fractures that may lead to severe paralysis. Few studies to date have examined the prevalence and distribution of OSIL in detail. This study is the first to define the concept of diffuse OSIL as bridging involving at least four sequential spinous processes, and in fact found 11.1% prevalence in patients with cervical OPLL. This rate may not be high, but when added to the rate of DISH (48.7%) shows that a large percentage of patients with cervical OPLL had spinal stiffening. Patients with cervical lesions must also be cautious to avoid traumatic incidents such as falls, but it is also necessary to look for concurrent OSIL and DISH at the thoracic vertebrae and beyond. These results indicate that patients with a grade 3 cervical OP-index are highly likely to have 360° spinal ligament ossification at the thoracolumbar vertebrae, and as such it is important to detect lesions of concern by CT evaluation of not only the cervical vertebrae but of the entire spine and to follow up on those lesions.

Orthopedic surgeons encounter ONL relatively frequently. However, its exact pathology is unclear because some studies propose that this ligament ossification develops due to trauma or repeated physical stress, whereas others consider it to be part of ligament ossification syndrome [5]. The prevalence of ONL in the Japanese population has been reported to be 23.3% [10], but we found a higher rate (65.5%) among patients with cervical OPLL in this study. We also found that patients with ONL had a significantly higher cervical-OP index and prevalence of DISH than patients without ONL. These findings demonstrate that ONL was closely related to spinal ligament ossification at other sites.

We also created a new DISH grouping system using clustering analysis. When we divided patients into six groups by this system, we found that the prevalence of DISH was a particularly high 84.2% at T3–10, mainly at the middle thoracic vertebrae. We also assigned one of three grades by the extent of DISH spread and found that a higher grade (i.e., greater cephalocaudal spread of ossification) was associated with older age. These two findings suggest that many cases of DISH start with bridging at the middle thoracic vertebrae, and then ossification spreads cephalocaudally with age.

Our study has a few limitations. First, it was not a population-based study and was conducted in a diseased population (i.e., patients with cervical OPLL), and so it is different from typical epidemiological studies. Second, we did not evaluate clinical aspects such as the relationship between progression of ossification relates and the presence or severity of symptoms, and we believe it is necessary to conduct a detailed prospective study on these aspects in the future. Nevertheless, we believe that the data from our large multicenter study provides beneficial information about patients with cervical OPLL such as the specific distribution of ossification [11], factors that predict severe ossification, and relationships with spinal ligament ossification at other sites.

18.5 Conclusion

In this study, basic data and whole-spine CT imaging data from patients with cervical OPLL were collected from 20 collaborating institutions and analyzed. Concurrent thoracolumbar OPLL was observed in 56.2% of patients with cervical OPLL. Multivariate analysis showed that the spinal OP-index, a measure of the extent of ossified lesion distribution across the entire spine, was strongly correlated with the number of cervical OPLL sites, female sex, and obesity. The severity of cervical OPLL ossification also showed positive correlations with prevalence of concurrent ONL, OSIL, and DISH. Furthermore, clustering analysis for DISH showed that DISH mostly occurred in the middle thoracic vertebrae and that ossification may spread cephalocaudally with age. We plan to conduct a prospective study to determine the association of clinical symptoms with ossification in the future.

Acknowledgments We would like to thank Dr. Akio Iwanami, Dr. Kanji Mori, Dr. Kazuhiro Takeuchi, Dr. Tsuyoshi Yamada, Dr. Soraya Nishimura, Dr. Narihito Nagoshi, Dr. Kanichiro Wada, Dr. Masao Koda, Dr. Yukihiro Matsuyama, Dr. Katsushi Takeshita, Dr. Masahiko Abematsu, Dr. Hirotaka Haro, Dr. Masahiko Watanabe, Dr. Kei Watanabe, Dr. Hiroshi Ozawa, Dr. Haruo Sugano, Dr. Shiro Imagama, Dr. Shunsuke Fujibayashi, Dr. Masashi Yamazaki, Dr. Morio Matsumoto, Dr. Masaya Nakamura, Dr. Shoji Seki, Dr. Takashi Tsuji, Dr. Kanehiro Fujiyoshi, Dr. Mitsuru Furukawa, Dr. Takeo Furuya, Dr. Tomohiko Hasegawa, Dr. Atsushi Kimura, Dr. Tetsuro Ohba, Dr. Hiroyuki Katoh, and Dr. Zenya Ito of the participating institutions in this study.

References

1. Fujimori T, Le H, Hu SS, et al. Ossification of the posterior longitudinal ligament of the cervical spine in 3161 patients: a CT-based study. Spine. 2015;40: E394–403.
2. Wada K, Terayama K, Ohtsuka K, et al. A radiological study on spinal and extraspinal ligamentous ossification in patients with cervical OPLL. Rinshoseikeigeka. 1988;23:489–94. (in Japanese)
3. Kawaguchi Y, Nakano M, Yasuda T, Seki S, Hori T, Kimura T. Ossification of the posterior longitudinal ligament in not only the cervical spine, but also other spinal regions: analysis using multidetector computed tomography of the whole spine. Spine. 2013;38(23):E1477–82. https://doi.org/10.1097/BRS.0b013e3182a54f00.
4. Hirai T, Yoshii T, Iwanami A, et al. Prevalence and distribution of ossified lesions in the whole spine of patients with cervical ossification of the posterior longitudinal ligament – JOSL CT study. PLoS One. 2016;11(8):e0160117.
5. Yoshii T, Hirai T, Iwanami A, et al. Co-occurrence of ossification of the nuchal ligament is associated with hyperostosis in the whole spine in patients with cervical ossification of the posterior longitudinal ligament CSRS-AP 2016, pp. 91.
6. Iwanami A, Nishimura S, Hirai T, et al. Incidence of OALL in Patients With Cervical OPLL Detected By Whole-Spine Computed Tomography: Multicenter Cross-Sectional Study. 7th annual meeting of the Cervical Spine Research Society– Asia Pacific Section, Seoul, Korea, April, 2016.
7. Mori K, Yoshii T, Hirai T, et al. Prevalence and distribution of ossification of the supra/interspinous ligaments in symptomatic patients with cervical ossification of the posterior longitudinal ligament of the spine: a CT-based multicenter cross-sectional study. BMC Musculoskelet Disord. 2016;17(1):492.
8. Mori K, Imai S, Kasahara T, et al. Prevalence, distribution, and morphology of thoracic ossification of the posterior longitudinal ligament in Japanese: results of CT-based cross-sectional study. Spine. 2014;39(5):394–9.
9. Fujimori T, Watabe T, Iwamoto Y, et al. Prevalence, concomitance, and distribution of ossification of the spinal ligaments results of whole spine CT scans in 1500 Japanese patients. Spine. 2016;41(21):1668–76.
10. Shingyouchi Y, Nagahama A, Niida M. Ligamentous ossification of the cervical spine in the late middle-aged Japanese men. Its relation to body mass index and glucose metabolism. Spine. 1996;21:2474–8.
11. Hirai T, Yoshii T, Nagoshi N, et al. Distribution of ossified spinal lesions in patients with severe ossification of the posterior longitudinal ligament and prediction of ossification at each segment based on the cervical OP index classification: a multicenter study (JOSL CT study). BMC Musculoskelet Disord. 2018;19(1):107.

Diagnostic Imaging of Thoracic OPLL and OLF

19

Kanji Mori

Abstract

The most standard diagnostic imaging modality for ossification of the posterior longitudinal ligament of the spine (OPLL) and ossification of the ligamentum flavum (OLF) is a plain radiography; however, standard plain radiography is not an adequate for diagnosis of thoracic OPLL (T-OPLL) and thoracic OLF (T-OLF) because of the characteristic anatomy of thoracic region. Computed tomography (CT) is probably the most suitable modality to identify the ossified lesions. It is especially useful for the precise evaluation of T-OPLL and T-OLF. Magnetic resonance (MR) imaging cannot distinguish between ossifications of the spinal ligaments and hypertrophied spinal ligaments; however, it helps us to evaluate not only the extent of spinal cord compression, but also the intensity change of spinal cord due to compression by T-OPLL and T-OLF. It is important to make correct diagnosis of T-OPLL as well as T-OLF using multiple diagnostic imaging modalities.

Keywords

OPLL · OLF · OYL · Diagnosis · Imaging Computed tomography · Myelography · CT myelography · Magnetic resonance imaging

The most standard diagnostic imaging modality for ossification of the posterior longitudinal ligament of the spine (OPLL) and ossification of the ligamentum flavum (OLF) synonymous with ossification of the yellow ligament (OYL) is a plain radiography. Plain lateral radiography can demonstrate OPLL as well as OLF; however, it is not an adequate for diagnosis of thoracic OPLL (T-OPLL) and thoracic OLF (T-OLF) because of the characteristic anatomy of thoracic region. The presence of T-OPLL and T-OLF can be masked by superimposed bony structures such as ribs and shoulder [1, 2].

The radiographic classification of cervical OPLL is as follows: *continuous*, *segmental*, *mixed*, and *localized or other* using a lateral standard radiograph is established by the Investigation Committee on OPLL of the Japanese Ministry of Health and Welfare [3]. In addition, T-OPLL is further classified into two subtypes: *flat*- or *beak*-type according to the form of T-OPLL [4]. *Flat*-type is a continuous- or mixed-type OPLL with a flat shape, and *beak*-type is a segmental OPLL with sharp protrusions located behind the disc spaces (Fig. 19.1) [4]. These two types were

K. Mori (✉)
Department of Orthopaedic Surgery, Shiga University of Medical Science, Shiga, Japan
e-mail: kanchi@belle.shiga-med.ac.jp

A. Okawa et al. (eds.), *OPLL*, https://doi.org/10.1007/978-981-15-3855-1_19

more evident on CT images. The small ossified lesion localized posterior vertebral body is sometimes difficult to differentiate from a posterior osteophyte [5].

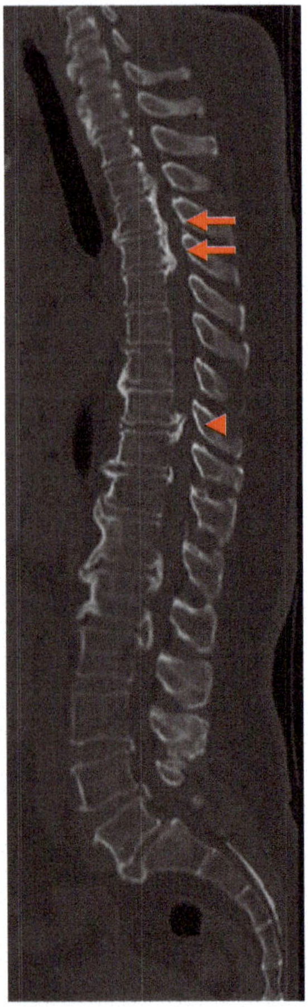

Fig. 19.1 Thoracic OPLL subtype by Matsuyama et al. Flat-type (double arrows) and beak-type (arrow head)

OLF is classified into four subtypes: *hook*, *beak*, *linear*, and *nodular* using a lateral standard radiograph (Fig. 19.2) [6]. *Hook*-type was the most frequently observed subtype followed by *beak*-type. *Linear-type* and *nodular*-type were relatively rare subtypes [6].

Computed tomography (CT), probably the most suitable modality to identify the ossified lesions, allows us precise evaluation of T-OPLL and T-OLF no matter what superimposition of the thoracic complexities [1, 2, 7].

The ligamentum flavum is a connective tissue that is attached to the posterior side of the caudal lamina and the anterior side of the rostrally adjacent lamina [8]. Therefore, when the ligamentum flavum is replaced by ectopic ossification (OLF), its morphology should be V-shaped or a part of V-shape on axial CT images. Thus, using preoperative CT images, OLF was classified into five subtypes: *lateral*, *extended*, *enlarged*, *fused*, and *tuberous* according to the morphological features of OLF (Fig. 19.3) [9, 10]. In addition to these ossified lesions, we sometimes encounter a mushroom-shaped ossification mimicking an osteochondroma localized at the center of laminae (Fig. 19.4). Mori et al. histologically revealed that this mushroom-shaped ossification localized at the center of lamina was OLF and designated it as *central* type [1]. Accordingly, OLF was classified into five subtypes: *small*, *medium*, *large*, *extra-large*, and *central* types according to the size and morphology (Fig. 19.5) [1].

In clinical practice, dural defect/ossification is one of the serious concerns. Two CT findings that seemed to indicate possible dural ossification in cervical OPLL were reported [11]. One

	Hook	Beak	Linear	Nodular
Typical appearance	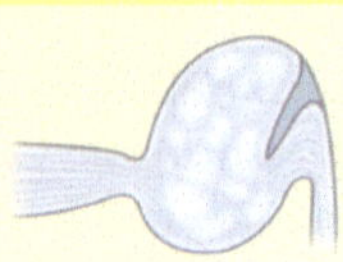	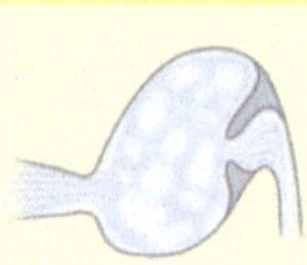	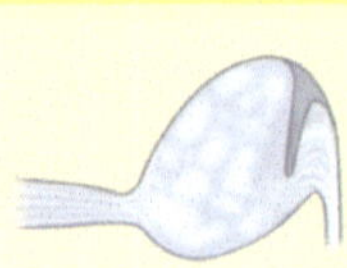	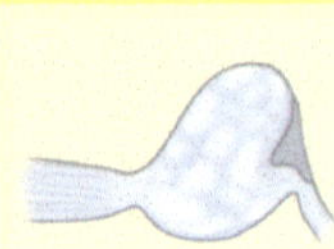
Percent	65.5	17.7	8.4	8.4

Fig. 19.2 OLF classification on X-ray

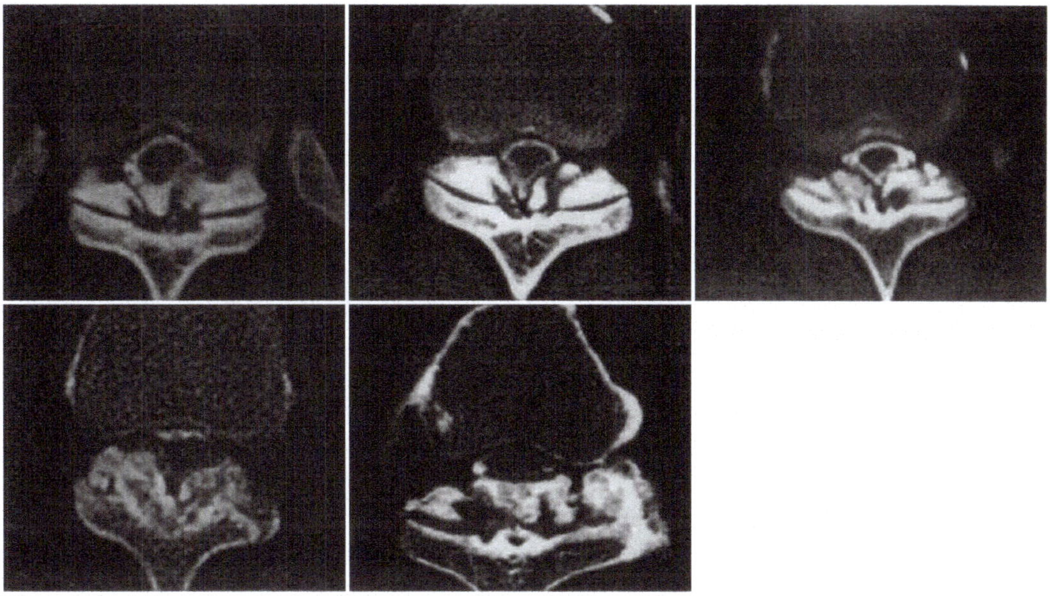

Fig. 19.3 Thoracic OLF classification on computed tomography

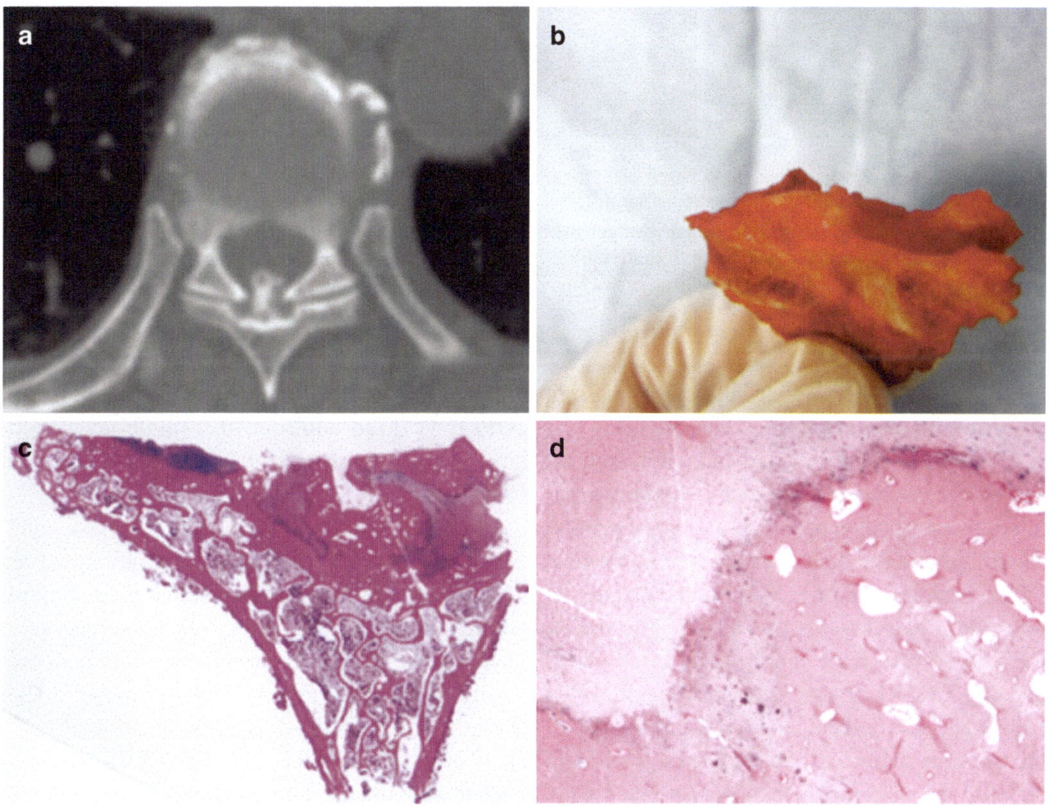

Fig. 19.4 Thoracic OLF classification (central type) by Mori et al. axial image of CT (**a**), macroscopic (**b**), and microscopic (**c**, **d**) images of resected central type OLF specimen

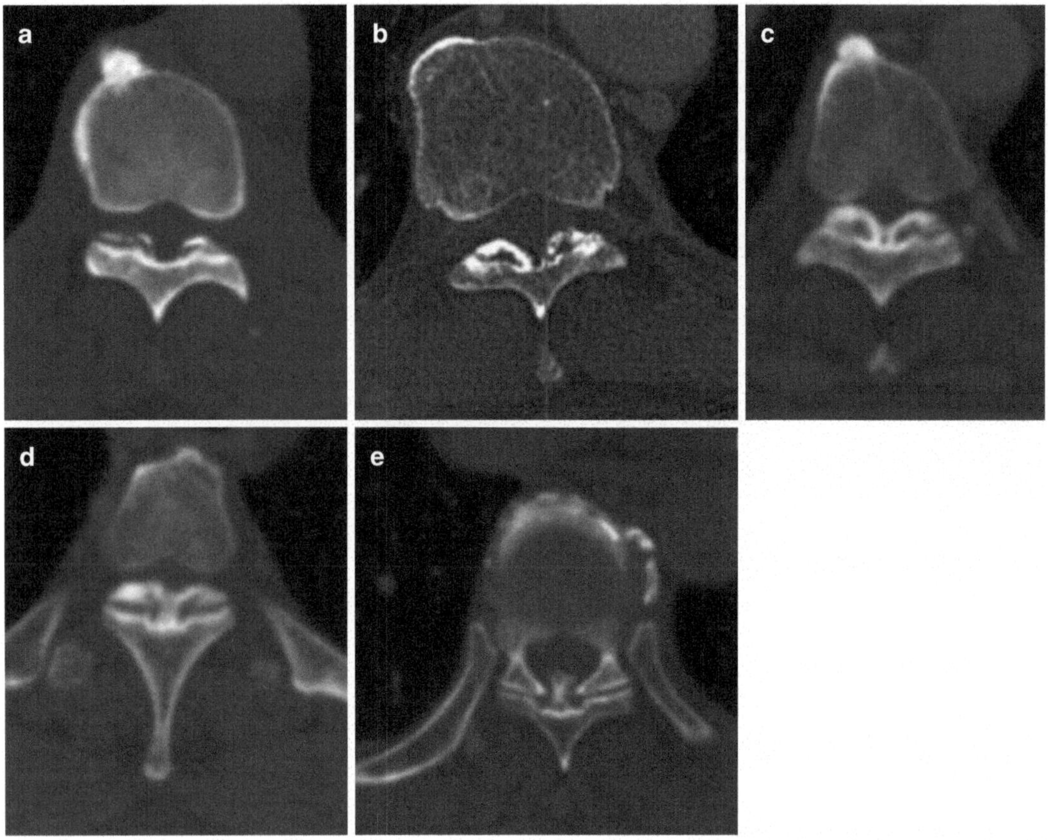

Fig. 19.5 Thoracic OLF classification based on CT. (**a**) *Small*: a clear ossification but smaller than 3 mm in its thickness. (**b**) *Medium*: an ossification that is larger than 3 mm in thickness but smaller than 1/4 of the anteroposterior diameter of the spinal canal. (**c**) *Large*: an ossification larger than one-fourth of the anteroposterior diameter of the spinal canal. (**d**) *Huge*: an ossification larger than half of the anteroposterior diameter. (**e**) *Central*: a mushroom-shaped ossification localized at the center of laminae

is the single-layer sign that indicates a mass of uniformly hyperdense OPLL and the other one is the double-layer sign that indicates anterior and posterior rims of hyperdense regions separated by a hypodense area. Previous reports suggested that the double-layer sign in cervical OPLL is more predictive of a focal dural defect than the single-layer sign [11–13]. However, these two signs have rarely been investigated into the T-OPLL. In the retrospective study by Min et al., dural defects were present in 60% of the patients with a double-layer sign and in 50% of the patients with a single-layer sign, respectively [13]. In T-OPLL, the incidences of these signs were higher than that of cervical OPLL [13]. In addition, the single-layer sign may be as important as the double-layer sign in T-OPLL.

In OLF, "tram tack sign" [14], "comma sign" [14], and "bridge sign" [15] were advocated as characteristic imaging findings that predict dural ossification. The tram tack sign is defined as a hyperdense bony excrescence with a hypodense center (Fig. 19.6; Fig. 19.1 of Li's paper). The comma sign is defined as an ossification of one-half of the dura mater (Fig. 19.6). Ossified dura mater and ligamentum flavum fused to be the head of the "comma" and its tail indicated the

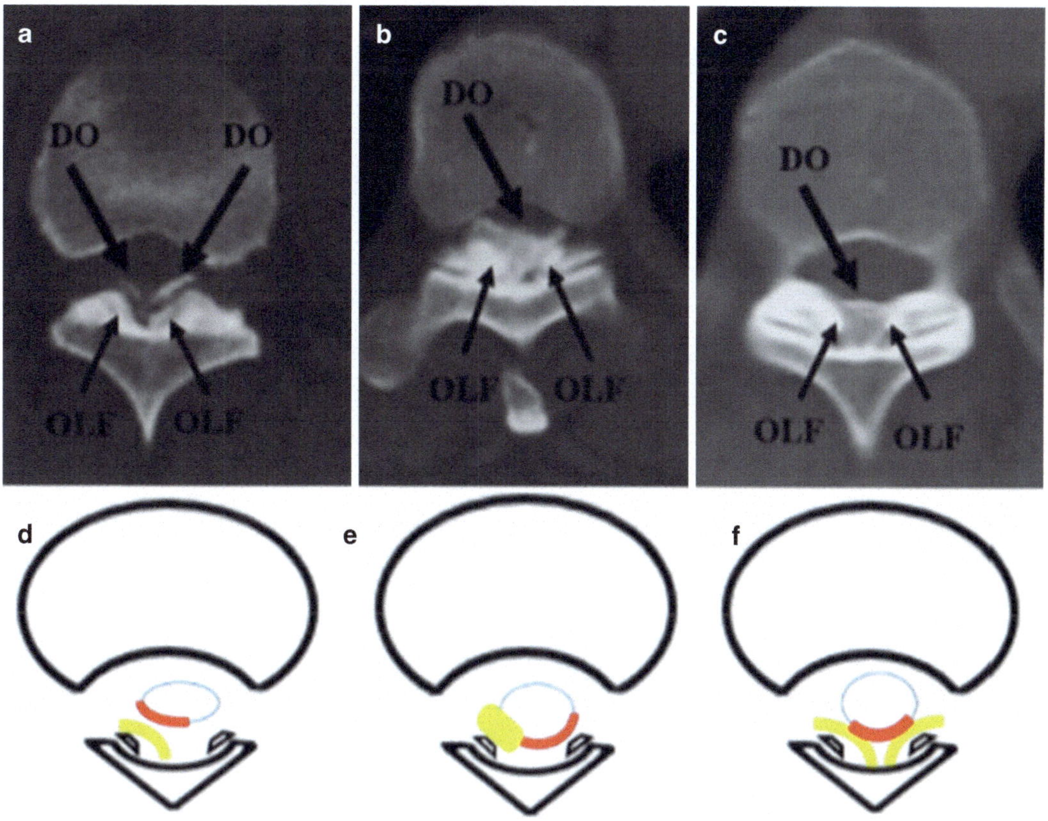

Fig. 19.6 CT imaging findings predicting dural ossification in OLF. (**a**, **d**) tram track sign, (**b**, **e**) comma sign and (**c**, **f**) bridge sign

dural ossification extended to the lateral and/or ventral side. The bridge sign is defined as a hyperdense bony bridge between bilateral OLF (Fig. 19.6).

Myelography is useful to evaluate spinal canal stenosis due to OPLL and/or OLF in the whole spine as well as the dynamic factor. Combination CT with myelography (CT-myelography) helps us for surgical planning of removal/floating of the ossified lesions.

Magnetic resonance (MR) imaging is useful to evaluate not only the extent of spinal cord compression, but also the intensity change of spinal cord due to compression by T-OPLL and T-OLF. However, MR imaging cannot distinguish between ossifications of the spinal ligaments and hypertrophied spinal ligaments.

Two types of intramedullary signal intensity changes were identified on MRI: one is normal intense in T1/hyperintense in T2-weighted image representing spinal cord edema, inflammation, ischemia, or myelomalacia (Fig. 19.7a) [16] and hypointense in T1/hyperintense in T2-weighted image representing cystic necrosis or syrinx (Fig. 19.7b) [17]. Several researchers advocated that the presence of signal intensity changes did not correlate with postoperative recovery [18–20]. However, the signal intensity ratio on T2-weighted image [21] and intramedullary signal size [22] are advocated as potentially useful for the prediction of surgical outcomes in patients with thoracic OLF.

It is important to make a correct diagnosis of T-OPLL as well as T-OLF using multiple diagnostic imaging modalities.

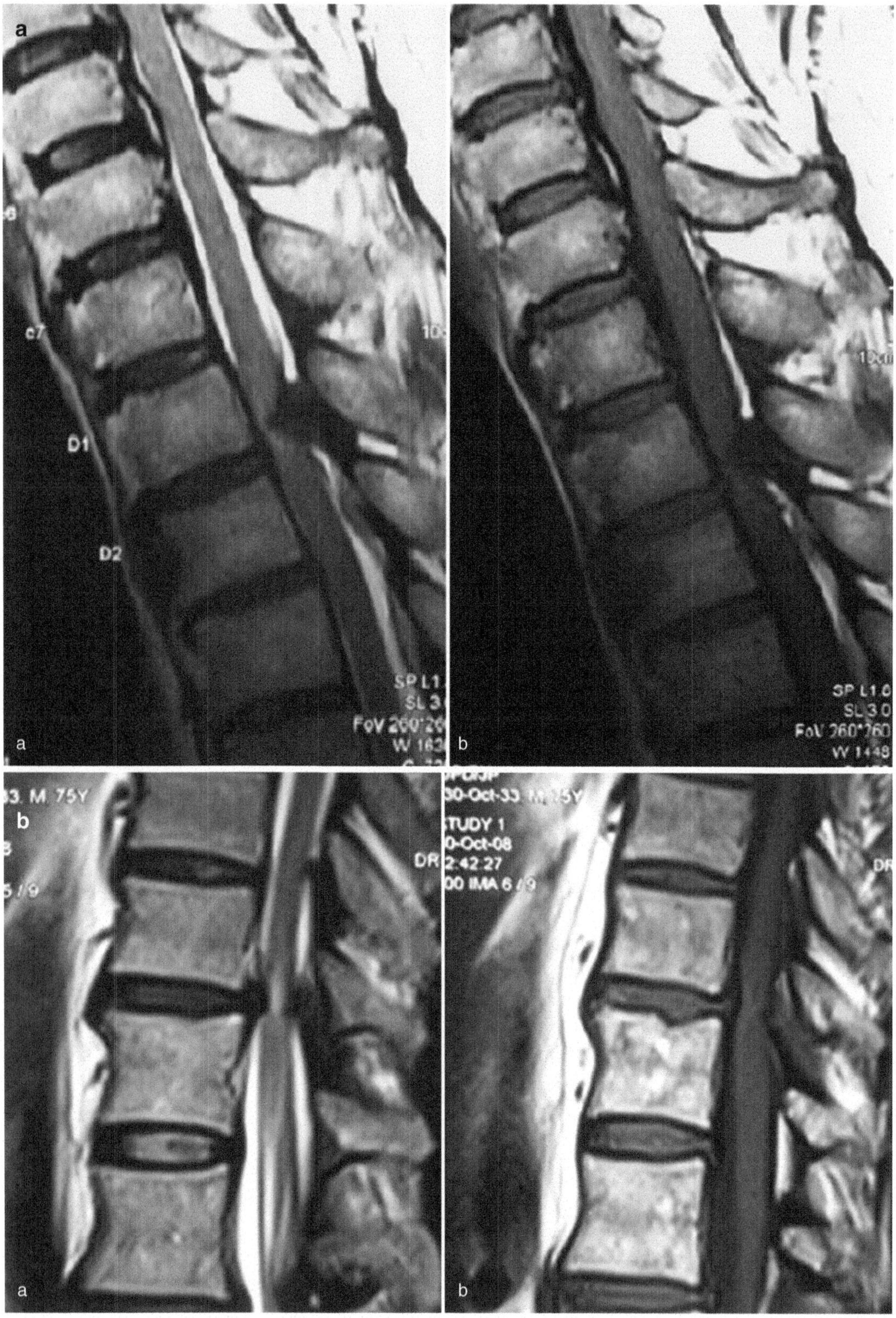

Fig. 19.7 Intramedullary intensity change due to thoracic OLF on magnetic resonance imaging. (**a**) Normal intense in T1/hyperintense in T2-weighted image representing spinal cord edema, inflammation, ischemia, or myelomalacia. (**b**) Hypointense in T1/hyperintense in T2-weighted image representing cystic necrosis or syrinx

References

1. Mori K, Kasahara T, Mimura T, Nishizawa K, Murakami Y, Matsusue Y, Imai S. Prevalence, distribution and morphology of thoracic ossification of the yellow ligament in Japanese: results of CT-based cross-sectional study. Spine (Phila Pa 1976). 2013;38(19):E1216–22.
2. Mori K, Imai S, Kasahara T, Nishizawa K, Mimura T, Matsusue Y. Prevalence, Distribution, and Morphology of Thoracic Ossification of the Posterior Longitudinal Ligament in Japanese: Results of CT-Based Cross-sectional Study. Spine (Phila Pa 1976). 2014;39(5):394–9.
3. Yonenobu K, Sakou T, Ono K, editors. OPLL. Tokyo: Springer–Verlag; 1997.
4. Matsuyama Y, Yoshihara H, Tsuji T, Sakai Y, Yukawa Y, Nakamura H, Ito K, Ishiguro N. Surgical outcome of ossification of the posterior longitudinal ligament (OPLL) of the thoracic spine: implication of the type of ossification and surgical options. J Spinal Disord Tech. 2005;18(6):492–7.. discussion 498
5. Epstein NE. The surgical management of ossification of the posterior longitudinal ligament in 43 North Americans. Spine (Phila Pa 1976). 1994;19(6):664–72.
6. Kudo S, Ono M, Russell WJ. Ossification of thoracic ligamenta flava. AJR Am J Roentgenol. 1983;141:117–21.
7. Hirai T, Yoshii T, Iwanami A, Takeuchi K, Mori K, Yamada T, Wada K, Koda M, Matsuyama Y, Takeshita K, Abematsu M, Haro H, Watanabe M, Watanabe K, Ozawa H, Kanno H, Imagama S, Fujibayashi S, Yamazaki M, Matsumoto M, Nakamura M, Okawa A, Kawaguchi Y. Prevalence and Distribution of Ossified Lesions in the Whole Spine of Patients with Cervical Ossification of the Posterior Longitudinal Ligament A Multicenter Study (JOSL CT study). PLoS One. 2016;11(8):e0160117.
8. Stollman A, Pinto R, Benjamin V, Kricheff I. Radiologic imaging of symptomatic ligamentum flavum thickening with and without ossification. AJNR Am J Neuroradiol. 1987;8(6):991–4.
9. Sato T, Kokubun S, Tanaka Y, Ishii Y. Thoracic myelopathy in the Japanese: epidemiological and clinical observations on the cases in Miyagi prefecture. Tohoku J Exp Med. 1998;184(1):1–11.
10. Miyakoshi N, Shimada Y, Suzuki T, Hongo M, Kasukawa Y, Okada K, Itoi E. Factors related to long-term outcome after decompressive surgery for ossification of the ligamentum flavum of the thoracic spine. J Neurosurg. 2003;99(3 Suppl):251–6.
11. Hida K, Iwasaki Y, Koyanagi I, Abe H. Bone window computed tomography for detection of dural defect associated with cervical ossified posterior longitudinal ligament. Neurol Med Chir (Tokyo). 1997;37:173–6.
12. Min JH, Jang JS, Lee SH. Significance of the double-layer and single-layer signs in the ossification of the posterior longitudinal ligament of the cervical spine. J Neurosurg Spine. 2007;6(4):309–12.
13. Min JH, Jang JS, Lee SH. Significance of the double- and single-layer signs in the ossification of the posterior longitudinal ligament of the thoracic spine. Neurosurgery. 2007;61(1):118–21.. discussion 121–122
14. Muthukumar N. Dural ossification in ossification of the ligamentum flavum: a preliminary report. Spine (Phila Pa 1976). 2009;34(24):2654–61.
15. Li B, Qiu G, Guo S, Li W, Li Y, Peng H, Wang C, Zhao Y. Dural ossification associated with ossification of ligamentum flavum in the thoracic spine: a retrospective analysis. BMJ Open. 2016;6(12):e013887.
16. Mehalic TF, Pezzuti RT, Applebaum BI. Magnetic resonance imaging and cervical spondylotic myelopathy. Neurosurgery. 1990;26(2):217–26.
17. Al-Mefty O, Harkey LH, Middleton TH, Smith RR, Fox JL. Myelopathic cervical spondylotic lesions demonstrated by magnetic resonance imaging. J Neurosurg. 1988;68(2):217–22.
18. Shiokawa K, Hanakita J, Suwa H, Saiki M, Oda M, Kajiwara M. Clinical analysis and prognostic study of ossified ligamentum flavum of the thoracic spine. J Neurosurg. 2001;94(2 Suppl):221–6.
19. Kuh SU, Kim YS, Cho YE, Jin BH, Kim KS, Yoon YS, et al. Contributing factors affecting the prognosis surgical outcome for thoracic OLF. Eur Spine J. 2006;15:485–91.
20. Kawaguchi Y, Yasuda T, Seki S, Nakano M, Kanamori M, Sumi S, Kimura T. Variables affecting postsurgical prognosis of thoracic myelopathy caused by ossification of the ligamentum flavum. Spine J. 2013;13(9):1095–107.
21. Zhang J, Wang L, Li J, et al. Predictors of surgical outcome in thoracic ossification of the ligamentum flavum: focusing on the quantitative signal intensity. Sci Rep. 2016;6:23019.
22. Sanghvi AV, Chhabra HS, Mascarenhas AA, Mittal VK, Sangondimath GM. Thoracic myelopathy due to ossification of ligamentum flavum: a retrospective analysis of predictors of surgical outcome and factors affecting preoperative neurological status. Eur Spine J. 2011;20(2):205–15.

20 Biomechanics of the Spinal Cord Compression Due to Cervical Ossification of the Posterior Longitudinal Ligament

Norihiro Nishida, Yasuaki Imajo, Hidenori Suzuki, Masahiro Funaba, and Takashi Sakai

Abstract

Cervical myelopathy due to ossification of the posterior longitudinal ligament (OPLL) is induced by static factors, dynamic factors, or a combination of both. And decompression procedures for cervical OPLL are anterior decompression with fusion, laminoplasty, and posterior decompression with fusion. We used a three-dimensional finite element method (3D-FEM) to analyze the stress distributions in the cervical spinal cord under static compression, dynamic compression, or a combination of both in the context of OPLL, and preoperative and postoperative stress analyses.

Keywords

Cervical ossification of the posterior longitudinal ligament (C-OPLL) · Dynamic factors
Static factors · Finite element method (FEM)
Intervertebral mobility

N. Nishida (✉) · Y. Imajo · H. Suzuki · M. Funaba
T. Sakai
Department of Orthopedic Surgery, Yamaguchi University Graduate School of Medicine, Yamaguchi, Japan
e-mail: nishida3@yamaguchi-u.ac.jp; i-yasuak@yamaguchi-u.ac.jp; hsuzuki@yamaguchi-u.ac.jp; cozy@yamaguchi-u.ac.jp

20.1 Introduction

Cervical ossification of the posterior longitudinal ligament (C-OPLL) is recognized as a common clinical entity that causes complicated myelopathy of the cervical spinal cord. It is believed that myelopathy develops due to compression of the spine by C-OPLL. However, some patients with little ossification exhibit myelopathy, whereas others with marked ossification do not. Thus, static factors alone cannot account for myelopathy [1]. Dynamic factors such as mobility of the spinal column are also important in the development of cervical myelopathy [1–4]. However, the contribution of dynamic factors to the development of myelopathy in C-OPLL patients has not been fully determined [5]. C-OPLL myelopathy is therefore likely to be induced by static factors, dynamic factors, or a combination of both [6, 7].

The surgical procedures applied to this disease are broadly divided into anterior decompression with fusion and posterior decompression, which is typified by laminoplasty [3, 8]. Anterior decompression with fusion is technically difficult and is also reported to cause complications, especially when multiple vertebrae are operated. However, because it technically facilitates laminoplasty and also achieves favorable outcomes in many cases, the procedure is often selected [5, 9–11]. Meanwhile, in cases of high residual anterior compression or a mobile spinal cord at the high level of cord compression, laminoplasty alone is not adequate to control postoperative

A. Okawa et al. (eds.), *OPLL*, https://doi.org/10.1007/978-981-15-3855-1_20

kyphotic changes. There are also reports that better outcomes are achieved by anterior decompression with fusion or posterior decompression combined with instrumented fusion [3, 5, 12, 13].

In the present study, we used a three-dimensional finite element method (3D-FEM) to analyze the stress distributions of cervical spinal cord under static compression, dynamic compression, and a combination of both in the context of OPLL. And, using the same models, the effects of posterior decompression for C-OPLL, as well as the effects of the presence of residual compression and instability on the cervical spinal cord, were evaluated.

20.2 Material and Methods

The ABAQUS 6.11 (Valley Street, Providence, RI, USA) finite element package was used for FEM simulation. The 3D-FEM spinal cord model used in this study consisted of gray matter, white matter, and pia mater (Fig. 20.1). In order to simplify calculation in the model, the denticulate ligament, dura, and nerve root sheaths were not included. The pia mater was included since it has been demonstrated that spinal cord with and without this component shows significantly different mechanical behavior [14]. The spinal cord was assumed to be symmetrical about the mid-sagittal plane, such that only half the spinal cord

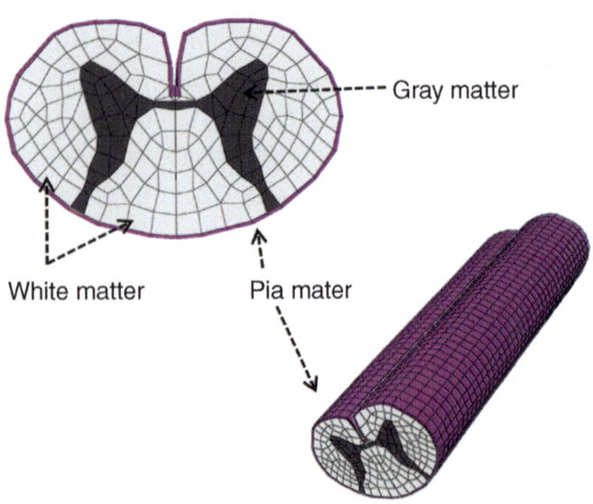

Fig. 20.1 The three-dimensional finite element method (3D-FEM) model of the spinal cord consists of gray matter, white matter, and pia mater

required reconstruction and the whole model could be integrated by a mirror image. The vertical length of spinal cord for CTM measurement was two vertebral bodies (about 40 mm).

Iwasaki et al. reported that neurological outcomes following laminoplasty for cervical OPLL were only poor or fair in patients with an occupying ratio > 60% and/or hill-shaped ossification [11]. The rigid, hill-shaped body with a slope of 30° was used to simulate C-OPLL by measuring paper (Fig. 20.2a) [11]. To assume a segmental range of motion (ROM) at the level of maximum cord compression, the center of the hill-shaped OPLL was established with discontinuity. In addition, upper and lower edges of the hill-shaped OPLL were matched to the posterior upper and lower edges of the vertebral body (Fig. 20.2a).

The lamina model was established by measuring CTM, MRI, and simulated C-OPLL (Fig. 20.2b).

The spinal cord consists of three distinct materials referred to as white matter, gray matter, and pia mater. The mechanical properties (Young's modulus and Poisson's ratio) of the gray and white matter were determined using data obtained by the tensile stress strain curve and stress relaxation under various strain rates [15, 16]. The mechanical properties of the pia mater were obtained from the literature [17]. The mechanical properties of the hill-shaped ossification and lamina were stiff enough for the spinal cord to be pressed. Based on the assumption that no slippage occurs at the interfaces of white matter, gray matter, and pia mater, these interfaces were glued together. Since there are no data on the friction coefficient between lamina and spinal cord, this was assumed to be frictionless. Similarly, the coefficient of friction between the hill-shaped ossification and spinal cord was assumed to be frictionless at the contact interfaces.

The spinal cord, hill-shaped ossification, and the lamina model were symmetrically meshed with 15- or 20-node elements. The total number of elements was 11,438, and the total number of nodes was 67,434.

For the static compression model (the preoperative model), compression was simulated by C-OPLL with a hill-shaped ossification. The top

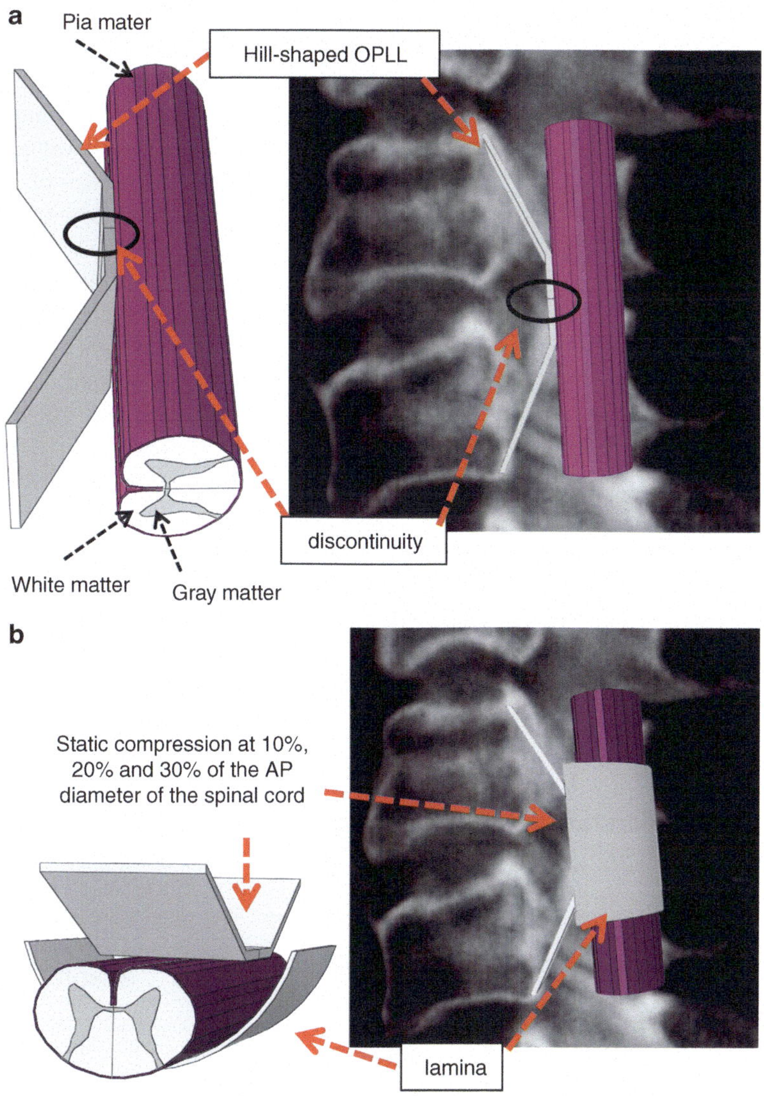

Fig. 20.2 (**a**) A rigid, hill-shaped body with a slope of 30° was used to simulate C-OPLL. The center of the hill-shaped OPLL established discontinuity. In addition, the upper and lower edges of the hill-shaped OPLL were set to match the posterior upper and lower edges of the vertebral body. The center of the hill-shaped OPLL showed an established discontinuity. (**b**) The lamina model was established at the rear of the spinal cord. For the static model (the preoperative model), anterior static compression at 10%, 20%, and 30% of the AP diameter of the spinal cord was applied to the spinal cord by the OPLL

and bottom of the spinal cord and the lamina were fixed in all directions and then the anterior static compression at 10%, 20%, and 30% of the anterior-posterior diameter of the spinal cord was applied by the OPLL (Fig. 20.2b).

For the dynamic compression model, the top and bottom of the spinal cord as well as the lamina were fixed. The lower and upper edges of the OPLL were rotated 2.5° (total 5°), 5° (total 10°), and 7.5° (total 15°) to the flexion direction as a segmental range of motion (ROM) to match the movement of the vertebral body without anterior static compression by OPLL (Fig. 20.3).

For the combined static (10%) and dynamic compression model under fixed of for the cranial and caudal of the spinal cord and lamina, static compression to the spinal cord of 10% of the anterior-posterior diameter of the spinal cord was applied by OPLL. In this state of compression, the lower and upper edges were rotated 2.5° (total 5°), 5° (total 10°), and 7.5° (total 15°) to the flexion direction as ROM (Fig. 20.4).

For the combined static (20%) and dynamic compression model under fixed of for the cranial and caudal of the spinal cord and lamina, static compression to the spinal cord of 20%

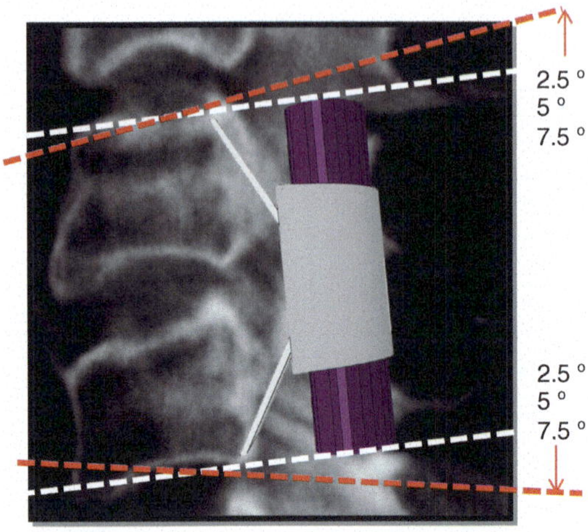

Fig. 20.3 For the dynamic compression model, the lower and upper edges of OPLL were rotated at 2.5° (total 5°), 5° (total 10°), and 7.5° (total 15°) to the flexion direction as the ROM

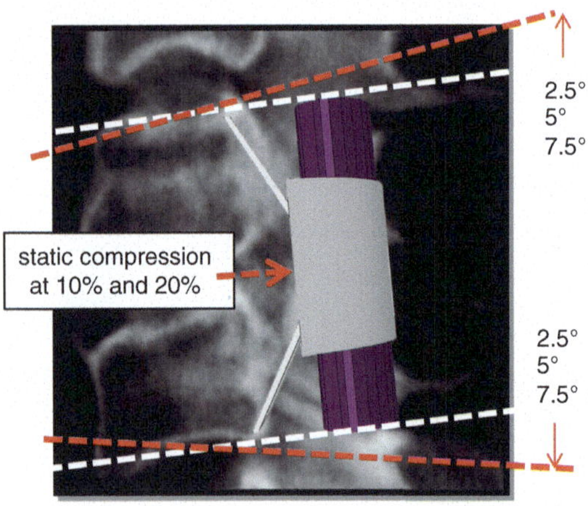

Fig. 20.4 For the combined static and dynamic model, anterior static compression was 10% and 20% of the AP diameter of the spinal cord and the lower and upper edges of OPLL were rotated at 2.5° (total 5°), 5° (total 10°), and 7.5° (total 15°) to the flexion direction as the ROM

of the anterior-posterior diameter of the spinal cord was applied by OPLL. In this state of compression, the lower and upper edges were rotated 2.5° (total 5°), 5° (total 10°), and 7.5° (total 15°) to the flexion direction as ROM (Fig. 20.4).

The posterior decompression with fusion model was developed by shifting the vertebral arch backwards, while 10%, 20%, or 30% compression was applied to the spinal cord, and the spinal cord was hypothesized not to move after surgery (Fig. 20.5a).

The post-decompression advanced kyphosis model was developed by displacing the spinal cord in kyphosis of 10°, while 10%, 20%, or 30% anterior compression was applied to the spinal cord after the vertebral arch was shifted. Because Henderson reported that stretch injury of the spinal cord is caused when it is displaced in kyphosis and stretched out, the spinal cord was stretched by 20% toward the head and in the direction of kyphosis (Fig. 20.5b) [18].

Furthermore, to develop the post-decompression advanced kyphosis+intervertebral mobility model, while 10%, 20%, or 30% anterior compression was applied to the spinal cord after the vertebral arch was shifted, the spinal cord was displaced in kyphosis of 10°. Then, to add mobility comparable to that of the vertebral body, each of the upper and lower margins of the OPLL site was moved in the direction of flexion by 2.5° (total 5°), 5° (total 10°), and 7.5° (total 15°) (Fig. 20.5c).

In total, 27 different compression combinations were evaluated and the average *von Mises* stress was recorded for each cross section.

20.3 Results

In the static compression model (the preoperative model), stresses were very low under the condition of 10% compression of the AP diameter of the spinal cord. At 20% compression, the stress distributions were confined to gray matter and the anterior funiculus. At 30% compression, the stresses on gray matter, anterior funiculus, lateral funiculus, and posterior funiculus were all increased (Fig. 20.6a).

For the dynamic compression model with 5° ROM, stresses on the spinal cord were very low. A 5° ROM corresponds to approximately 9% compression of the AP diameter of the spinal cord at the maximal compression site. At 10° ROM, stress distributions were confined to the gray matter and the anterior funiculus. A 10°

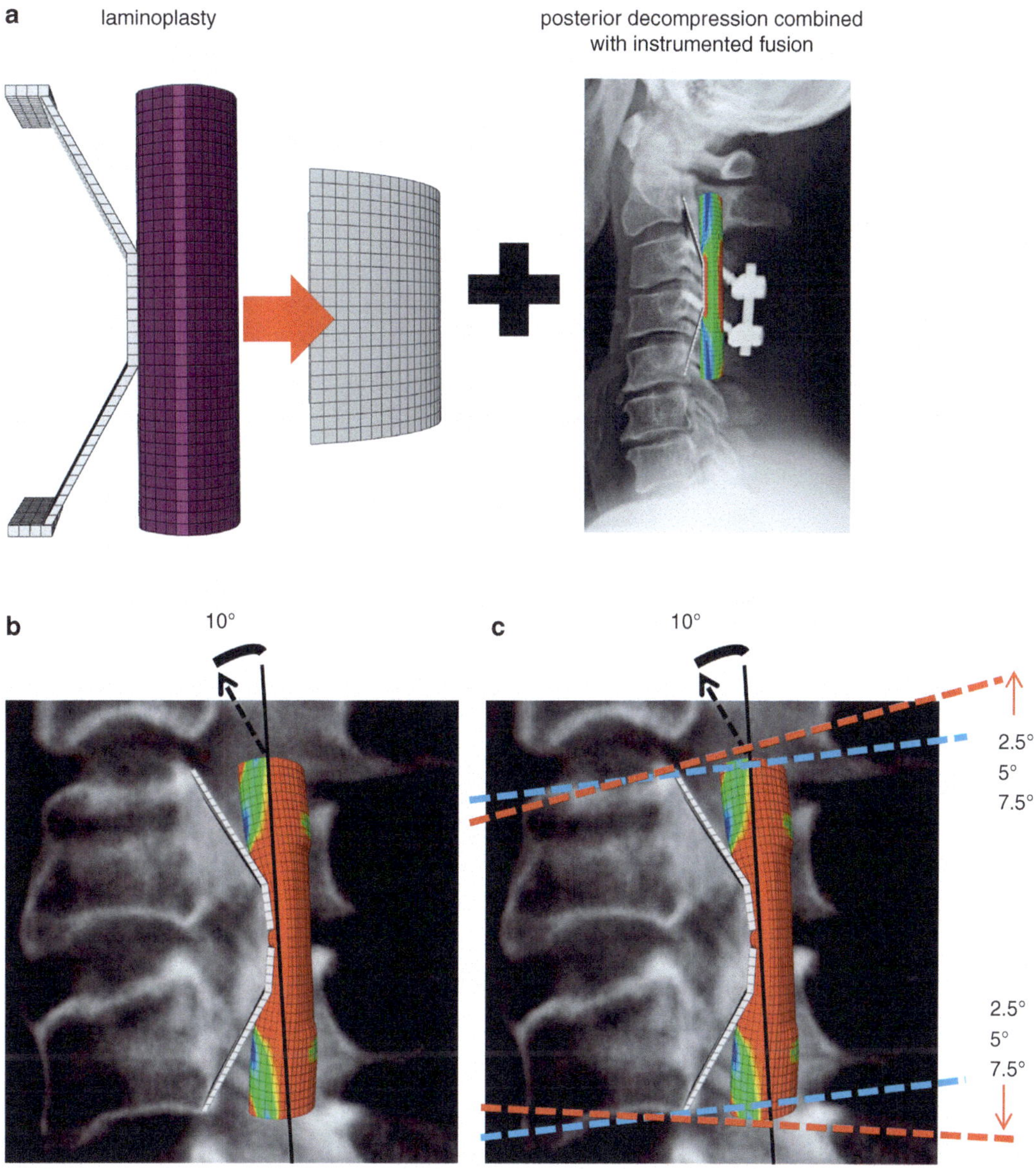

Fig. 20.5 The posterior decompression with fusion model was developed by shifting the vertebral arch backwards, while 10%, 20%, or 30% compression was applied to the spinal cord, and the spinal cord was hypothesized not to move after surgery (**a**). The post-decompression advanced kyphosis model was developed by displacing the spinal cord in kyphosis of 10°, while 10%, 20%, or 30% anterior compression was applied to the spinal cord after the vertebral arch was shifted (**b**). Furthermore, to develop the post-decompression advanced kyphosis+intervertebral mobility model, while 10%, 20%, or 30% anterior compression was applied to the spinal cord after the vertebral arch was shifted, the spinal cord was displaced in kyphosis of 10°. Then, to add mobility comparable to that of the vertebral body, each of the upper and lower margins of the OPLL site was moved in the direction of flexion by 2.5° (total 5°), 5° (total 10°), and 7.5° (total 15°) (**c**)

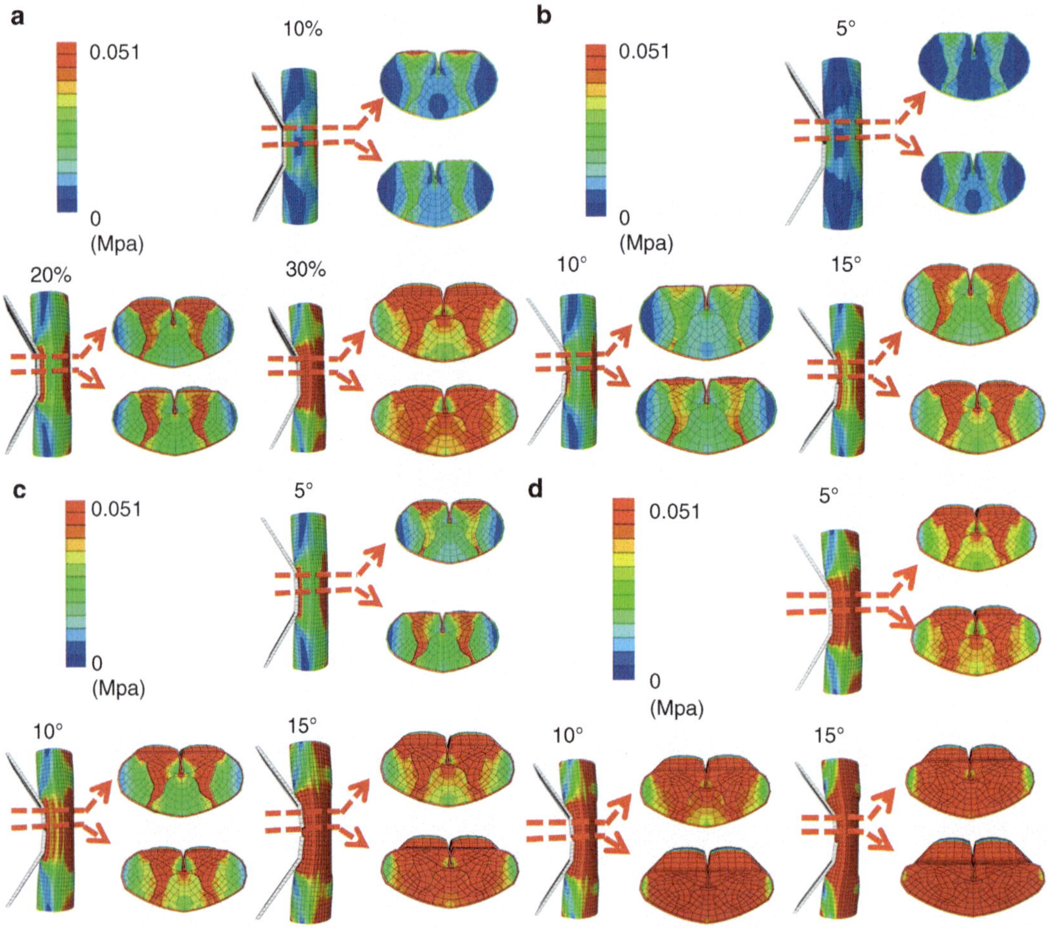

Fig. 20.6 Stress distributions in proximal and central area of compression by C-OPLL are shown for the static compression model (**a**), the dynamic compression model (**b**), the combined static (10%) and dynamic compression model (**c**), and the combined static (20%) and dynamic compression model (**d**)

ROM corresponds to about 16% compression of the AP diameter of the spinal cord at the maximal compression site. The stresses increased at 15° ROM, which corresponds to about 25% compression of the AP diameter of the spinal cord at the maximal compression site (Fig. 20.6b).

For the combined static (10%) and dynamic compression model, at 5° ROM, the stress distributions were higher than for 10% static compression alone, but were still quite low. This corresponded to about 19% compression of the AP diameter of the spinal cord at the maximal compression site. At 10° ROM, stress appeared in the gray matter and anterior funiculus, while at 15° ROM the stresses on gray matter, anterior funiculus, lateral funiculus, and posterior funiculus all increased. A 10° ROM corresponds to approximately 26% compression of the AP diameter of the spinal cord at the maximal compression site while a 15° ROM corresponds to about 35% compression (Fig. 20.6c).

For the combined static (20%) and dynamic compression model, at 5° ROM the stress distributions were higher than for 20% static compression alone. At 10° ROM, stresses appeared in the spinal cord and increased further at 15° ROM (Fig. 20.6d). A 5° ROM corresponds to about 29% compression of the AP diameter of the spinal cord at the maximal compression site, 10° ROM corresponds to about 36% compression, and 15° ROM corresponds to about 45% compression.

In the posterior decompression with fusion model, stress decreased in comparison to the preoperative compression model. However, when 20% and 30% compression persisted in the spinal cord, stress persisted at the ventral and dorsal sides of the spinal cord (Fig. 20.7a).

In the kyphosis model, only a mild increase in stress was observed in the gray matter and the posterior funiculus when 10% compression was applied to the spinal cord. However, stress increased in the anterior and posterior funiculus when 20% compression was applied to the spinal cord. When 30% compression was applied, stress also increased in the lateral funiculus (Fig. 20.7b).

In the post-decompression advanced kyphosis+intervertebral mobility model (5°), stress increased in the gray matter and the posterior funiculus when 10% compression was applied to the spinal cord, and intraspinal stress increased more than in the advanced kyphosis model when 20% and 30% compression was applied (Fig. 20.8a). As intervertebral mobility increased to 10° and 15°, intraspinal stress increased even with 10% residual compression in the spinal cord. Intraspinal stress increased according to degrees of residual compression and intervertebral mobility (Fig. 20.8b, c).

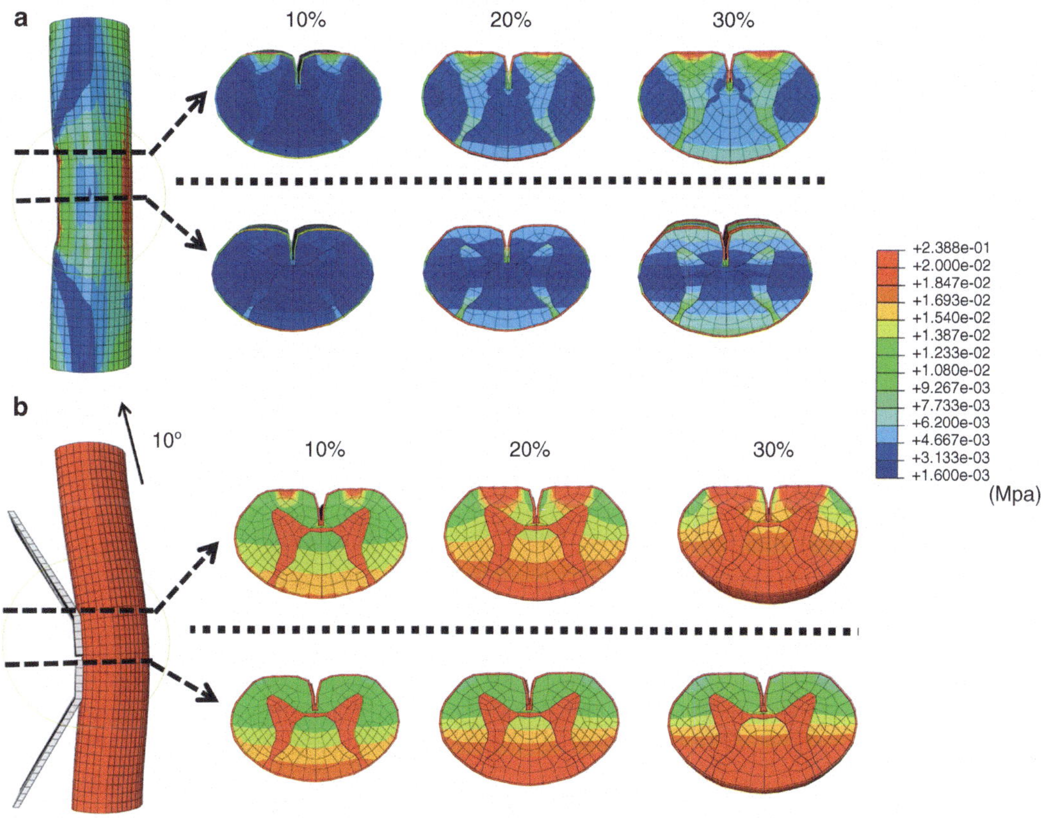

Fig. 20.7 (**a**) Posterior decompression with fusion model. With posterior decompression, the stress in the spinal cord decreased, but the stress distribution still remained under a compression of 20% and 30%. (**b**) Post-decompression advanced kyphosis model. With advancing kyphosis, the stress distribution in the posterior fuliculus and in the gray matter of the spinal cord increased. Intraspinal stress increased according to the degree of residual compression

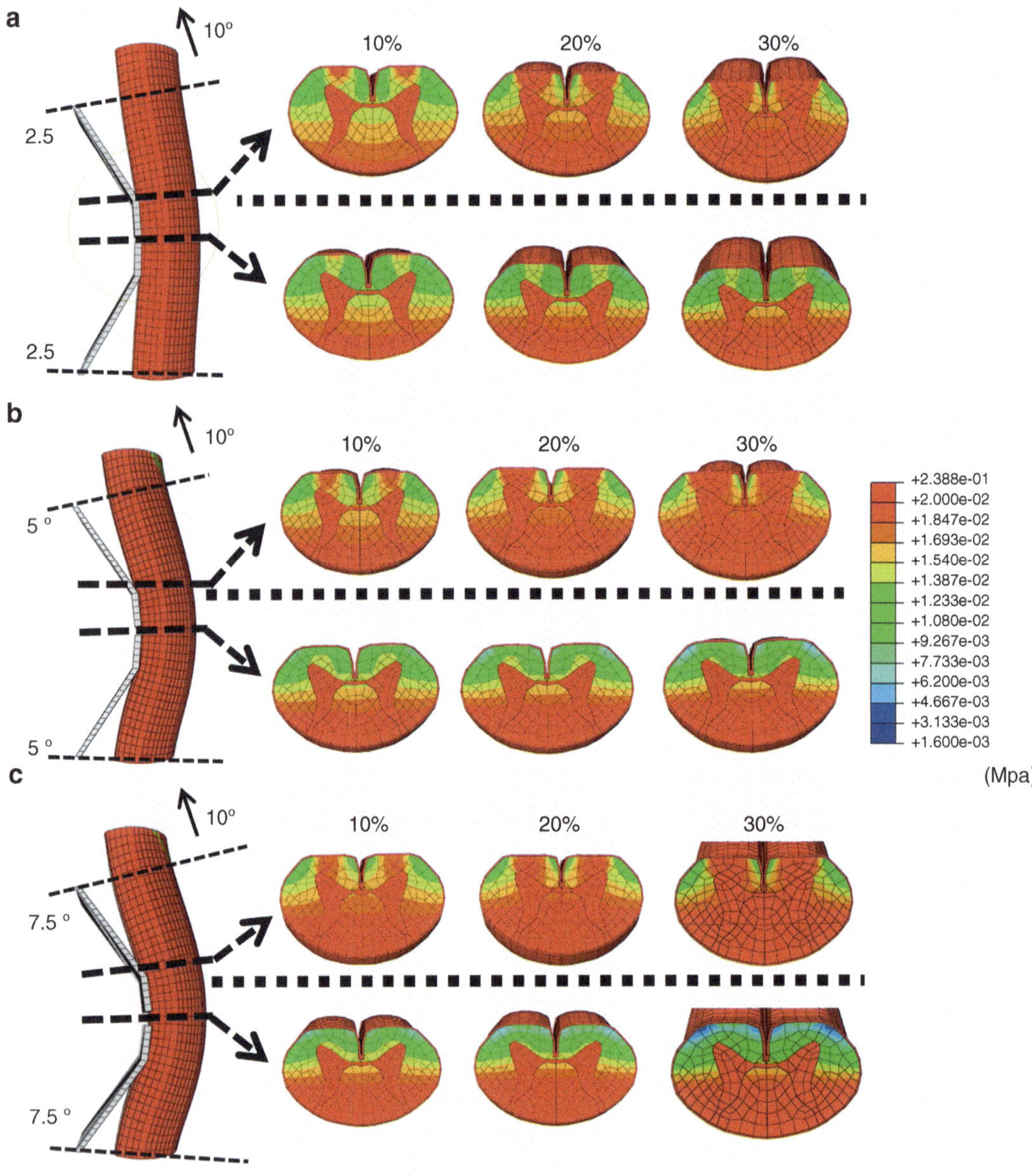

Fig. 20.8 (**a**). Post-decompression advanced kyphosis+intervertebral mobility model (5°). (**b**) Post-decompression advanced kyphosis+intervertebral mobility model (10°). (**c**) Post-decompression advanced kyphosis+intervertebral mobility model (15°). Intraspinal stress increased more than in the advanced kyphosis model. As intervertebral mobility increased to 10° and 15°, the intraspinal stress increased even with 10% residual compression in the spinal cord. Intraspinal stress increased according to the extent of residual compression and intervertebral mobility

20.4 Discussion

The development of myelopathy significantly affects the prognosis of patients with OPLL in the cervical spine. Matsunaga et al. reported that when the space available for the spinal cord (SAC, static compression factor) was <6 mm, this could induce myelopathy of the cervical spine [1]. Koyanagi et al. reported that the proportion of patients showing motor deficits of the lower extremities increased significantly when the sagittal canal diameter of CT was narrowed to <8 mm [19]. Matsunaga et al. further reported that all patients with >60% spinal canal stenosis due to OPLL exhibited myelopathy [7]. These findings indicate that static compression is an important factor in myelopathy associated with C-OPLL and that pathologic compression beyond a certain critical point may indeed be the most significant causal factor. Prior to these studies it was believed that dynamic factors were largely responsible for the development of myelopathy associated with C-OPLL. Matsunaga et al. found that ROM of the cervical spine was significantly greater in patients with myelopathy and whose SAC diameter was >6 mm [1]. Azuma et al. concluded that C-OPLL myelopathy was induced by static factors, dynamic factors, or a combination of both. To evaluate the contribution of each factor and the responsible level, they measured SAC and ROM at each vertebral and intervertebral level and determined the responsible level by spinal cord-evoked potentials (SCEPs) [6]. Fujiyoshi et al. reported that patients with massive OPLL did not develop myelopathy and the mobility of their cervical spine was highly restricted [5]. These workers concluded that dynamic factors such as segmental ROM preferentially contributed to the development of myelopathy in patients with C-OPLL.

In general, three types of surgical procedures are mainly performed for the treatment of C-OPLL: anterior decompression with fusion, laminoplasty, and posterior decompression with fusion. Because compression caused by C-OPLL is located in an ossification lesion in the anterior part, anterior decompression with fusion, in which complete decompression is attempted, is theoretically the best option [20, 21]. However, because it is technically difficult and also causes complications, such as airway edema, displacement of a bone graft, and pain at the site of bone graft harvest, the technically easier laminoplasty is selected more often [3, 22]. Laminoplasty is a procedure to indirectly decompress the posterior part, but there are also reports that outcomes are poor in some cases of OPLL with an occupying ratio of 50% or more, and some cases of high intervertebral mobility at the level of maximum cord compression [3, 12]. The poor outcomes may be due to failure to relieve residual anterior compression or because the presence of residual mobility after the procedure leads to repeated occurrence of injury to the spinal cord or enhanced kyphosis [3, 5]. Fujiyoshi et al. defined the line connecting the center of the vertebral canal to cervical vertebrae 2–7 as the K-line on a lateral cervical radiograph and regarded a case of OPLL exceeding the K-line as K-line (−). When posterior decompression is performed in cases of residual compression, K-line (-) cases, residual intervertebral mobility at a high level of cord compression, and advanced kyphosis, addition of posterior fusion is reported to yield favorable outcomes, which are still inferior to those of anterior decompression with fusion [5].

Using this prior knowledge, we investigated effect of static factors and dynamic factor for spinal cord of OPLL. And we analyzed intraspinal stress for fusion model, kyphosis model, and an increased kyphosis model with intervertebral mobility.

Our study was limited to the investigation of stress distribution caused by compression. Other causal factors that can contribute to C-OPLL include ischemia. With respect to blood flow, Ono et al. reported ischemic changes in the white matter and gray matter at the stenosis level [23]. In addition, the effect of the speed of compression of components and the impact of aging were not considered [24]. Discontinuity was set in the middle of OPLL. Deformity of the spinal cord by long-term compression of C-OPLL and apoptotic factors were not considered in the FEM analysis. Moreover, the FEM model used here was simplified in order to facilitate the calculations. Analysis errors were reduced by using a FEM mesh by assuming the spinal cord was symmetric and by not including the vertebral body, the denticulate ligament, cerebrospinal fluid, dura, and nerve root. Furthermore, because there are no data on distance between the spinal cord, OPLL lesions, and the vertebral arch, it remains unknown how much the occupying ratio and compression degree are associated. In order for future models to address these various factors, it will be necessary to design models according to specific cases or conditions. We have now emphasized the simplicity of the analysis model, without blood and other components, however, so that it may fully reflect the clinical features of cervical myelopathy for C-OPLL patients.

In the present study, the stress distribution in the spinal cord increased following static compression and dynamic compression by C-OPLL with hill-shaped ossification. However, the stress distribution did not increase throughout the entire spinal cord. Under combined static and dynamic compression, the stress distribution increased in the entire spinal cord at a ROM of >10° even at a static compression of 10% of the AP diameter of the spinal cord. Stress increased in the entire spinal cord under static compression of 20% and dynamic compression at a ROM of >5°. As static compression increases, the stress distribution increases, even with a mild ROM. Thus, when both static compression and dynamic compression such as segmental ROM occur, damage to the spinal cord and the progression of symptoms are likely to arise.

Also, analyses revealed that intraspinal stress is increased by compression due to C-OPLL with hill-shaped ossification and decreased by posterior decompression with fusion. Although the usefulness of posterior decompression with fusion was demonstrated, intraspinal stress more frequently persisted with higher residual compression. It was assumed that if compression were higher, stress would be more likely to persist. Both the usefulness and limitations of posterior decompression with fusion were suggested. Moreover, intraspinal stress increased again in cases of advanced kyphosis after only posterior decompression was performed and in cases of OPLL with discontinuous lesions and intervertebral mobility at a high level of cord compression.

20.5 Conclusion

We conducted stress analyses in a static compression model, dynamic compression model, combination static and dynamic compression model, a decompression with fusion model, and a combined model of postoperative residual compression and residual instability in C-OPLL with hill-shaped ossification of C-OPLL [25, 26].

It is possible that symptoms occur under static compression only or under dynamic compression only. However, under static compression the stress distribution increases with the ROM at the responsible level and this makes it very likely that symptoms will worsen. We conclude that C-OPLL myelopathy is induced by static factors, dynamic factors, and a combination of both. When ROM is large, careful attention must be paid in case the symptoms worsen, even if static compression is small. And, although instrumented fusion after posterior decompression is useful, stress to the spinal cord tended to persist in cases of high residual compression. Moreover, it was found that when fusing is not performed and results in instability, intraspinal stress increases again. Thus, in cases of high residual compression and instability after posterior decompression, anterior decompression with fusion or posterior decompression with instrumented fusion should be considered as previously reported.

Acknowledgement This is an accepted manuscript of an article published by Taylor & Francis in [Cervical ossification of the posterior longitudinal ligament: factors affecting the effect of posterior decompression] on [2017], available online: http://www.tandfonline.com/[Article DOI:https://doi.org/10.1080/10790268.2016.1140392] and [Cervical ossification of the posterior longitudinal ligament: Biomechanical analysis of the influence of static and dynamic factors] on [2015], available online: http://www.tandfonline.com/[Article DOI:https://doi.org/10.1179/2045772314Y.0000000221].

References

1. Matsunaga S, Kukita M, Hayashi K, Shinkura R, Koriyama C, Sakou T, et al. Pathogenesis of myelopathy in patients with ossification of the posterior longitudinal ligament. J Neurosurg. 2002;96:168–72.
2. Matsunaga S, Sakou T, Hayashi K, Ishidou Y, Hirotsu M, Komiya S. Trauma-induced myelopathy in patients with ossification of the posterior longitudinal ligament. J Neurosurg. 2002;97(2):172–5.
3. Masaki Y, Yamazaki M, Okawa A, Aramomi M, Hashimoto M, Koda M, et al. An analysis of factors causing poor surgical outcome in patients with cervical myelopathy due to ossification of the posterior

longitudinal ligament: anterior decompression with spinal fusion versus laminoplasty. J Spinal Disord Tech. 2007;20(1):7–13.
4. Morio Y, Nagashima H, Teshima R, Nawata K. Radiological pathogenesis of cervical myelopathy in 60 consecutive patients with cervical ossification of the posterior longitudinal ligament. Spinal Cord. 1999;37(12):853–7.
5. Fujiyoshi T, Yamazaki M, Okawa A, Kawabe J, Hayashi K, Endo T, et al. Static versus dynamic factors for the development of myelopathy in patients with cervical ossification of the posterior longitudinal ligament. J Clin Neurosci. 2010;17(3):320–4.
6. Azuma Y, Kato Y, Taguchi T. Etiology of cervical myelopathy induced by ossification of the posterior longitudinal ligament: determining the responsible level of OPLL myelopathy by correlating static compression and dynamic factors. J Spinal Disord Tech. 2010;23(3):166–9.
7. Matsunaga S, Nakamura K, Seichi A, Yokoyama T, Toh S, Ichimura S, et al. Radiographic predictors for the development of myelopathy in patients with ossification of the posterior longitudinal ligament: a multicenter cohort study. Spine. 2008;33(24):2648–50.
8. Tsuyama N. Ossification of the posterior longitudinal ligament of the spine. Clin Orthop Relat Res. 1984;184:71–84.
9. Shinomiya K, Okamoto A, Kamikozuru M, Furuya K, Yamaura I. An analysis of failures in primary cervical anterior spinal cord decompression and fusion. J Spinal Disord. 1993;6(4):277–88.
10. Matsumoto M, Chiba K, Toyama Y. Surgical treatment of ossification of the posterior longitudinal ligament and its outcomes: posterior surgery by laminoplasty. Spine. 2012;37(5):E303–8.
11. Iwasaki M, Okuda S, Miyauchi A, Sakaura H, Mukai Y, Yonenobu K, et al. Surgical strategy for cervical myelopathy due to ossification of the posterior longitudinal ligament: part 1: clinical results and limitations of laminoplasty. Spine. 2007;32(6):647–53.
12. Tani T, Ushida T, Ishida K, Iai H, Noguchi T, Yamamoto H. Relative safety of anterior microsurgical decompression versus laminoplasty for cervical myelopathy with a massive ossified posterior longitudinal ligament. Spine. 2002;27(22):2491–8.
13. Iwasaki M, Okuda S, Miyauchi A, Sakaura H, Mukai Y, Yonenobu K, et al. Surgical strategy for cervical myelopathy due to ossification of the posterior longitudinal ligament: part 2: advantages of anterior decompression and fusion over laminoplasty. Spine. 2007;32(6):654–60.
14. Cecilia P, Jon S, Richard M. The importance of fluid-structure interaction in spinal trauma models. J Neurotrauma. 2011;28:113–25.
15. Ichihara K, Taguchi T, Yoshinori S, Ituo S, Shunichi K, Shinya K. Gray matter of the bovine cervical spinal cord is mechanically more rigid and fragile than the white matter. J Neurotrauma. 2001;18(3):361–7.
16. Ichihara K, Taguchi T, Sakuramoto I, Kawano S, Kawai S. Mechanism of the spinal cord injury and the cervical spondylotic myelopathy: new approach based on the mechanical features of the spinal cord white and gray matter. J Neurosurg. 2003;99(3 suppl):278–85.
17. Tunturi AR. Elasticity of the spinal cord, pia and denticulate ligament in the dog. J Neurosurg. 1978;48:975–9.
18. Henderson FC, Geddes JF, Vaccaro AR, Woodard E, Berry KJ, Benzel EC. Stretch-associated injury in cervical spondyloticmyelopathy: new concept and review. Neurosurgery. 2005;56(5):1101–13.
19. Koyanagi I, Imamura H, Fujimoto S, Hida K, Iwasaki Y, Houkin K. Spinal canal size in ossification of the posterior longitudinal ligament of the cervical spine. Surg Neurol. 2004;62(4):286–91.
20. Mochizuki M, Aiba A, Hashimoto M, Fujiyoshi T, Yamazaki M. Cervical myelopathy in patients with ossification of the posterior longitudinal ligament. J Neurosurg Spine. 2009;10(2):122–8.
21. Yamaura I, Kurosa Y, Matuoka T, Shindo S. Anterior floating method for cervical myelopathy caused by ossification of the posterior longitudinal ligament. Clin Orthop Relat Res. 1999;359:27–34.
22. Seichi A, Hoshino Y, Kimura A, Nakahara S, Watanabe M, Kato T, et al. Neurological complications of cervical laminoplasty for patients with ossification of the posterior longitudinal ligament-a multi-institutional retrospective study. Spine. 2011;36(15):E998–1003.
23. Ono K, Ota H, Tada K, Yamamoto T. Cervical myelopathy secondary to multiple spondylotic protrusions. A clinicopathologic study. Spine. 1977;2(2):109–25.
24. Sparrey CJ, Manley GT, Keaveny TM. Effects of white, grey, and pia mater properties on tissue level stresses and strains in the compressed spinal cord. J Neurotrauma. 2009;26(4):585–25.
25. Nishida N, Kanchiku T, Kato Y, Imajo Y, Yoshida Y, Kawano S, et al. Cervical ossification of the posterior longitudinal ligament: biomechanical analysis of the influence of static and dynamic factors. J Spinal Cord Med. 2015;38(5):593–8.
26. Nishida N, Kanchiku T, Kato Y, Imajo Y, Suzuki H, Yoshida Y, et al. Cervical ossification of the posterior longitudinal ligament: factors affecting the effect of posterior decompression. J Spinal Cord Med. 2017;40(1):93–9.

Part V

Treatment

Surgical Indications and Choice of Surgical Procedure for Cervical Ossification of the Longitudinal Ligament

21

Yukitaka Nagamoto and Motoki Iwasaki

Abstract

Patients with cervical ossification of the longitudinal ligament (OPLL) who have myelopathy usually require surgery. There are two main options in the surgical procedure: anterior decompression and fusion (ADF), or the posterior approach including various types of laminoplasty. ADF can achieve good surgical results by direct decompression; however, many spine surgeons often feel hesitant performing ADF due to its technical difficulties and high incidence of surgery-related complications. In contrast, the posterior approach has been widely used since it is less technically demanding and less frequently associated with serious complications. Nevertheless, there are several limiting factors for the indication of posterior approach because of its nature of indirect decompression. Thus, each procedure has both advantages and disadvantages. The choice of surgical procedure has always been controversy and there has been no clear guideline for choosing surgical procedures. Several studies, such as meta-analysis, recently have been published. Based on the accumulation of research over many years, it is recommended that spine surgeons make a more appropriate decision about choice of the procedure for each pathomechanism, if not enough evidence is found. In this chapter, we summarize the long-time controversy over the issue and discuss the choice of procedure based on the latest information.

Keywords

Ossification of the posterior longitudinal ligament (OPLL) · Myelopathy · Anterior decompression and fusion · Laminoplasty Posterior decompression and fusion

Abbreviations

ADF	Anterior decompression and fusion
CT	Computed tomography
JOA	Japan Orthopaedic Association
MRI	Magnetic resonance imaging
OPLL	Ossification of the longitudinal ligament
PDF	Posterior decompression and fusion
SCI	Spinal cord injury
ULP	Upper limp palsy

21.1 Surgical Indications

21.1.1 Cervical Myelopathy Due to OPLL

Persistent compression of the spinal cord by ossification may lead to the onset of myelopathy.

Y. Nagamoto (✉) · M. Iwasaki
Department of Orthopaedic Surgery, Osaka Rosai Hospital, Osaka, Japan

A. Okawa et al. (eds.), *OPLL*, https://doi.org/10.1007/978-981-15-3855-1_21

However, the development of ossification does not always lead to myelopathy. In a study of the natural history of 323 patients with OPLL, the myelopathy-free rate in patients without myelopathy at presentation was 71% at 30-year follow-up examination [1]. In addition to the static compression factor, dynamic factor is considered to play an important role in developing myelopathy. Matsunaga et al. [2] elucidated that all patients with space available for the spinal cord less than 6 mm suffered myelopathy. Among patients with moderate stenosis, the range of motion of the cervical spine is significantly larger in patients with myelopathy than in those without myelopathy. These results indicated that the static compression above a certain critical point may be the most significant factor in inducing myelopathy, whereas below that point dynamic factors may be largely involved in myelopathy.

21.1.2 Surgical Indications for Cervical OPLL

Surgical decompression of the spinal cord should be considered for patients who had apparent symptoms of myelopathy, such as spastic gait disturbance and clumsiness of the hands. Many literatures have reported the effectiveness of surgery for myelopathy with approximately 50% recovery rate (range, 45–62%) [3–11] whereas it is not always effective for pain relief in patients whose predominant complaint is neck-shoulder pain and so it is generally not recommended.

For patients with moderate or severe myelopathy, early surgical decompression is generally recommended. Matsunaga et al. reported that quality of life, including life prognosis, is poor unless surgical treatment is performed at an appropriate time for patients with moderate myelopathy (Nurick Grade 3 or 4), and a good effect of surgery was not expected for patients with severe myelopathy (Nurick Grade 5) [12]. Iwasaki et al. reported that a better neurological recovery was associated with younger age at operation and milder myelopathy [5]. For patients with mild myelopathy, surgical indication is still controversial. Qizhi et al. elucidated the risk factors affecting signal changes for the patients with OPLL as follows: prolonged symptoms, high occupying ratio, low preoperative modified Japan Orthopaedic Association (mJOA) score, kyphosis, or instability of the cervical spine [13]. Signal changes of the spinal cord on magnetic resonance imaging (MRI) reflect pathological changes in the spinal cord, indicative of the prognosis although there are still some controversies. Early surgery would be recommended for patients with one of those factors before developing intramedullary spinal cord changes. Other than these factors, even if the myelopathy is mild, surgery should be indicated more aggressively in cases with known poor prognostic factors such as elder patients and diabetes [14]. On the other hand, a prospective randomized controlled study comparing surgery with conservative treatment for patients with mild myelopathy (mJOA score of 12 points or more) due to cervical spondylosis explained that surgery is not superior to conservative treatment in scores for daily activities and subjective evaluation over 2-year follow-up [15].

For patients who have cord compression due to OPLL but no symptoms of myelopathy, there are concerns that sudden onset or deterioration of myelopathy sometimes occurs by minor trauma with hyperextension of the neck. However, there is no evidence in the effectiveness of prophylactic surgical decompression. The incidence of myelopathy and trauma-induced cervical spinal cord injury (SCI) in patients with OPLL are reported to be both low [1, 16]. In a minimum 10-year prospective cohort study, of the 368 patients without myelopathy at the time of initial consultation, only six patients (2%) subsequently developed trauma-induced myelopathy [16]. On the other hand, OPLL is highly prevalent (34–38%) in cervical SCI patients without bone injuries [17, 18] and is considered to be one of major risk factors for the development of acute cervical SCI. Considering these, the prophylactic surgery should be indicated carefully. The vast majority of cervical SCI patients with OPLL were unaware of OPLL before injury [17]. A previous study suggested that once patients are made aware of OPLL and its potential risk, they generally are more careful to avoid high-risk behaviors, such as walking on slippery slopes, bicycling, or drinking too much alcohol [16]. For patients who suffered cervical SCI without any radiographic abnormality commonly found in the elderly, emergency surgery is not commonly indicated in Japan because there is no evidence in the effectiveness of emergent decompression of the spinal cord. To clarify the effectiveness of the emergency surgery, a nationwide randomized controlled trial comparing emergency surgery within 24 h versus delayed surgery is currently in progress [19].

21.2 Choice of Surgical Procedure

21.2.1 Surgical Options for Cervical OPLL

To resolve myelopathy due to cervical OPLL, surgery is widely accepted as a treatment option. Although various surgical approaches have been used, the main question has always been which of the anterior approach including anterior decompression and fusion (ADF) or posterior approach including laminoplasty is more optimal.

ADF can ideally resolve spinal cord compression by direct removal of ossified lesions and can stabilize involved segments. Given the benefits of its theoretical advantages, many studies have shown that surgical outcomes following ADF are superior to any other procedures [7, 20–30] especially in patients with an occupying ratio of 60% or more [7, 21, 24, 28]. On the other hand, the procedure that includes corpectomies and resection or floating of the ossified lesion followed by strut graft fusion is complex and technically demanding. As a result, high incidence of surgery-related complications has been reported. According to the latest meta-analysis comparing ADF and laminoplasty, the incidence of surgical complications in ADF ranged from 20 to 24% and was significantly higher compared with laminoplasty [21, 28]. Among the complications, cerebrospinal fluid leak was the most common with 8.1%, followed dysphagia/dysphonia (5.7%), and implant dislocation (1.6%) in this order [28]. Less commonly, vertebral artery or esophageal injury may occur [31]. Reoperation rate was also significantly higher in ADF compared to that in laminoplasty [21, 28]. The major reason for revision was implant complications, such as bone graft dislodgement and pseudoarthrosis [21, 32]. Therefore, ADF has a tendency to fall into disfavor despite its theoretical advantage.

On the contrary, laminoplasty has been widely accepted for the treatment of not only OPLL but also spondylotic myelopathy because the procedure is safer and easier than ADF and also can be indicated in patients with multi-level OPLL, especially plateau type. The mechanism of decompression is posterior shift of the spinal cord by enlargement of the posterior elements and is therefore indirect. Since the ossification remains ventral to the spinal cord after laminoplasty, neurological recovery is poor in patients with massive ossification, kyphotic alignment, or segmental motion between interrupted ossified lesions. Iwasaki et al. found that the surgical outcome was significantly poorer in patients with ≥60% canal-occupying ratio of OPLL, and the most significant predictor of poor outcome was "hill-shaped" ossification [6]. Hill-shaped ossification reflects severe compression of the spinal cord at localized levels with sharp angulation of the spinal cord. Fujiyoshi et al. advocated the K-line, which is defined as the line that connects the midpoints of the spinal canal at C2 and C7 [24]. The patients are classified K-line (−) if the K-line is involved in the ossification. Both cervical kyphosis and canal compromise by OPLL can be simply evaluated using the index. They found that neurological recovery was obtained insufficiently after posterior decompression in patients with K-line (−). Complications after laminoplasty peculiar to OPLL include postoperative upper limb palsy (ULP), also referred as C5 palsy, and progression of ossification. Takenaka et al. reported that the prevalence of ULP after laminoplasty was significantly higher with OPLL than without OPLL in their meta-analysis (early-onset ULP, 5.2% vs. 2.5%; late-onset ULP, 5.1% vs. 2.3%) [33]. In terms of progression of ossification, higher risks were shown in younger patients (< 60 years) and patients with continuous and mixed-type OPLL [5, 34, 35]. However, there are many reports of low prevalence of symptomatic OPLL progression after laminoplasty although the frequency of OPLL progression has been reported to be as high as 70% [5, 36–38]. Lee et al. elucidated that laminoplasty frequently induces progression of OPLL compared with fusion surgery (laminoplasty; 62.5%, fusion surgery; 7.6%) but does not make significant clinical deterioration in their meta-analysis [39]. Meanwhile, Odate et al. speculated it is one of the possible causes of postoperative neurological deterioration based on their novel experience of 19 consecutive revision cases after posterior decompression for cervical OPLL [40]. Nevertheless, long-term outcomes of laminoplasty are favorable with an acceptable complication rate in majority of patients [41]. Among posterior approaches, laminectomy was previously used for cervical OPLL [37], but laminoplasty has become the current major treatment of posterior approach for not only OPLL but also cervical spondylotic myelopathy [5] since laminoplasty has biomechanical and clinical advantages over laminectomy [42–45].

Both anterior and posterior approaches have their advantages and disadvantages. To avoid disadvantages of both approaches as much as possible, recently posterior decompression and fusion using instrumentation (PDF) is becoming one of the surgical options for cervical OPLL. PDF can provide immediate and long-term stability of the cervical spine and can prevent the development of kyphosis. Several studies have revealed its achieved favorable results [46, 47]. In studies compared with other approaches for OPLL, Yoshii et al. explained that the postoperative recovery rates of PDF and ADF were similar for a $\geq$ 50% canal occupying ratio [48]. Koda et al. reported that PDF had a recovery rate of JOA midway between ADF and laminoplasty in patients with K-line (−) [25]. Although PDF can be an effective alternative option, especially in patients with massive OPLL or mild kyphosis (flexible), there are several disadvantages. Some previous studies have shown a high incidence of upper limb palsy after PDF ranged from 11.9 to 50% [33, 47, 49]. Takemitsu et al. reported that the risk of developing the palsy with PDF was 11.6-fold greater than laminoplasty alone [50]. Takenaka et al. reported that the onset of the palsy after PDF is more frequent within two days than at three days or more with the pooled prevalence being 9.0% and 4.3%, respectively [33]. They speculated the cause of the early-onset palsy after PDF is that the lag correction effect, which is defined as iatrogenic foraminal stenosis or tension on the nerve roots with posterior instrumented fusion, occurs immediately after surgery. Another disadvantage of PDF is neck pain after surgery [51, 52]. Detaching the paraspinal muscles widely is necessary to place the posterior instrument. Injury to the paraspinal muscles causes postoperative neck pain after the posterior procedure.

21.2.2 Current Surgical Strategy for Cervical OPLL

As mentioned above, all current surgical options including laminoplasty, ADF, and PDF have both their advantages and disadvantages. Our proposed surgical strategy for cervical myelopathy due to OPLL is shown in Fig. 21.1. Laminoplasty would be our preference for patients with occupying ratio less than 50%, plateau-shaped ossification, without apparent cervical kyphosis (30-degree or more lordosis is ideal). For patients with occupying ratio between 50% and 60%, ADF or alternatives to laminoplasty including PDF would be recommended if one of following characteristics reported to contribute poor clinical outcomes was present: (1) Hill-shaped ossification; (2) kyphosis or malalignment of the cervical spine or the spinal cord; (3) segmental motion between the interrupted ossified lesions [6]. Regarding the segmental motion, Fujimori et al. elucidated that a minute gap in sagittal computed tomography (CT) between the interrupted ossified lesions always have intervertebral motion using three-dimensional motion analysis method [53]. Therefore, segmental motion can be judged by the absence of bony bridge on sagittal CT (existence of the gap of ossified lesion). For patients

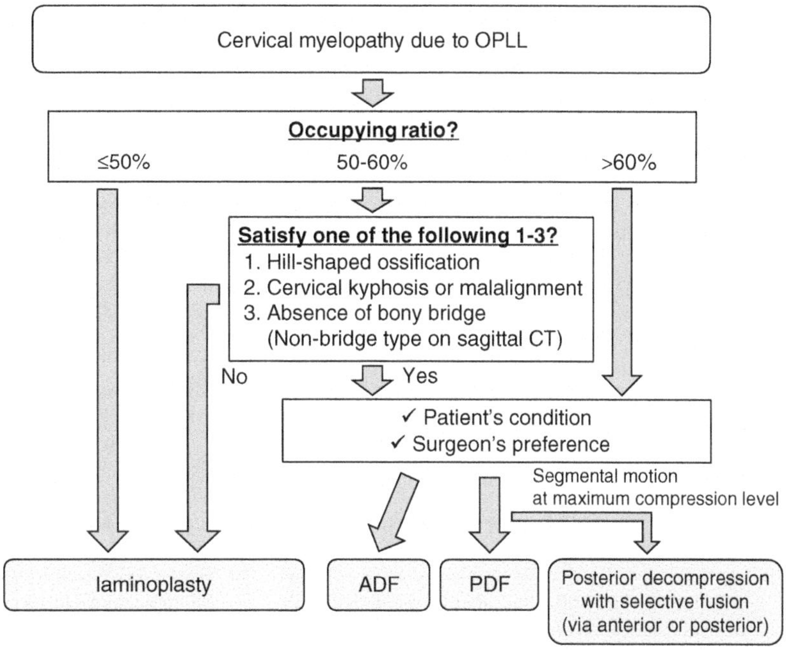

Fig. 21.1 Our proposed surgical strategy

with occupying ratio greater than 60%, ADF or alternatives to laminoplasty would also be recommended. Although ADF would be our preference for massive OPLL with occupying ratio greater than 50% because of its theoretical advantage and its good results, PDF should be considered according to surgeon's preference and/or patient's condition. However, complications in PDF, such as segmental motor palsy, neck stiffness and pain, also should not be overlooked. Recently, posterior decompression with selective fusion was advocated for patients who have segmental motion at the maximal compression level in order to avoid the disadvantages of PDF [54]. We have performed posterior decompression with anterior selective stabilization at the maximal compression level in patients with massive OPLL and reported succcessful clinical results [54]. As a same concept of surgery, Onari et al. are the pioneers [55]. They performed anterior fusion without resecting the ossification as the first choice treatment of OPLL since the early 1960s and reported the effectiveness of the surgery in more than 10-year follow-up. Their results suggested that dynamic factor is essential pathomechanism of myelopathy in cervical OPLL. Based on these findings and our clinical experiences, we consider that immobilization and minute dekyphosis at the maximal compression segment are essential in successful neurological recovery after surgery for patients with massive OPLL.

References

1. Matsunaga S, Sakou T, Taketomi E, Komiya S. Clinical course of patients with ossification of the posterior longitudinal ligament: a minimum 10-year cohort study. J Neurosurg Spine. 2004;100(3):245–8.
2. Matsunaga S, Kukita M, Hayashi K, Shinkura R, Koriyama C, Sakou T, Komiya S. Pathogenesis of myelopathy in patients with ossification of the posterior longitudinal ligament. J Neurosurg Spine. 2002a;96(2):168–72.
3. Goto S, Kita T. Long-term follow-up evaluation of surgery for ossification of the posterior longitudinal ligament. Spine. 1995;20(20):2247–56.
4. Hou Y, Liang L, Shi G, Xu P, Xu G, Shi J, Yuan W. Comparing effects of cervical anterior approach and laminoplasty in surgical management of cervical ossification of posterior longitudinal ligament by a prospective nonrandomized controlled study. Orthop Traumatol Surg Res. 2017;103(5):733–40.
5. Iwasaki M, Kawaguchi Y, Kimura T, Yonenobu K. Long-term results of expansive laminoplasty for ossification of the posterior longitudinal ligament of the cervical spine: more than 10 years follow up. J Neurosurg Spine. 2002;96(2):180–9.

6. Iwasaki M, Sy O, Miyauchi A, Sakaura H, Mukai Y, Yonenobu K, Yoshikawa H. Surgical strategy for cervical myelopathy due to ossification of the posterior longitudinal ligament: part 1: clinical results and limitations of laminoplasty. Spine. 2007a;32(6):647–53.
7. Iwasaki M, Sy O, Miyauchi A, Sakaura H, Mukai Y, Yonenobu K, Yoshikawa H. Surgical strategy for cervical myelopathy due to ossification of the posterior longitudinal ligament: part 2: advantages of anterior decompression and fusion over laminoplasty. Spine. 2007b;32(6):654–60.
8. Kawaguchi Y, Nakano M, Yasuda T, Seki S, Hori T, Kimura T. Anterior decompressive surgery after cervical laminoplasty in patients with ossification of the posterior longitudinal ligament. Spine J. 2014;14(6):955–63.
9. Kim B, Shin HC, Kim KN, Yi S, Shin DA, Ha Y. Surgical outcome and prognostic factors of anterior decompression and fusion for cervical compressive myelopathy due to ossification of the posterior longitudinal ligament. Spine J. 2015;15(5):875–84.
10. Liu K, Shi J, Jia L, Yuan W. Surgical technique: hemilaminectomy and unilateral lateral mass fixation for cervical ossification of the posterior longitudinal ligament. Clin Orthop Relat Res. 2013;471(7):2219–24.
11. Yamaura I, Kurosa Y, Matuoka T, Shindo S. Anterior floating method for cervical myelopathy caused by ossification of the posterior longitudinal ligament. Clin Orthop Relat Res. 1999;359:27–34.
12. Matsunaga S, Sakou T, Arishima Y, Koga H, Hayashi K, Komiya S. Quality of life in elderly patients with ossification of the posterior longitudinal ligament. Spine. 2001;26(5):494–8.
13. Qizhi S, Lili Y, Ce W, Yu C, Wen Y. Factors associated with intramedullary MRI abnormalities in patients with ossification of the posterior longitudinal ligament. J Spinal Disord Tech. 2015;28(5):E304–9.
14. Gu Y, Shi J, Cao P, Yuan W, Wu H, Yang L, Tian Y, Liang L. Clinical and imaging predictors of surgical outcome in multilevel cervical ossification of posterior longitudinal ligament: an analysis of 184 patients. PLoS One. 2015;10(9):e0136042.
15. Kadaňka Z, Bednařík J, Voháňka S, Vlach O, Stejskal L, Chaloupka R, Filipovičová D, Šurelová D, Adamová B, Novotný O. Conservative treatment versus surgery in spondylotic cervical myelopathy: a prospective randomised study. Eur Spine J. 2000;9(6):538–44.
16. Matsunaga S, Sakou T, Hayashi K, Ishidou Y, Hirotsu M, Komiya S. Trauma-induced myelopathy in patients with ossification of the posterior longitudinal ligament. J Neurosurg Spine. 2002b;97(2):172–5.
17. Chikuda H, Seichi A, Takeshita K, Matsunaga S, Watanabe M, Nakagawa Y, Oshima K, Sasao Y, Tokuhashi Y, Nakahara S. Acute cervical spinal cord injury complicated by preexisting ossification of the posterior longitudinal ligament: a multicenter study. Spine. 2011;36(18):1453–8.
18. Koyanagi I, Iwasaki Y, Hida K, Akino M, Imamura H, Abe H. Acute cervical cord injury without fracture or dislocation of the spinal column. J Neurosurg Spine. 2000;93(1):15–20.
19. Chikuda H, Ohtsu H, Ogata T, Sugita S, Sumitani M, Koyama Y, Matsumoto M, Toyama Y. Optimal treatment for spinal cord injury associated with cervical canal stenosis (OSCIS): a study protocol for a randomized controlled trial comparing early versus delayed surgery. Trials. 2013;14(1):245.
20. Chen Y, Guo Y, Lu X, Chen D, Song D, Shi J, Yuan W. Surgical strategy for multilevel severe ossification of posterior longitudinal ligament in the cervical spine. Clin Spine Surg. 2011;24(1):24–30.
21. Chen Z, Liu B, Dong J, Feng F, Chen R, Xie P, Zhang L, Rong L. Comparison of anterior corpectomy and fusion versus laminoplasty for the treatment of cervical ossification of posterior longitudinal ligament: a meta-analysis. Neurosurg Focus. 2016;40(6):E8.
22. Epstein N. The surgical management of ossification of the posterior longitudinal ligament in 51 patients. J Spinal Disord. 1993;6(5):432–54.. discussion 454-435
23. Fessler RG, Steck JC, Giovanini MA. Anterior cervical corpectomy for cervical spondylotic myelopathy. Neurosurgery. 1998;43(2):257–65.
24. Fujimori T, Iwasaki M, Okuda S, Takenaka S, Kashii M, Kaito T, Yoshikawa H. Long-term results of cervical myelopathy due to ossification of the posterior longitudinal ligament with an occupying ratio of 60% or more. Spine. 2014;39(1):58–67.
25. Koda M, Mochizuki M, Konishi H, Aiba A, Kadota R, Inada T, Kamiya K, Ota M, Maki S, Takahashi K. Comparison of clinical outcomes between laminoplasty, posterior decompression with instrumented fusion, and anterior decompression with fusion for K-line (−) cervical ossification of the posterior longitudinal ligament. Eur Spine J. 2016;25(7):2294–301.
26. Liu T, Xu W, Cheng T, Yang H-L. Anterior versus posterior surgery for multilevel cervical myelopathy, which one is better? A systematic review. Eur Spine J. 2011;20(2):224–35.
27. Masaki Y, Yamazaki M, Okawa A, Aramomi M, Hashimoto M, Koda M, Mochizuki M, Moriya H. An analysis of factors causing poor surgical outcome in patients with cervical myelopathy due to ossification of the posterior longitudinal ligament: anterior decompression with spinal fusion versus laminoplasty. Clin Spine Surg. 2007;20(1):7–13.
28. Qin R, Chen X, Zhou P, Li M, Hao J, Zhang F. Anterior cervical corpectomy and fusion versus posterior laminoplasty for the treatment of oppressive myelopathy owing to cervical ossification of posterior longitudinal ligament: a meta-analysis. Eur Spine J. 2018;27(6):1375–87.
29. Sakai K, Okawa A, Takahashi M, Arai Y, Kawabata S, Enomoto M, Kato T, Hirai T, Shinomiya K. Five-year follow-up evaluation of surgical treatment for cervical myelopathy caused by ossification of the posterior longitudinal ligament: a prospective comparative study of anterior decompression and fusion

with floating method versus laminoplasty. Spine. 2012;37(5):367–76.
30. Tani T, Ushida T, Ishida K, Iai H, Noguchi T, Yamamoto H. Relative safety of anterior microsurgical decompression versus laminoplasty for cervical myelopathy with a massive ossified posterior longitudinal ligament. Spine. 2002;27(22):2491–8.
31. Smith ZA, Buchanan CC, Raphael D, Khoo LT. Ossification of the posterior longitudinal ligament: pathogenesis, management, and current surgical approaches: a review. Neurosurg Focus. 2011;30(3):E10.
32. Li H, Dai L-Y. A systematic review of complications in cervical spine surgery for ossification of the posterior longitudinal ligament. Spine J. 2011;11(11):1049–57.
33. Takenaka S, Nagamoto Y, Aono H, Kaito T, Hosono N. Differences in the time of onset of postoperative upper limb palsy among surgical procedures: a meta-analysis. Spine J. 2016;16(12):1486–99.
34. Chiba K, Yamamoto I, Hirabayashi H, Iwasaki M, Goto H, Yonenobu K, Toyama Y. Multicenter study investigating the postoperative progression of ossification of the posterior longitudinal ligament in the cervical spine: a new computer-assisted measurement. J Neurosurg Spine. 2005;3(1):17–23.
35. Kawaguchi Y, Kanamori M, Ishihara H, Nakamura H, Sugimori K, Tsuji H, Kimura T. Progression of ossification of the posterior longitudinal ligament following en bloc cervical laminoplasty. JBJS. 2001;83(12):1798–802.
36. Kalb S, Martirosyan NL, Perez-Orribo L, Kalani MYS, Theodore N. Analysis of demographics, risk factors, clinical presentation, and surgical treatment modalities for the ossified posterior longitudinal ligament. Neurosurg Focus. 2011;30(3):E11.
37. Kato Y, Iwasaki M, Fuji T, Yonenobu K, Ochi T. Long-term follow-up results of laminectomy for cervical myelopathy caused by ossification of the posterior longitudinal ligament. J Neurosurg. 1998;89(2):217–23.
38. Ogawa Y, Toyama Y, Chiba K, Matsumoto M, Nakamura M, Takaishi H, Hirabayashi H, Hirabayashi K. Long-term results of expansive open-door laminoplasty for ossification of the posterior longitudinal ligament of the cervical spine. J Neurosurg Spine. 2004;1(2):168–74.
39. Lee C-H, Sohn M-J, Lee CH, Choi CY, Han SR, Choi B-W. Are there differences in the progression of ossification of the posterior longitudinal ligament following laminoplasty versus fusion?: a meta-analysis. Spine. 2017;42(12):887–94.
40. Odate S, Shikata J, Soeda T, Yamamura S, Kawaguchi S. Surgical results and complications of anterior decompression and fusion as a revision surgery after initial posterior surgery for cervical myelopathy due to ossification of the posterior longitudinal ligament. J Neurosurg Spine. 2017;26(4):466–73.
41. Matsumoto M, Chiba K, Toyama Y. Surgical treatment of ossification of the posterior longitudinal ligament and its outcomes: posterior surgery by laminoplasty. Spine. 2012;37(5):E303–8.
42. Baisden J, Voo LM, Cusick JF, Pintar FA, Yoganandan N. Evaluation of cervical laminectomy and laminoplasty: a longitudinal study in the goat model. Spine. 1999;24(13):1283.
43. Fields MJ, Hoshijima K, Feng AH, Richardson WJ, Myers BS. A biomechanical, radiologic, and clinical comparison of outcome after multilevel cervical laminectomy or laminoplasty in the rabbit. Spine. 2000;25(22):2925–31.
44. Heller JG, Edwards CC, Murakami H, Rodts GE. Laminoplasty versus laminectomy and fusion for multilevel cervical myelopathy: an independent matched cohort analysis. Spine. 2001;26(12):1330–6.
45. Herkowitz HN. A comparison of anterior cervical fusion, cervical laminectomy, and cervical laminoplasty for the surgical management of multiple level spondylotic radiculopathy. Spine. 1988;13(7):774–80.
46. Anderson PA, Matz PG, Groff MW, Heary RF, Holly LT, Kaiser MG, Mummaneni PV, Ryken TC, Choudhri TF, Vresilovic EJ. Laminectomy and fusion for the treatment of cervical degenerative myelopathy. J Neurosurg Spine. 2009;11(2):150–6.
47. Chen Y, Guo Y, Chen D, Wang X, Lu X, Yuan W. Long-term outcome of laminectomy and instrumented fusion for cervical ossification of the posterior longitudinal ligament. Int Orthop. 2009;33(4):1075.
48. Yoshii T, Sakai K, Hirai T, Yamada T, Inose H, Kato T, Enomoto M, Tomizawa S, Kawabata S, Arai Y. Anterior decompression with fusion versus posterior decompression with fusion for massive cervical ossification of the posterior longitudinal ligament with a≥ 50% canal occupying ratio: a multicenter retrospective study. Spine J. 2016;16(11):1351–7.
49. Nakashima H, Imagama S, Yukawa Y, Kanemura T, Kamiya M, Yanase M, Ito K, Machino M, Yoshida G, Ishikawa Y. Multivariate analysis of C-5 palsy incidence after cervical posterior fusion with instrumentation. J Neurosurg Spine. 2012;17(2):103–10.
50. Takemitsu M, Cheung KM, Wong YW, Cheung W-Y, Luk KD. C5 nerve root palsy after cervical laminoplasty and posterior fusion with instrumentation. Clin Spine Surg. 2008;21(4):267–72.
51. Liu X, Chen Y, Yang H, Li T, Xu B, Chen D. Expansive open-door laminoplasty versus laminectomy and instrumented fusion for cases with cervical ossification of the posterior longitudinal ligament and straight lordosis. Eur Spine J. 2017;26(4):1173–80.
52. Yang L, Gu Y, Shi J, Gao R, Liu Y, Li J, Yuan W. Modified plate-only open-door laminoplasty versus laminectomy and fusion for the treatment of cervical stenotic myelopathy. Orthopedics. 2013;36(1):e79–87.
53. Fujimori T, Iwasaki M, Nagamoto Y, Kashii M, Ishii T, Sakaura H, Sugamoto K, Yoshikawa H. Three-dimensional measurement of intervertebral range of motion in ossification of the posterior longitudinal ligament: are there mobile segments in the continuous type? J Neurosurg Spine. 2012;17(1):74–81.

54. Nagamoto Y, Iwasaki M, Okuda S, Matsumoto T, Sugiura T, Takahashi Y, Furuya M. Anterior selective stabilization combined with laminoplasty for cervical myelopathy due to massive ossification of the posterior longitudinal ligament: report of early outcomes in 14 patients. J Neurosurg Spine. 2020;13:1–7.
55. Onari K, Akiyama N, Kondo S, Toguchi A, Mihara H, Tsuchiya T. Long-term follow-up results of anterior interbody fusion applied for cervical myelopathy due to ossification of the posterior longitudinal ligament. Spine. 2001;26(5):488–93.

22 Overview of Laminoplasty

Kazuhiro Chiba

Abstract

Anterior cervical decompression and fusion (ACDF) and laminectomy used to be the only available surgical options for patients with myelopathy caused by ossification of posterior longitudinal ligament (OPLL). Laminoplasty was devised to address problems associated with ACDF; i.e., intraoperative nerve injury, cerebrospinal fluid leakage, pseudarthrosis, and other graft-related complications, and those associated with laminectomy; i.e., development of postoperative instability and kyphosis, and recurrent myelopathy due to scar formation. This simple, less invasive, yet innovative, procedure obtained widespread acceptance, initially in Japan, and gradually spread out to the world. There are many modified procedures available but can ultimately be summarized into two basic techniques: open-door and spinous process splitting laminoplasty. There is no significant difference in clinical outcomes between the two, and it is the surgeon's preference whether to choose one or the other. Best candidates for laminoplasty are those with multilevel OPLL and developmental spinal stenosis whose cervical alignment is lordosis. Because OPLL itself remains inside the spinal canal, the type, size, and shape of the ossified mass should also be taken into account when deciding indications. Through continuous efforts to establish the definite indications and to improve and refine the surgical techniques, surgical outcomes have improved significantly and issues such as postoperative axial pain, development of kyphosis, and segmental motor weakness have partly been resolved but not completely. Postoperative progression of OPLL remains as an unsolved problem, and indications of prophylactic decompression are still under debate.

Keywords

Ossification of the posterior longitudinal ligament (OPLL) · Laminoplasty · Open-door laminoplasty · Spinous processes splitting laminoplasty · Anterior cervical decompression and fusion (ACDF) · Laminectomy · Axial pain · Kyphosis · Segmental motor weakness · Prophylactic decompression

K. Chiba (✉)
Department of Orthopaedic Surgery, National Defense Medical College, Saitama, Japan
e-mail: kchiba@ndmc.ac.jp

Anterior cervical decompression and fusion (ACDF) was the preferred treatment for patients with ossification of the posterior longitudinal ligament (OPLL) among the majority of surgeons because it was considered logical to address the anteriorly placed pathology directly from an

A. Okawa et al. (eds.), *OPLL*, https://doi.org/10.1007/978-981-15-3855-1_22

anterior approach. The biggest advantage of ACDF is that ossified ligaments can be extirpated or floated anteriorly to obtain direct spinal cord decompression [1, 2]. However, anterior procedures are technically demanding especially when OPLL involves multiple levels, and perioperative complications; e.g., intraoperative nerve injury, cerebrospinal fluid leakage, airway obstruction, pseudoarthrosis with or without dislodgement of the grafted bone, have been reported [3, 4]. The long-term results of ACDF also revealed that recurrent myelopathy due to the development of adjacent segment pathology was not uncommon, especially in those with developmental spinal stenosis [5].

Until late 1960s, conventional laminectomy that totally removes laminae with attached ligamentous structures was the only available posterior procedure for cervical myelopathy caused by multilevel OPLL; however, surgical outcomes were not always satisfactory due to inherent traumatic nature of laminectomy using rongeurs [6]. After the introduction of a high-speed drill, a Japanese spine surgeon, Kirita devised a sophisticated technique in which the laminae were thinned and divided at the midline followed by total resection of the laminae to achieve safe and simultaneous decompression of the spinal cord [7]. This procedure brought significant improvement in the surgical results and reduced the rate of postoperative complications; however, problems inherent to total removal of the posterior anatomical structures, e.g., the development of postoperative kyphosis, vulnerability of the exposed spinal cord, and recurrent stenosis due to scar formation, remained unsolved [8].

Laminoplasty has evolved in Japan to address such problems by preserving the laminae to cover the spinal cord and retain stability. In 1973, Hattori and his coworkers devised an expansive Z-plasty of the laminae in which the spinal canal was reconstructed by the preserved laminae; however, this procedure did not gain widespread acceptance because of its technical complexity [9]. Inspired by Kirita's method, Hirabayashi developed his own en bloc laminectomy in which bony gutters were made at the bilateral junction of the laminae and facet joints using a high-speed drill followed by en bloc resection of the laminar block. During this procedure, Hirabayashi noticed that the dural pulsation was already present when he lifted one side of the lamina, even before removing the whole lamina. This observation has led to the advent of "expansive open-door laminoplasty" in which the ventral cortex of the gutter at one side was left to act as a hinge and the other side was lifted, similar to opening a book cover [10–12].

Laminoplasty has a biomechanical advantage over laminectomy because it leaves most part of the laminae and the spinous processes with the supra- and interspinous ligaments intact contributing to postoperative stability [13]. Moreover, laminoplasty has less surgical impact on the patient resulting in fewer complications [3, 14, 15]. Instability, disc herniation, and spondylotic changes in the adjacent levels, which are often seen 10–20 years after ACDF that occasionally require salvage surgeries, are seldom seen after laminoplasty [12]. This simple and safe procedure gradually gained advocacy among Japanese spine surgeons.

Provoked by Hirabayashi's concept of laminoplasty, development of various modified procedures has followed. Among them, the spinous process splitting laminoplasty devised by Kurokawa also gained widespread popularity because secure reconstruction of the spinal canal could be achieved by placing the bone grafts between the opened laminae, thereby reinforcing stability of the cervical spine [16]. There are several modifications of the open-door procedure using a bone graft, bone graft substitutes, or miniplates in the opened space [17, 18]. Spinous process splitting laminoplasty has also been modified by placing a long strut bone graft or bone graft substitutes [19]. Tomita, et al. used threaded wire saw, which they devised for total spondylectomy, to split the spinous processes [20]. All these various laminoplasty procedures can be classified into three types: Z-plasty, open door, and midsagittal splitting, but currently, open-door and midsagittal splitting types are mainly performed. There are advocates for both types, some claiming that the midsagittal splitting type has less epidural bleeding, whereas others stated that open-door type is safer because the gutters are formed at the lateral portions of the spinal canal where spinal cord compression is milder than the central portion [12]. However, no significant difference has been reported in the surgical outcomes between the two procedures to date and it is mostly the surgeons' preference whether to choose one or the other [21]. Even though numerous modified techniques have been devised to date, it should always be reminded that these two fundamental yet innovative techniques, open-door laminoplasty by Hirabayashi and spinous process splitting laminoplasty by Kurokawa, form the basis of the following modified procedures and yet remain as the most viable options.

Overall clinical results of expansive laminoplasty for OPLL have been reported to be 40–60% expressed by the recovery rate calculated using the Japanese Orthopaedic Association scoring system for the treatment of cervical myelopathy [12, 21]. Such favorable postoperative results brought a remarkable increase in the number of patients undergoing laminoplasty. However, to obtain favorable results, patient selection is the key. Some problems including postoperative axial pain, development of postoperative kyphosis, and segmental motor weakness have partly been resolved although not completely. Other problems are yet to be solved, i.e., postoperative progression of ossification and indications of prophylactic decompression.

22.1 Indications of Laminoplasty for OPLL

Best candidates of laminoplasty are those who have multilevel OPLL with developmental spinal stenosis and lordosis in whom sufficient posterior shift of the spinal cord is expected [12]. The biggest concern of laminoplasty for OPLL is the fact that the ossified mass remains intact inside the spinal canal, and, therefore, the type (continuous, segmental, mixed), size, and shape of OPLL must also be taken into account. If the ossified mass is large (canal occupying ratio >60%, thickness >7.2 mm) or a beak type with a sharp tip, optimal decompression may not be expected [22, 23]. In patients with segmental or mixed type OPLL, in whom ROM is preserved, the dynamic factor may lead later to neurological deterioration [24]. For these patients, ACDF or posterior instrumented fusion with pedicle screws or lateral mass screws may be considered. Fujiyoshi, et al. recommended to use K-line, which is the line connecting the midpoints of the spinal canal AP diameters at C2 and C7, to determine whether the patients should be treated anteriorly or posteriorly. If a patient has kyphosis and the tip of ossification extends beyond the K-line, the patient should be treated anteriorly or if treated posteriorly, fusion should be supplemented [25].

22.2 Axial Pain

Severe axial pain that occurs immediately after surgery is a common problem after laminoplasty. Although, in most cases, the symptom is alleviated spontaneously or by conservative treatments, such as injection of local anesthetics into the region of tenderness or an external support by a brace, some patients complain prolonged pain [26]. Preservation of the C7 spinous process where several paraspinal muscles attach has been reported to result in decrease of axial pain [27]. Shiraishi, et al. devised a sophisticated technique in which selected laminae are removed after minimal detachment of the muscles yet providing adequate decompression of the spinal cord and named it "skip laminectomy" although this technique is indicated mainly for spondylotic myelopathy [28]. After the report by Shiraishi, many studies on similar less invasive techniques followed in an attempt to reduce postoperative pain and preserve neck motion [29, 30].

22.3 Postoperative Kyphosis

In addition to the direct decompression effect by the posterior displacement of the laminae, laminoplasty has an indirect total decompression effect resulting from the dorsal shift of the spinal cord as long as patient's cervical alignment is maintained in lordosis [31]. In such case, the decompression effect of laminoplasty is equivalent to laminectomy and is comparable to ACDF [13, 15]. In patients with kyphosis, recovery of myelopathy was unfavorable than that in patients with lordotic curvature [32]. Baba, et al. reported that neurologic improvement was associated with the degree of posterior cord migration on MR images and postoperative neurologic improvement was correlated to the volume of the enlarged bony canal, which was predominant in patients with lordosis [33]. Sodeyama, et al. also reported that critical value of posterior cord migration for good recovery of myelopathy was 3 mm on average [34]. All these studies emphasize the importance of preserving the lordotic curvature in patients undergoing laminoplasty.

Continuous efforts have been made to preserve preoperative lordosis and to prevent postoperative kyphosis. Insertion of the semispinalis cervicis muscle to the C2 spinous processes should be preserved whenever possible because this muscle has a crucial role in preserving the postoperative lordosis [35, 36]. If decompression at C3/4 segment is necessary, C3 dome laminoplasty is recommended instead of expanding the C3 lamina to leave the C2 spinous process untouched.

In CSM patients, development of mild postoperative kyphosis is acceptable because in CSM patients redundancy of the spinal cord induced by multilevel disc space narrowing attenuate compression force on the spinal cord thereby providing acceptable results. However, in OPLL patients, because the ossified ligaments often hold the disc space and the spinal cord remains in tension and is, therefore, more vulnerable to compression induced by kyphosis [37].

However, Hirabayashi also stated that severe kyphotic deformity or instability after expansive laminoplasty requiring salvage anterior fusion has never been experienced in their clinic although postoperative reduction in lordosis, which may be the consequence of progressive atrophy of the nuchal muscles, was seen in 5% of the patients after expansive laminoplasty [12]. The exact impact of the cervical alignment on the clinical results of laminoplasty should be determined in future studies.

22.4 Segmental Motor Weakness

Motor weakness that occurs mainly in C5 or C6 segments, usually without sensory disturbance, is the most common neurological complication after any type of laminoplasty. Friction heat generated by drilling of the gutters, a traumatic use of surgical instruments including air drills and Kerrison rongeurs, and the fall of the laminae into the canal after hinge breakage, a stretch of the nerve roots by the tethering effect induced by the posterior shift of the spinal cord, have been the proposed causes of this palsy [38, 39]. Involvement of micro-circulatory events has also been implied in the literature [40]. Although there is no established way to prevent this palsy, spontaneous recovery can be expected in most cases within 2 years after surgery. Tsuji, et al. have reported that selected laminoplasty in which the reduced number of levels was decompressed has led to the decrease in the incidence of C5 segmental palsy maybe due to limited posterior shift of the spinal cord, resulting in less tethering effect of the nerve roots [41].

22.5 Postoperative Progression of OPLL

OPLL itself is not removed after expansive laminoplasty, and there remains a possibility of postoperative progression of the ossified lesion, possibly due to biologic stimulation attributable to surgical invasion, biomechanical stresses, and hereditary disposition [42]. Therefore, when performing laminoplasty in patients with OPLL, it is necessary to expand the sagittal spinal canal sufficiently over the range of one vertebral level above and below the stenotic level and, at the same time, to obtain enough width of the expansion of the spinal canal [11].

22.6 Prophylactic Decompression

So far, there is no effective way to regenerate the spinal cord once it is damaged beyond its healing capacity. The only available solution presently is to operate on a patient with myelopathy before the spinal cord is damaged irreversibly [12, 43]. Therefore, to obtain better surgical outcomes, early surgical decompression is recommended before the spinal cord deteriorates irreversibly, especially in young patients with a narrow spinal canal even if their myelopathy is not severe. This early-stage surgery is made possible by the reliability of the surgery. Laminoplasty is a reliable procedure, which has an equivalent decompression effect as ACDF and laminectomy, and is considered to maintain a more stable spine than laminectomy. It is also much safer and easier than ACDF against severely deteriorated spinal cord resulting in fewer complications. There is, however, no consensus on whether prophylactic decompression is justified for a patient with mild myelopathy or even before one develops myelopathy. This needs to be further discussed in future studies [44–46].

References

1. Epstein N. The surgical management of ossification of the posterior longitudinal ligament in 51 patients. J Spinal Disord. 1993;6(5):432–54.
2. Yamaura I, Kurosa Y, Matuoka T, Shindo S. Anterior floating method for cervical myelopathy caused by ossification of the posterior longitudinal ligament. Clin Orthop Relat Res. 1999;359:27–34.
3. Yonenobu K, Fuji T, Ono K, Okada K, Yamamoto T, Harada N. Choice of surgical treatment for multisegmental cervical spondylotic myelopathy. Spine (Phila Pa 1976). 1985;10(8):710–6.
4. Shinomiya K, Okamoto A, Kamikozuru M, Furuya K, Yamaura I. An analysis of failures in primary cervical anterior spinal cord decompression and fusion. J Spinal Disord. 1993;6(4):277–88.
5. Song JS, Choi BW, Song KJ. Risk factors for the development of adjacent segment disease following anterior cervical arthrodesis for degenerative cervical disease: comparison between fusion methods. J Clin Neurosci. 2014;21(5):794–8.
6. Mayfield FH. Complications of laminectomy. Clin Neurosurg. 1976;23:435–9.
7. Miyazaki K, Kirita Y. Extensive simultaneous multisegment laminectomy for myelopathy due to the ossification of the posterior longitudinal ligament in the cervical region. Spine (Phila Pa 1976). 1986;11(6):531–42.
8. Cattell HS, Clark GL Jr. Cervical kyphosis and instability following multiple laminectomies in children. J Bone Joint Surg Am. 1967;49(4):713–20.
9. Kawai S, Sunago K, Doi K, Saika M, Taguchi T. Cervical laminoplasty (Hattori's method). Procedure and follow-up results. Spine (Phila Pa 1976). 1988;13(11):1245–50.
10. Hirabayashi K. Expansive open-door laminoplasty for cervical spondylotic myelopathy. Shujutsu (Operation). 1978;32:1159–2263. (in Japanese)
11. Hirabayashi K, Miyakawa J, Satomi K, Maruyama T, Wakano K. Operative results and postoperative progression of ossification among patients with ossification of cervical posterior longitudinal ligament. Spine (Phila Pa 1976). 1981;6(4):354–64.
12. Hirabayashi K, Toyama Y, Chiba K. Expansive laminoplasty for myelopathy in ossification of the longitudinal ligament. Clin Orthop Relat Res. 1999;359:35–48.
13. Herkowitz HN. A comparison of anterior cervical fusion, cervical laminectomy, and cervical laminoplasty for the surgical management of multiple level spondylotic radiculopathy. Spine (Phila Pa 1976). 1988;13(7):774–80.
14. Yonenobu K, Hosono N, Iwasaki M, Asano M, Ono K. Neurologic complications of surgery for cervical compression myelopathy. Spine (Phila Pa 1976). 1991;16(11):1277–82.
15. Iwasaki M, Ebara S, Miyamoto S, Wada E, Yonenobu K. Expansive laminoplasty for cervical radiculomyelopathy due to soft disc herniation. Spine (Phila Pa 1976). 1996;21(1):32–8.
16. Kurokawa T, Tsuyama N, Tanaka H. Enlargement of spinal canal by the sagittal splitting of the spinous process. Bessatsu Seikeigeka (Orthop Surg). 1982;2:234–40. (in Japanese)
17. Itoh T, Tsuji H. Technical improvements and results of laminoplasty for compressive myelopathy in the cervical spine. Spine (Phila Pa 1976). 1985;10(8):729–36.
18. Park AE, Heller JG. Cervical laminoplasty: use of a novel titanium plate to maintain canal expansion--surgical technique. J Spinal Disord Tech. 2004;17(4):265–71.
19. Hoshi K, Kurokawa T, Nakamura K, Hoshino Y, Saita K, Miyoshi K. Expansive cervical laminoplasties--observations on comparative changes in spinous process lengths following longitudinal laminal divisions using autogenous bone or hydroxyapatite spacers. Spinal Cord. 1996;34(12):725–8.
20. Tomita K, Kawahara N, Toribatake Y, Heller JG. Expansive midline T-saw laminoplasty (modified spinous process-splitting) for the management of cervical myelopathy. Spine (Phila Pa 1976). 1998;23(1):32–7.
21. Matsumoto M, Chiba K, Toyama Y. Surgical treatment of ossification of the posterior longitudinal ligament and its outcomes: posterior surgery by laminoplasty. Spine (Phila Pa 1976). 2012;37(5):E303–8.
22. Iwasaki M, Okuda S, Miyauchi A, Sakaura H, Mukai Y, Yonenobu K, et al. Surgical strategy for cervical myelopathy due to ossification of the posterior longitudinal ligament: part 1: clinical results and

limitations of laminoplasty. Spine (Phila Pa 1976). 2007;32(6):647–53.
23. Seichi A, Chikuda H, Kimura A, Takeshita K, Sugita S, Hoshino Y, et al. Intraoperative ultrasonographic evaluation of posterior decompression via laminoplasty in patients with cervical ossification of the posterior longitudinal ligament: correlation with 2-year follow-up results. J Neurosurg Spine. 2010;13(1):47–51.
24. Ogawa Y, Chiba K, Matsumoto M, Nakamura M, Takaishi H, Hirabayashi H, et al. Long-term results after expansive open-door laminoplasty for the segmental-type of ossification of the posterior longitudinal ligament of the cervical spine: a comparison with nonsegmental-type lesions. J Neurosurg Spine. 2005;3(3):198–204.
25. Fujiyoshi T, Yamazaki M, Kawabe J, Endo T, Furuya T, Koda M, et al. A new concept for making decisions regarding the surgical approach for cervical ossification of the posterior longitudinal ligament: the K-line. Spine (Phila Pa 1976). 2008;33(26):E990–3.
26. Hosono N, Yonenobu K, Ono K. Neck and shoulder pain after laminoplasty. A noticeable complication. Spine (Phila Pa 1976). 1996;21(17):1969–73.
27. Hosono N, Sakaura H, Mukai Y, Yoshikawa H. The source of axial pain after cervical laminoplasty-C7 is more crucial than deep extensor muscles. Spine (Phila Pa 1976). 2007;32(26):2985–8.
28. Shiraishi T, Fukuda K, Yato Y, Nakamura M, Ikegami T. Results of skip laminectomy-minimum 2-year follow-up study compared with open-door laminoplasty. Spine (Phila Pa 1976). 2003;28(24):2667–72.
29. Kotani Y, Abumi K, Ito M, Sudo H, Takahata M, Nagahama K, et al. Impact of deep extensor muscle-preserving approach on clinical outcome of laminoplasty for cervical spondylotic myelopathy: comparative cohort study. Eur Spine J. 2012;21(8):1536–44.
30. Riew KD, Raich AL, Dettori JR, Heller JG. Neck pain following cervical laminoplasty: does preservation of the C2 muscle attachments and/or C7 matter? Evid Based Spine Care J. 2013;4(1):42–53.
31. Fujimura Y, Nishi Y, Nakamura M. Dorsal shift and expansion of the spinal cord after expansive open-door laminoplasty. J Spinal Disord. 1997;10(4):282–7.
32. Batzdorf U, Batzdorff A. Analysis of cervical spine curvature in patients with cervical spondylosis. Neurosurgery. 1988;22(5):827–36.
33. Baba H, Uchida K, Maezawa Y, Furusawa N, Azuchi M, Imura S. Lordotic alignment and posterior migration of the spinal cord following en bloc open-door laminoplasty for cervical myelopathy: a magnetic resonance imaging study. J Neurol. 1996;243(9):626–32.
34. Sodeyama T, Goto S, Mochizuki M, Takahashi J, Moriya H. Effect of decompression enlargement laminoplasty for posterior shifting of the spinal cord. Spine (Phila Pa 1976). 1999;24(15):1527–31. discussion 31-2
35. Takeshita K, Seichi A, Akune T, Kawamura N, Kawaguchi H, Nakamura K. Can laminoplasty maintain the cervical alignment even when the C2 lamina is contained? Spine (Phila Pa 1976). 2005;30(11):1294–8.
36. Sakaura H, Hosono N, Mukai Y, Fujimori T, Iwasaki M, Yoshikawa H. Preservation of muscles attached to the C2 and C7 spinous processes rather than subaxial deep extensors reduces adverse effects after cervical laminoplasty. Spine (Phila Pa 1976). 2010;35(16):E782–6.
37. Chiba K, Toyama Y, Watanabe M, Maruiwa H, Matsumoto M, Hirabayashi K. Impact of longitudinal distance of the cervical spine on the results of expansive open-door laminoplasty. Spine (Phila Pa 1976). 2000;25(22):2893–8.
38. Chen Y, Chen D, Wang X, Guo Y, He Z. C5 palsy after laminectomy and posterior cervical fixation for ossification of posterior longitudinal ligament. J Spinal Disord Tech. 2007;20(7):533–5.
39. Imagama S, Matsuyama Y, Yukawa Y, Kawakami N, Kamiya M, Kanemura T, et al. C5 palsy after cervical laminoplasty: a multicentre study. J Bone Joint Surg Br. 2010;92(3):393–400.
40. Chiba K, Toyama Y, Matsumoto M, Maruiwa H, Watanabe M, Hirabayashi K. Segmental motor paralysis after expansive open-door laminoplasty. Spine (Phila Pa 1976). 2002;27(19):2108–15.
41. Tsuji T, Asazuma T, Masuoka K, Yasuoka H, Motosuneya T, Sakai T, et al. Retrospective cohort study between selective and standard C3-7 laminoplasty. Minimum 2-year follow-up study. Eur Spine J. 2007;16(12):2072–7.
42. Chiba K, Yamamoto I, Hirabayashi H, Iwasaki M, Goto H, Yonenobu K, et al. Multicenter study investigating the postoperative progression of ossification of the posterior longitudinal ligament in the cervical spine: a new computer-assisted measurement. J Neurosurg Spine. 2005;3(1):17–23.
43. Ogawa Y, Toyama Y, Chiba K, Matsumoto M, Nakamura M, Takaishi H, et al. Long-term results of expansive open-door laminoplasty for ossification of the posterior longitudinal ligament of the cervical spine. J Neurosurg Spine. 2004;1(2):168–74.
44. Yonenobu K. Is surgery indicated for asymptomatic or mildly myelopathic patients with significant ossification of the posterior longitudinal ligament? Spine (Phila Pa 1976). 2012;37(5):E315–7.
45. Lee SE, Jahng TA, Kim HJ. Surgical outcomes in patients with mild symptoms, but severely compressed spinal cord from cervical ossification of the posterior longitudinal ligament. J Clin Neurosci. 2016;33:163–8.
46. Cheung JPY, Cheung PWH, Chiu CK, Chan CYW, Kwan MK. Variations in practice among Asia-Pacific surgeons and recommendations for managing cervical myelopathy: the first Asia-Pacific spine society collaborative study. Asian Spine J. 2019;13(1):45–55.

23 Open-Door Laminoplasty for Cervical OPLL: Technique, Long-Term Results, and Complications

Yoshiharu Kawaguchi

Abstract

Cervical laminoplasty has become a standard procedure for the posterior decompression of the cervical cord, as ossification of the posterior longitudinal ligament (OPLL) a potential of cervical cord compression at multisegmental levels. We developed en bloc cervical laminoplasty, an open-door type procedure in 1981. The long-term (>20 years) outcome of this procedure is favorable without any major complications. However, postoperative radiculopathy, postoperative axial pain, and neurological deterioration due to the progression of OPLL must be considered after cervical laminoplasty.

Keywords

OPLL · Cervical myelopathy · Cervical laminoplasty · Long-term follow-up · Surgical outcome · Radiological result · Complication

Y. Kawaguchi (✉)
Department of Orthopaedic Surgery, Toyama University Hospital, Toyama, Japan
e-mail: zenji@med.u-toyama.ac.jp

23.1 Introduction

Ossification of the posterior longitudinal ligament (OPLL) is characterized by the replacement of the ligamentous tissue with ectopic new bone formation [1, 2]. OPLL commonly results in the narrowing of the spinal canal and is recognized as a cause of cervical myelopathy. As OPLL has a potential of cervical cord compression at multisegmental levels, cervical laminoplasty has become a standard procedure for the posterior decompression of the cervical cord [3]. In the early 1970s, cervical laminoplasty was developed in Japan to resolve postoperative problems after conventional laminectomy [4]. Conventional laminectomy often caused instability and deformity that caused recurrent cervical myelopathy. Cervical laminoplasty has undergone several modifications that were proposed in the 1980s. Although there are two types of cervical laminoplasty, the expansive open-door type [5] and the double-door by splitting spinous process type [6]; the concept of both the procedures is the same. Laminoplasty is a posterior decompression surgery that preserves the structural mechanics of the posterior element in the cervical spine. Many studies have reported that cervical laminoplasty yields favorable surgical outcomes; thus, the concept of cervical laminoplasty has been widely accepted and has spread not only in Japan, but also throughout the world [7–14]. Our institute developed en bloc cervical laminoplasty, an open-door type procedure in 1981 [15, 16]. We

A. Okawa et al. (eds.), *OPLL*, https://doi.org/10.1007/978-981-15-3855-1_23

still perform the same procedure in clinical practice. In this chapter, we describe the clinical outcomes and potential risks of en bloc cervical laminoplasty based on long-term follow-up.

23.2 Operative Procedure of En Bloc Laminoplasty

En bloc laminoplasty, as proposed by Itoh and Tsuji [15, 16], has been utilized for the decompression of the spinal cord in patients with multilevel OPLL. The details of this procedure have been previously reported in the literature [13–16]. The method is briefly described here. The laminae are exposed from the caudal half of C2 to the cranial half of T1. Decompression of the spinal canal via en bloc laminoplasty is performed from C3 to C7 or T1. The levels of decompression are determined using imaging studies, including plain radiography, CT, myelography, and MRI. One side of the laminae was opened, and the other side served as the hinge. Bone grafts from the dissected spinous processes or a molded hydroxyapatite (HA) block are put in the opened laminae and fixed with braded wires or nylon threads. Bone grafts or HA blocks in the open gap are placed at 3–5 levels as per cervical instability. Bone chips are also placed in the hinged side. Recently, we do not apply bone graft at the hinge side to preserve the mobility in the cervical spine. Attention is paid to avoid destroying the bilateral facet joints. Spinal cord shifts posteriorly by expanding the spinal canal. After decompressing the spinal cord, the paravertebral muscle and the nuchal ligament are sutured at the original portion. The patients are required to stay in bed for 1 day postoperatively; thereafter, walking is allowed with a neck collar. A neck collar is recommended for 1 month after the surgery.

23.3 Long-Term Results

We have reported the long-term (>20 years) results of en bloc cervical laminoplasty [14]. The data are summarized below. Totally 216 patients underwent en bloc cervical laminoplasty for the treatment of cervical compressive myelopathy due to cervical spondylosis (CS) or OPLL between 1981 and 1994. One hundred and forty-eight patients who were followed up for >20 years were analyzed. With respect to the survivors, there were 68 patients (45 men and 23 women) with an average age of 51.7 years at the time of the operation (range: 24–70 years). There were 26 patients with CS and 42 with OPLL. The average age at the last follow-up was 77.2 years (range: 45–95 years). The average length of follow-up was 25.5 years with a range of 20–32 years. At the time of this study, 80 patients had already died. We were unable to contact the remaining 68 patients. Thus, the follow-up rate, including the survivors and the dead patients, was 68.5% (148/216).

23.3.1 Clinical Results

23.3.1.1 Survivors

Data of 65 patients were available. There were 24 patients (16 men and 9 women) with CS and 41 patients (27 men and 14 women) with OPLL. The average preoperative JOA score was 9.5 ± 2.5 out of 17 points (range 6–15) in patients with CS and 9.3 ± 2.7 (range 4–17) in patients with OPLL. The JOA score in both the CS and OPLL groups improved rapidly within a year and continued to improve until 5 years postoperatively. The JOA score and recovery rate increased to 14.2% and 64.9%, respectively at 5 years after surgery. The mean JOA score and recovery rate were maintained at 13.9% and 61.6% at 10 years, respectively. The JOA score was decreased to 11.4 at the final follow-up. The maximum score and recovery rate during the follow-up were 14.3% and 67.8%, respectively, in CS and 14.6% and 70.3%, respectively, in OPLL. The average recovery rate at the final follow-up was 22.6% ± 69.1% in CS and 37.1% ± 56.7% in OPLL. There was no difference in the postoperative JOA score and recovery rate between CS and OPLL.

In 32 out of 65 patients (49.2%), the JOA scores worsened during the follow-up period. This group consisted of 11 patients (7 men and 4 women) with CS and 21 (12 men and 9 women) with OPLL. The additional spine surgeries were conducted between 10 and 30 years after cervical laminoplasty.

There was no major general complication after laminoplasty. Although 11 patients (2 with CS and 9 with OPLL) (11/65, 17%) complained of axial neck pain at the final follow-up, this was not the chief complaint, except in 1 patient with OPLL. Two patients with OPLL experienced postoperative radiculopathy in the unilateral upper extremity and required additional corpectomy and anterior interbody fusion.

23.3.1.2 Patients Who Died during Follow-Up [17]

With respect to the 80 patients who died during the follow-up, the mean age at death was 78.2 ± 8.6 years. There were 44 patients with CS (31 men and 13 women) and 36 patients with OPLL (30 men and 6 women). The mean period between surgery and death was 13.4 ± 7.4 years (range: 1–31 years). The family members of 5 patients were unable to report the exact year when the patient died. Twelve patients died within 5 years of surgery, 14 died between 6 and 10 years of surgery, 34 died between 11 and 20 years, while 15 died more than 21 years postoperatively. No patient died from complications related to the operation. The most frequent cause of death was malignant tumor (23 cases) followed by ischemic heart disease (13 cases) and cerebral infarction (6 cases). There was no obvious relationship between the cause of death and the spinal cord lesion.

23.3.1.3 Radiological Evaluation

Radiological evaluation was performed for 48 patients using radiography more than 10 years after cervical laminoplasty. There were 14 patients with CS (10 men and 4 women) and 34 with OPLL (23 men and 11 women).

The average sagittal diameter of the spinal canal in the patients with CS was increased from 12.8 mm to 17.8 mm at the bone-grafted level (C5) and from 13.8 mm to 18.1 mm at the non-bone-grafted level (C6) at the last follow-up. In the patients with OPLL, it was increased from 10.1 mm to 13.7 mm at the narrowest level. However, the recovery rate was not related to the distance of the space available for the spinal cord. There were no patients with lamina closure during the follow-up. The mean preoperative angle of cervical alignment in the neutral position was 15.7° ± 12.2° in the patients with CS and 11.0° ± 8.9° in those with OPLL. Cervical alignment became kyphotic after the surgery. There was no relationship between pre- and postoperative cervical alignment and the recovery of the JOA score after laminoplasty. The mean preoperative ROM of the cervical spine was 40.9° ± 16.0° in CS and 30.9° ± 16.6° in the OPLL group. The ROM decreased to 13.6° ± 10.9° in the CS group and 4.4 ± 5.7° in the OPLL group at the final follow-up. The postoperative ROM in the OPLL group was lower than that in the CS group. One of the causes of ROM reduction was postoperative interlaminar fusion because the decrease in postoperative ROM was more marked in patients with longer laminar fusion. The number of fused laminae was 3.0 ± 1.4 in the CS group and 4.0 ± 1.1 in the OPLL group, postoperatively. The number of fused laminae was higher in the OPLL group than in the CS group.

23.4 Problems Regarding Cervical Laminoplasty in the Long-Term Follow-Up

There was no major general complication after laminoplasty. Although postoperative radiculopathy, including C5 palsy, is a complication of cervical laminoplasty, few patients complained of postoperative radiculopathy in the long-term follow-up [18–21]. Postoperative neck pain was observed in 17% of the patients who underwent en bloc laminoplasty [22–26]. Limited range of motion after cervical laminoplasty was commonly observed [27].

23.4.1 Progression of OPLL [28–31]

Postoperative progression of OPLL is one of the main problems observed in the long-term follow-up. In our recent study [31], 9 out of 167 patients (5.4%) underwent the second additional surgery because of neurological deterioration due to

OPLL progression. In this study, the age of the second surgery group was lower than that of the controls who did not require the second surgery. More subjects in the second surgery group had mixed type of OPLL than in the control group. Six patients achieved neurological recovery after the second surgery; however, three patients still had a neurological deficit. The patients who showed poor recovery had clear T2 high intensity zone on MR image in the spinal cord. Thus, early additional decompression might be considered in patients at risk of OPLL progression.

23.5 Conclusion

En bloc laminoplasty is a safe procedure without major general complications for treating cervical OPLL. This operation achieves favorable neurological recovery in the long-term (>20 years). In spite of several complications, including postoperative radiculopathy and neurological deterioration due to the progression of OPLL, cervical laminoplasty is indicated in patients with multilevel cervical cord compression by OPLL.

References

1. Tsukimoto H. On an autopsied case of compression myelopathy with a callus formation in the cervical spinal canal. Nihon-Geka-Hokan. 1960;29:1003–7.
2. Onji Y, Akiyama H, Shimomura Y, Ono K, Hukuda S, Mizuno S. Posterior paravertebral ossification causing cervical myelopathy. J Bone Joint Surg Am. 1967;49:1314–28.
3. Matsumoto M, Chiba K, Toyama Y. Surgical treatment of ossification of the posterior longitudinal ligament and its outcomes: posterior surgery by laminoplasty. Spine (Phila Pa 1976). 2012;37(5):E303–8.
4. Nakamura K, Seichi A. History of laminoplasty. In: Cervical Laminoplasty. Tokyo: Springer-Verlag; 2003. p. 3–11.
5. Chiba K, Maruiwa H, Matsumoto M, Hirabayashi K, Toyama Y. Expansive open-door laminoplasty. Tokyo: Springer-Verlag; 2003. p. 27–45.
6. Seichi A, Iwasaki M, Nakamura K. Double-door laminoplasty by splitting spinous processes. Tokyo: Springer-Verlag; 2003. p. 47–62.
7. Seichi A, Takeshita K, Ohishi I, Kawaguchi H, Akune T, Anamizu Y, Kitagawa T, Nakamura K. Long-term results of double-door laminoplasty for cervical stenotic myelopathy. Spine (Phila Pa 1976). 2011;26(5):479–87.
8. Kimura A, Seichi A, Inoue H, Hoshino Y. Long-term results of double-door laminoplasty using hydroxyapatite spacers in patients with compressive cervical myelopathy. Eur Spine J. 2011;20(9):1560–6.
9. Motosuneya T, Maruyama T, Yamada H, Tsuzuki N, Sakai H. Long-term results of tension-band laminoplasty for cervical stenotic myelopathy: a ten-year follow-up. J Bone Joint Surg Br. 2011;93(1):68–72.
10. Ogawa Y, Chiba K, Matsumoto M, Nakamura M, Takaishi H, Hirabayashi H, Hirabayashi K, Nishiwaki Y, Toyama Y. Long-term results after expansive open-door laminoplasty for the segmental-type of ossification of the posterior longitudinal ligament of the cervical spine: a comparison with nonsegmental-type lesions. J Neurosurg Spine. 2005;3(3):198–204.
11. Chiba K, Ogawa Y, Ishii K, Takaishi H, Nakamura M, Maruiwa H, Matsumoto M, Toyama Y. Long-term results of expansive open-door laminoplasty for cervical myelopathy--average 14-year follow-up study. Spine (Phila Pa 1976). 2006;31(26):2998–3005.
12. Iwasaki M, Kawaguchi Y. Kimura, Yonenobu K. Long-term results of expansive laminoplasty for ossification of the posterior longitudinal ligament of the cervical spine: more than 10 years follow up. J Neurosurg. 2002;96(2 Suppl):180–9.
13. Kawaguchi Y, Kanamori M, Ishihara H, Ohmori K, Nakamura H, Kimura T. Minimum 10-year followup after en bloc cervical laminoplasty. Clin Orthop Relat Res. 2003;411:129–39.
14. Kawaguchi Y, Nakano M, Yasuda T, Seki S, Hori T, Suzuki K, Makino H, Kimura T. More than 20 years follow-up after en bloc cervical laminoplasty. Spine (Phila Pa 1976). 2016;41(20):1570–9.
15. Ito T, Tsuji H. Technical improvements and results of laminoplasty for compressive myelopathy in the cervical spine. Spine (Phila Pa 1976). 1985;10(8):729–36.
16. Tsuji H. Laminoplasty for patients with compressive myelopathy due to so-called spinal canal stenosis in cervical and thoracic regions. Spine (Phila Pa 1976). 1982;7(1):28–34.
17. Kawaguchi Y, Nakano M, Yasuda T, Seki S, Hori T, Suzuki K, Makino H, Kimura T. Life expectancy after cervical en bloc laminoplasty: analysis of data following more than 20 years. Spine (Phila Pa 1976). 2017;42(7):450–5.
18. Sakaura H, Hosono N, Mukai Y, Ishii T, Yoshikawa H. C5 palsy after decompression surgery for cervical myelopathy: review of the literature. Spine (Phila Pa 1976). 2003;28(21):2447–51.
19. Gu Y, Cao P, Gao R, Tian Y, Liang L, Wang C, Yang L, Yuan W. Incidence and risk factors of C5 palsy following posterior cervical decompression: a systematic review. PLoS One. 2014;9(8):e101933.
20. Nassr A, Nassr A, Eck JC, Ponnappan RK, Zanoun RR, Donaldson WF 3rd, Kang JD. The incidence of C5 palsy after multilevel cervical decompression procedures: a review of 750 consecutive cases. Spine (Phila Pa 1976). 2012;37(3):174–8.

21. Imagama S, Matsuyama Y, Yukawa Y, Kawakami N, Kamiya M, Kanemura T, Ishiguro N, Nagoya Spine Group. C5 palsy after cervical laminoplasty: a multicentre study. J Bone Joint Surg Br. 2010;92(3):393–400.
22. Hosono N, Yonenobu K, Ono K. Neck and shoulder pain after laminoplasty. A noticeable complication. Spine (Phila Pa 1976). 1996;21(17):1969–73.
23. Kawaguchi Y, Matsui H, Ishihara H, Gejo R, Yoshino O. Axial symptoms following en bloc cervical laminoplasty. J Spinal Disord. 1999;12(5):392–5.
24. Riew KD, Raich AL, Dettori JR, Heller JG. Neck Pain Following Cervical Laminoplasty: Does Preservation of the C2 Muscle Attachments and/or C7 Matter? Evid Based Spine Care J. 2013;4(1):42–53.
25. Wang SJ, Jiang SD, Jiang LS, Dai LY. Axial pain after posterior cervical spine surgery: a systematic review. Eur Spine J. 2011;20(2):185–94.
26. Kawaguchi Y, Kanamori M, Ishiara H, Nobukiyo M, Seki S, Kimura T. Preventive measures for axial symptoms following cervical laminoplasty. J Spinal Disord Tech. 2003;16(6):497–501.
27. Machino M, Yukawa Y, Hida T, Ito K, Nakashima H, Kanbara S, Morita D, Kato F. Cervical alignment and range of motion after laminoplasty: radiographical data from more than 500 cases with cervical spondylotic myelopathy and a review of the literature. Spine (Phila Pa 1976). 2012;37(20):E1243–50.
28. Kawaguchi Y, Kanamori M, Ishihara H, Nakamura H, Sugimori K, Tsuji H, Kimura T. Progression of ossification of the posterior longitudinal ligament following en bloc cervical laminoplasty. J Bone Joint Surg Am. 2001;83(12):1798–802.
29. Hori T, Kawaguchi Y, Kimura T. How does the ossification area of the posterior longitudinal ligament progress after cervical laminoplasty? Spine (Phila Pa 1976). 2006;31(24):2807–12.
30. Hori T, Kawaguchi Y, Kimura T. How does the ossification area of the posterior longitudinal ligament thicken following cervical laminoplasty? Spine (Phila Pa 1976). 2007;32(19):E551–6.
31. Kawaguchi Y, Nakano M, Yasuda T, Seki S, Suzuki K, Yahara Y, Makino H, Kobayashi K, Kimura T. Clinical impact of ossification of the posterior longitudinal ligament progression after cervical laminoplasty. Clin Spine Surg. 2019;32(3):E133–E9.

Double-Door Laminoplasty for Cervical OPLL: Technique, Complications, and Long-Term Results

24

Katsushi Takeshita

Abstract

Double-door laminoplasty, one of the two fundamental laminoplasties, is performed by splitting the spinous process and widening the split laminae, which are held by spacers. Surgical outcome of cervical laminoplasty is satisfactory except cases with the massive OPLL and kyphotic alignment. C5-nerve root palsy as well as massive bleeding is a complication of laminoplasty in OPLL patients. Surgical recovery is maintained over 10 years.

Keywords

Double-door laminoplasty · OPLL · JOA score · C5-nerve root palsy · Hydroxyapatite spacer · K-line · Lateral gutter · Kyphosis

24.1 History

Laminoplasty has been the main surgical technique for cervical OPLL even after modern instrumentation was applied to cervical disorders.

There are two types of laminoplasties: unilateral laminoplasty and double-door laminoplasty. Unilateral laminoplasty, first reported by Hirabayashi [1], was also called open-door laminoplasty. Double-door laminoplasty, first reported by Kurokawa, [2] was also called French-door or mid-sagittal spinous-splitting method.

24.2 Surgical Techniques

A patient is flipped over carefully to the supine position after intubation. The prone position is kept by a four-poster Hall frame or a Jackson® (Mizuho/OSI) table. The head is fixed by Mayfield or is placed on a soft pad such as Prone View® (Dupaco). The mild reversed Trendelenburg position is preferable to decrease intraoperative bleeding.

The incision is mid-central, and the posterior cervical spine is exposed down to the lamina. The lamina is explored to the medial edge of facet, which is identical to the line of lateral gutters. Attachment of muscles and ligaments, which anchor to the spinous processes and laminae, is kept intact as much as possible (Fig. 24.1) [3]. Especially, the significance of C2 to prevent kyphotic change is well-known. When laminoplasty needs to go up to C2, detached muscles of greater posterior rectus capitis muscle, inferior obliquus capitis muscle, and cervical semispinalis need to be sutured before closing (Fig. 24.2) [4].

K. Takeshita (✉)
Department of Orthopaedics, Jichi Medical University, Tochigi, Japan
e-mail: dtstake@jichi.ac.jp

A. Okawa et al. (eds.), *OPLL*, https://doi.org/10.1007/978-981-15-3855-1_24

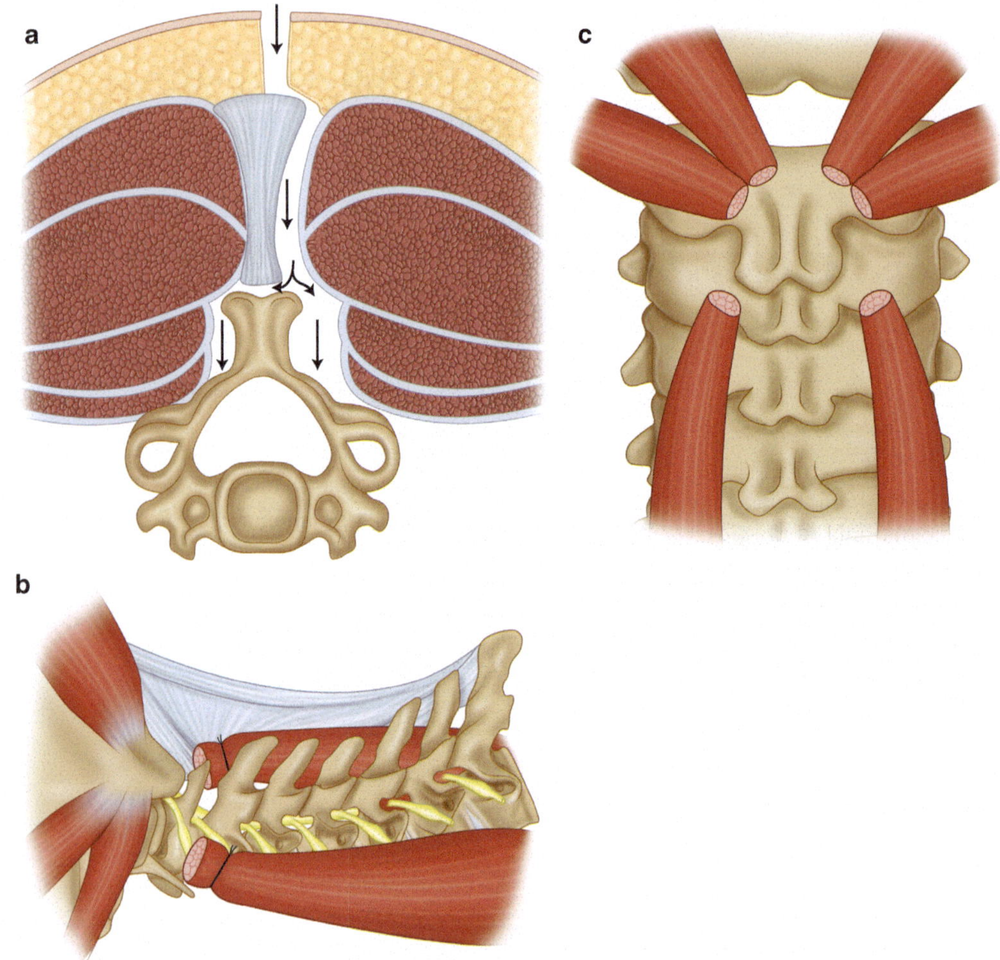

Fig. 24.1 (**a**) The arrows show the posterior approach to the cervical laminae. The approach is made along the edge of the nuchal ligament. The most superficial muscle, the trapezius, is separated from the superior nuchal ligament and the spinous process of C7. The splenius capitis muscles are also detached from the nuchal ligament. This approach preserves the continuity of the nuchal ligament. (**b**) The nuchal ligament is preserved. The semispinalis cervicis is transiently detached from the C2 spinous process to allow access from C3 to C7. (**c**) When C1 and C2 are included in the decompressive area, rectus capitis posterior major and obliqus capitis inferior muscles are detached. Reused with permission from [3]

For double-door laminoplasty, burring bilateral lateral gutters and mid-sagittal splitting of the spinous process are main procedures (Fig. 24.3). Firstly, the spinous process is cut by a thin diamond burr, which is confirmed by direct vision or trial spreading of split laminae. Cutting the inner cortex of spinous process should be performed carefully to avoid the iatrogenic neurological deterioration. Some surgeons prefer to preserve a thin cortex in this stage and break it during the splitting maneuver. An alternative method for cutting the spinous process is the inside-out technique by a threaded saw such as T-saw® (DePuy Spine), which was originally developed for total spondylectomy. Compared to the cutting of every spinous process by a burr one by one, the inside-out technique by a threaded saw can cut all spinous processes altogether. However, passing a threaded saw and initial cutting should be performed carefully in a case with severe stenosis [5]. Secondly, both sides of lateral gutters are created by the burr. Excessive burring

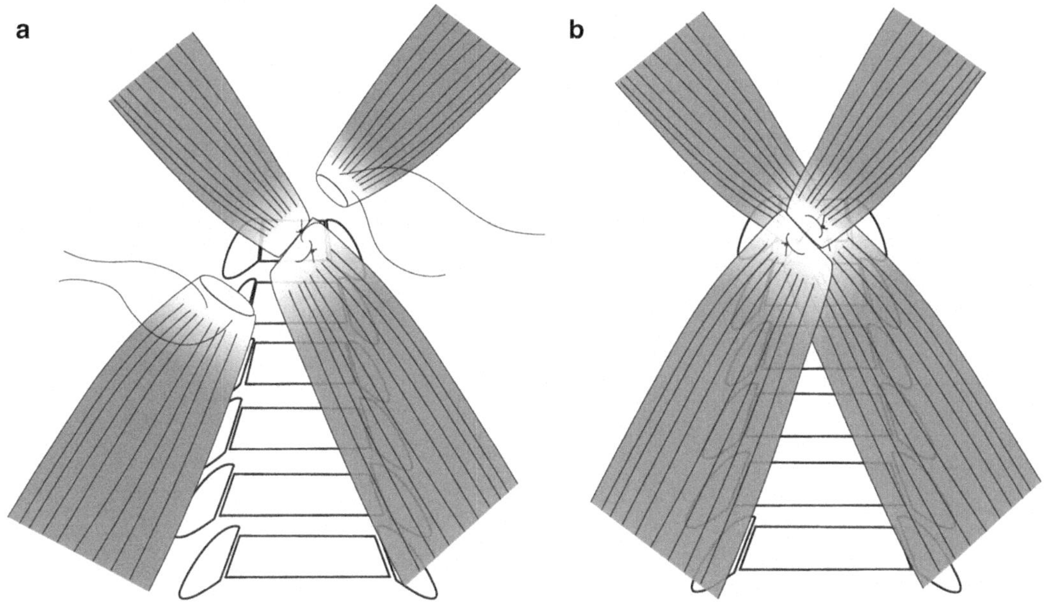

Fig. 24.2 Muscles attaching the C2 lamina are approximated after all spacers of spinous processes are held in position with threads. (**a**) One side of the rectus capitis posterior major and the inferior oblique are sutured to the contralateral semispinalis cervicis, followed by the other side. (**b**) Reused with permission from [4]

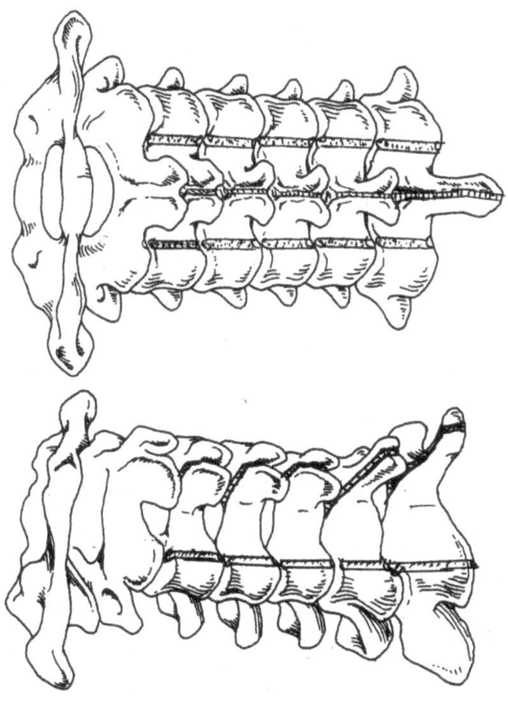

Fig. 24.3 Spinous processes are sagitally split and bilateral troughs (bony grooves) for the hinges are made at the transitional area between the facet joint and the laminae. Reused with permission from [3]

leads to unstable laminae and ends with laminectomy. The position of the lateral gutter is crucial. Preoperative assessment of the spinal canal by computed tomography is preferable. Too far-lateral gutters mean invasion of facet joints as well as pedicles. Too far-lateral gutters are not only hard to be completed but could lead to injury of a cervical nerve root and the vertebral artery. Too far-medical gutters make narrow spinal canal widening and sometimes lead to pinched dura and the spinal cord between gutters. In this stage, gutters need not be completed because during the procedure of spreading spit laminae, the yellow ligament is dissected between adjacent laminae, and split laminae get more movable. When decompression needs to be addressed up to the axial lesion, typical laminoplasty is hard to perform. C1 lamina is usually dealt with laminectomy though laminoplasty of C1 is technically feasible. Because of the thickness of lamina, lateral groove of C2 should be created as a triangular shape for widening.

Both ends of decompression can be dealt with partial laminectomy to minimize the soft tissue containment. C2 can be decompressed with the

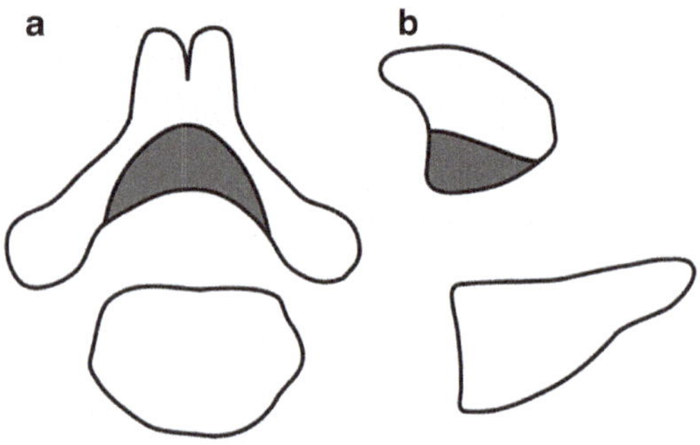

Fig. 24.4 The C2 dome-like laminotomy. (**a**) Axial view. (**b**) Sagittal view. Reused with permission from [4]

surface of the lamina intact by a dome-shaped decompression (Fig. 24.4).

Successively, split laminae are gradually spread. A designated tool called a laminae spreader facilitates this maneuver. Stiffness of laminae are dealt by additional burring and often relieved by cutting the yellow ligament. Epidural bleeding should be controlled. Epidural soft tissue hindering the expansion of the dura should be released.

To finish the laminoplasty, spacers to prevent the closure of split laminae need to be placed (Fig. 24.5). Autologous bone from the tip of C6 or C7 spinous process or from the iliac crest is often used to achieve bone union between a spacer and split laminae. Artificial materials especially hydroxyapatite spacers are usually used (Fig. 24.6).

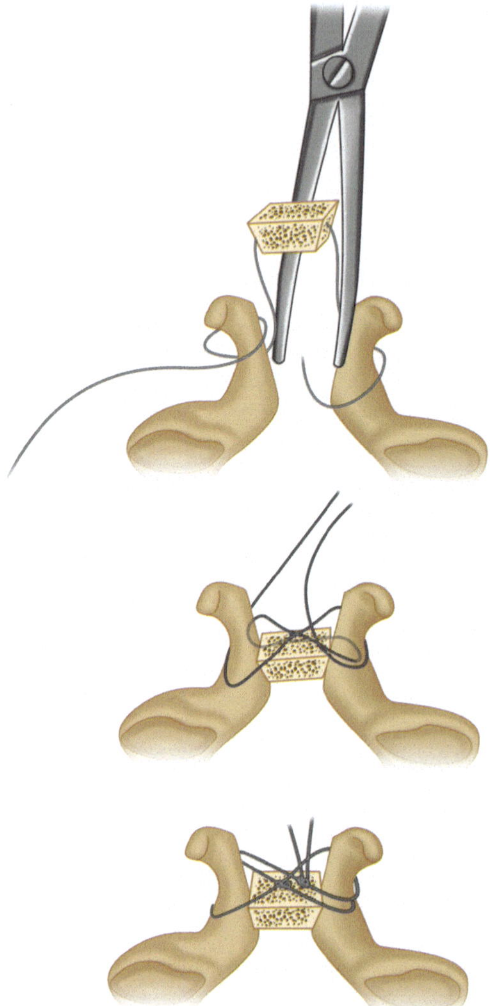

Fig. 24.5 A hydroxyapatite spacer or iliac bone block is held in place with sutures passing through holes made in the spinous process. Reused with permission from [3]

24.3 Short-Term Results, Complications, and Satisfaction

Surgical outcome of cervical laminoplasty is satisfactory except for cases with the massive OPLL and kyphotic alignment [6]. Thickness of the OPLL, cervical alignment, and the range of motion are significant radiographic parameters relevant with surgical outcome. The K-line, which can assess the thickness of the OPLL and cervical alignment simultaneously, is a useful tool to determine the surgical approach for patients with OPLL [7, 8]. Selective laminoplasty compared with traditional double-door laminoplasty showed no difference in clinical outcome from a retrospective study of 190 patients with cervical myelopathy [9].

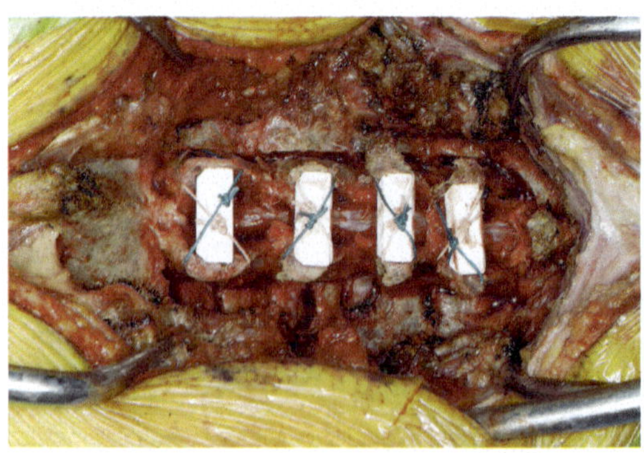

Fig. 24.6 Laminoplasty was completed just after spacers were held in place with sutures between the split spinous processes

The overall complication rate was 22.5% in the United State from an analysis by national administrative database [10]. The most notorious complication of cervical laminoplasty is C5-nerve root palsy though recent studies tend to show its decreasing rate. Rodriguez-Feo et al. from the United States reported that the C5 palsy rate was 8.1% from 222 myelopathic patients who experienced cervical open-door laminoplasty. They also reported that the reoperation rate was 13.5% [11]. In addition, deterioration of lower-extremity function can occur. Seichi et al. reported a retrospective multicenter study of 581 patients who had undergone laminoplasty for cervical OPLL. Among 581 patients, 311 patients had undergone double-door laminoplasty. They found 3.1% of patients experienced worsening of low-extremity function [12]. Massive bleeding during laminoplasty in OPLL patients is not rare. Kato et al. analyzed the risk factors of massive bleeding during laminoplasty from 545 OPLL patients and found that an occupying ratio of 60% or greater is a risk factor for major blood loss [13].

The satisfaction rate was 65.9% from a retrospective study of 44 patients with cervical OPLL. The dissatisfied patients had a hill-shaped ossification [14].

24.4 Long-Term Results

Kimura et al. reported long-term results of double-door laminoplasty with hydroxyapatite spacers. Sixty-eight patients consisted of 39 spondylotic myelopathy and 29 OPLL patients followed up over 10 years. Clinical assessment by JOA score demonstrated that the surgical effect had generally maintained till final follow-up with a gradual decline of the lower-limb motor score because of other musculoskeletal disorders (Fig. 24.7) [15].

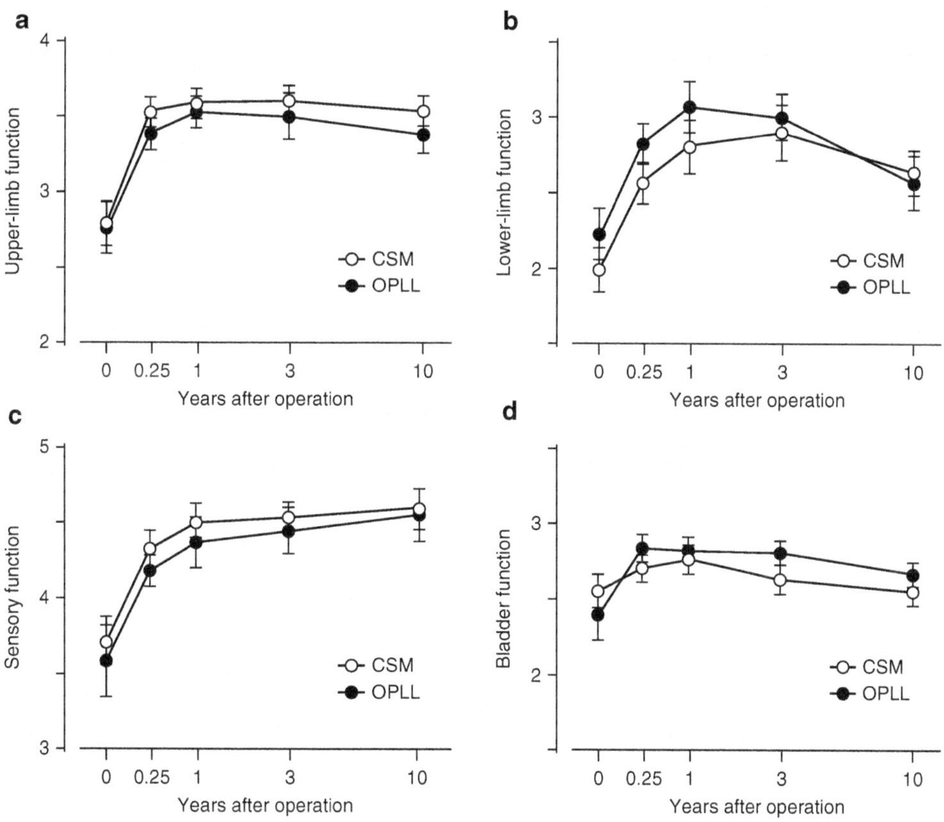

Fig. 24.7 Time course of JOA score for each category of function. The average upper limb motor and sensory scores improved significantly after surgery and were maintained almost until the final follow-up in both the CSM and OPLL groups. The lower-limb motor scores improved significantly, but gradually deteriorated after the third postoperative year in both groups. *Burrs* indicate standard errors. Reused with permission from [15]

References

1. Hirabayashi K, Miyakawa J, Satomi K, Maruyama T, Wakano K. Operative results and postoperative progression of ossification among patients with ossification of cervical posterior longitudinal ligament. Spine (Phila Pa 1976). 1981;6(4):354–64.
2. Kurokawa T, Tanaka H, Nakamura K, et al. Double door laminoplasty through longitudinal splitting of the spinal process [in Japanese]. Bessatsu Seikeigeka. 1986;9:128–9.
3. Seichi A, Iwasaki M, Nakamura K. Double-door laminoplasty by splitting spinous processes. In: Nakamura K, Toyama Y, Hoshino Y, editors. Cervical laminoplasty. Tokyo: Springer; 2003.
4. Katsushi T., ;Atsushi S., Toru A., et al. Can laminoplasty maintain the cervical alignment even when the C2 lamina is contained? Spine. 30(11):1294–1298 2005.
5. Tomita K, Kawahara N, Toribatake Y, et al. Expansive midline T-saw laminoplasty (modified spinous process-splitting) for the management of cervical myelopathy. Spine (Phila Pa 1976). 1998;23(1):32–7.
6. Yoshii T, Egawa S, Hirai T, et al. A systematic review and meta-analysis comparing anterior decompression with fusion and posterior laminoplasty for cervical ossification of the posterior longitudinal ligament. J Orthop Sci. 2019. pii: S0949-2658(19)300739
7. Fujiyoshi T, Yamazaki M, Kawabe J, et al. A new concept for making decisions regarding the surgical approach for cervical ossification of the posterior longitudinal ligament: the K-line. Spine (Phila Pa 1976). 2008;33(26):E990–3.
8. Kanbara S, Imagama S, Ito K, et al. A retrospective imaging study of surgical outcomes and range of motion in patients with cervical ossification of the posterior longitudinal ligament. Eur Spine J. 2018;27(6):1416–22.
9. Hirota R, Miyakoshi N, Yoshimoto M, et al. Comparison of health-related quality of life between double-door laminoplasty and selective laminoplasty for degenerative cervical myelopathy, with a minimum follow-up of 5 years. Spine (Phila Pa 1976). 2019;44(4):E211–8.
10. Veeravagu A, Azad TD, Zhang M, et al. Outcomes of cervical laminoplasty—population-level analysis of a national longitudinal database. J Clin Neurosci. 2018;48:66–70.
11. Rodriguez-Feo JA, Leas D, Odum SM, et al. Reoperation rates following open-door cervical Laminoplasty. Int J Spine Surg. 2018;12(6):751–6.
12. Seichi A, Hoshino Y, Kimura A, et al. Neurological complications of cervical laminoplasty for patients with ossification of the posterior longitudinal ligament-a multi-institutional retrospective study. Spine (Phila Pa 1976). 2011;36(15):E998–1003.
13. Kato S, Chikuda H, Seichi A, et al. Radiographical risk factors for major intraoperative blood loss during laminoplasty in patients with ossification of the posterior longitudinal ligament. Spine (Phila Pa 1976). 2012;37(25):E1588–93.
14. Ohya J, Oshima Y, Oka H, et al. Patient satisfaction with posterior decompression surgery for cervical ossification of the posterior longitudinal ligament: prognostic radiographic factors and patient-reported outcomes for the effectiveness of surgical treatment. World Neurosurg. 2016;96:272–9.
15. Kimura A, Seichi A, Inoue H, Hoshino Y. Long-term results of double-door laminoplasty using hydroxyapatite spacers in patients with compressive cervical myelopathy. Eur Spine J. 2011;20(9):1560–6. https://doi.org/10.1007/s00586-011-1724-7.. Epub 2011 Feb 19

25 Posterior Decompression and Fusion for Cervical OPLL: Indication and Technique

Masao Koda, Tetsuya Abe, Takeo Furuya, Toru Funayama, Hiroshi Takahashi, Hiroshi Noguchi, Kousei Miura, Katsuya Nagashima, Yosuke Shibao, and Masashi Yamazaki

Abstract

Surgical indication of posterior decompression and fusion (PDF) for cervical OPLL in mainly based on K-line, which is defined as that which connects the midpoints of the spinal canal at C2 and C7 in a plain lateral radiogram of the cervical spine. We defined K-line (+) as cases where the peak of ossification foci does not exceed the K-line and K-line (−) as cases where the peak of ossification foci exceeds the K-line. Previous reports revealed that laminoplasty produces a poor outcome in K-line (−) OPLL. One of the surgical options is PDF.

Generally, fixation from C2 to C7 or T1 is applied because the C2 pedicle screw is the most reliable anchor in the cervical spine, and the C7 and/or T1 pedicle screw can be inserted without risk of vertebral artery violation. A lateral mass screw is generally used as a mid-cervical fixation anchor.

PDF surgery is an option for cervical OPLL. PDF might improve the clinical outcome of OPLL patients with K-line (−).

Keywords

OPLL · Posterior surgery · Fusion surgery · Spinal instrumentation · K-line

M. Koda (✉) · T. Abe · T. Funayama
H. Takahashi · H. Noguchi · K. Miura · K. Nagashima
Y. Shibao · M. Yamazaki
Department of Orthopedic Surgery, University of Tsukuba, Ibaraki, Japan

T. Furuya
Department of Orthopedic Surgery, Graduate School of Medicine, Chiba University, Chiba, Japan

25.1 Introduction

Instrumentation surgery for the cervical spine has become widely used because of recent marked development of its technique and various kinds of instruments. Currently, we apply posterior decompression and fusion (PDF) surgery for selected patients with cervical ossification of the posterior longitudinal ligament (OPLL) in addition to conventional surgical procedures including laminoplasty and anterior decompression and fusion surgeries. We will discuss the indications for surgery and technique for PDF surgery for cervical OPLL.

A. Okawa et al. (eds.), *OPLL*, https://doi.org/10.1007/978-981-15-3855-1_25

25.2 Surgical Indication of PDF for Cervical OPLL

25.2.1 K-line (−)

OPLL can cause spinal cord compression, resulting in progressive myelopathy that often needs surgical intervention to resolve myelopathic symptoms [1]. Among the various surgical procedures for cervical OPLL, laminoplasty is the most prevalent in Japan because it can be performed via a posterior approach, which is familiar to most spinal surgeons [2]. Simultaneous decompression can be accomplished by laminoplasty for multilevel spinal canal stenosis caused by OPLL, and the technique for laminoplasty is relatively straightforward compared with that for anterior surgery, which directly approaches the ossification foci. There are many reports describing the favorable clinical outcome of laminoplasty for cervical OPLL [2–5].

The rationale for spinal cord decompression by laminoplasty is indirect spinal cord decompression induced by a posterior shift of the spinal cord through a bowstringing effect [6, 7]. After the release of posterior structures by elevating laminae, the spinal cord can be shifted posteriorly like a bowstring where the cervical spine is lordotic. However, laminoplasty may often result in insufficient spinal cord decompression and poor neurological recovery in patients with thick ossification foci and/or kyphotic alignment, because the bowstringing effect is not effective in those types of OPLL [5–10].

The K-line was first introduced [11] as a practical indicator for application to surgical procedures for OPLL. The K-line is defined as that which connects the midpoints of the spinal canal at C2 and C7 in a plain lateral radiogram of the cervical spine. We defined K-line (+) as cases where the peak of ossification foci does not exceed the K-line and K-line (−) as cases where the peak of ossification foci exceeds the K-line. We stress that the K-line does not simply reflect the alignment of the cervical spine but can reflect both the alignment and the thickness of ossification foci. Comparison of clinical outcome after laminoplasty between K-line (+) and K-line (−) OPLL patients revealed that laminoplasty showed a favorable outcome for K-line (+) OPLL, whereas laminoplasty produces a poor outcome in K-line (−) OPLL [11].

Thus, laminoplasty is indicated for K-line (+) OPLL but should not be applied to K-line (−) OPLL. Ideally, anterior decompression and fusion (ADF) can resolve spinal cord compression by direct removal of an OPLL, even in K-line (−) patients [12, 13]. However, ADF for OPLL has tended to fall into disfavor because of its technical complexity and troublesome perioperative management including upper airway management, cerebrospinal fluid leakage, and graft-related complications [14]. Another surgical option is addition of the instrumented fusion to laminoplasty, namely posterior decompression and fusion surgery (PDF). The rationale of PDF surgery for K-line (−) OPLL is as follows: removal of the residual segmental motion that has negative impact on neurological recovery and prevents progression of postoperative kyphosis, which can induce latent neurological deterioration [15–18].

25.3 Surgical Technique of PDF for Cervical OPLL

A Mayfield skull clamp should be used to obtain optimal alignment during the surgery. We set the cervical spine alignment to match the neutral position seen in preoperative cervical X-ray images. Excessive postural alignment correction might induce iatrogenic foraminal stenosis and/or deterioration of spinal cord compression.

Our routine set-up is shown in Fig. 25.1. Patients are positioned prone with their head stabilized in a Mayfield skull clamp, and the apparatus for anesthesia is moved caudally to obtain a wide space around the head of the patients. Fluoroscopy is obtained cranially. The operator stands on the left side of the patient's head, and the first assistant stands on the opposite side. In some cases, the operator can stand above the patient's head to see the screw insertion angle without parallax error. Precise intraoperative lateral fluoroscopic images are essential for safe and

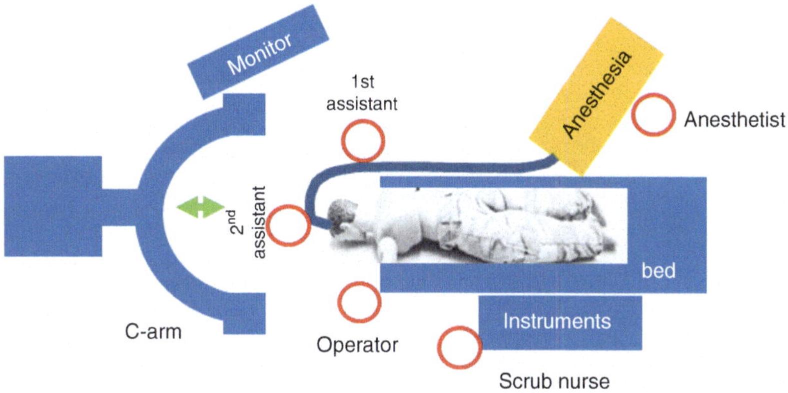

Fig. 25.1 Surgical set-up for posterior decompression and fusion surgery for cervical OPLL. Patients are positioned prone with their head stabilized in a Mayfield skull clamp, and apparatus for anesthesia is moved caudally to obtain a wide space around the head of the patients. Fluoroscopy is obtained cranially. The operator stands on the left side of the patient's head and the first assistant stands on the opposite side. In some cases, the operator can stand above the patient's head to see the screw insertion angle without parallax error

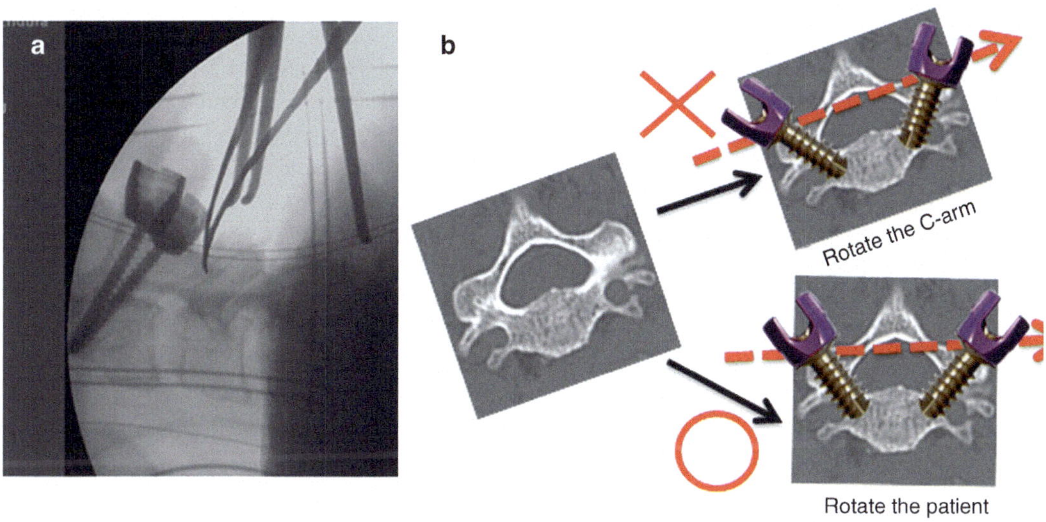

Fig. 25.2 Method to obtain true lateral fluoroscopic image. Precise intraoperative lateral fluoroscopic images are essential for safe and accurate insertion of the screws. Two Penfield nerve spatulas are set to the inferior border of the corresponding facets bilaterally (**a**). The fluoroscope is adjusted so that the position of the two spatulas coincide. Care must be taken to adjust the rotation image by rotating the patients, not by rotating the image intensifier, because the rotation of the image intensifier can lead to an inappropriate medial-lateral insertion angle for the screw (**b**)

accurate insertion of the screws. Two Penfield nerve spatulas are set to the inferior border of the corresponding facets bilaterally (Fig. 25.2a). The fluoroscope is adjusted so that the position of the two spatulas coincide. Care must be taken to adjust the rotation image by rotating the patients, not by rotating the image intensifier because the rotation of the image intensifier can lead to an inappropriate medial-lateral insertion angle for the screw (Fig. 25.2b). The use of navigation is recommended for safer screw insertion.

Electrophysiological monitoring is recommended to detect and avoid any neurological deterioration during the surgery.

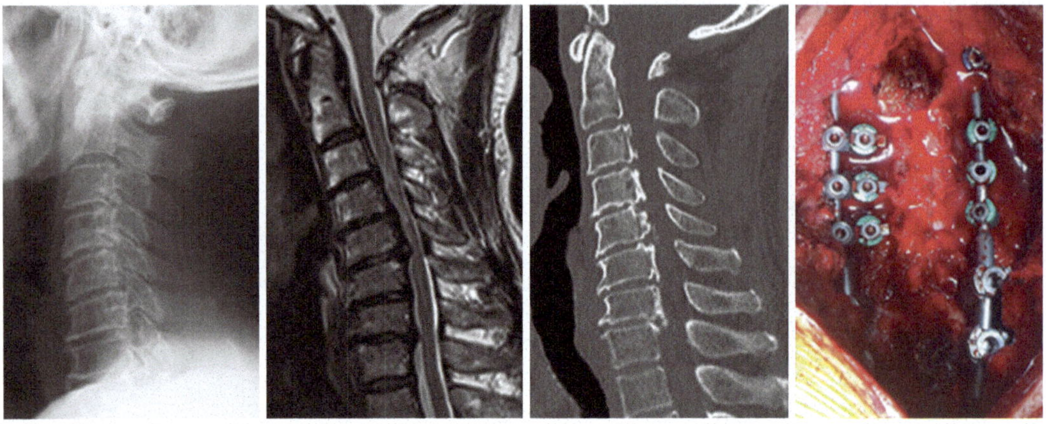

Fig. 25.3 Posterior decompression and fusion surgery for cervical OPLL

Generally, fixation from C2 to C7 or T1 is applied because the C2 pedicle screw is the most reliable anchor in the cervical spine and the C7 and/or T1 pedicle screw can be inserted without risk of vertebral artery violation. A lateral mass screw is generally used as a mid-cervical fixation anchor. A lateral mass screw can obtain sufficient fixation because patients with OPLL usually have good bone quality. We insert C2 and C7/T1 screws and make screw holes in mid-cervical levels for lateral mass screws under fluoroscopic imaging before spinal cord decompression. Lateral mass screws are inserted after decompression because the screw head can interfere with the spinal decompression procedure. After spinal cord decompression, we apply fixation in situ according to the neutral cervical spine alignment set by posture without excessive intraoperative alignment correction (Fig. 25.3).

25.4 Surgical Outcome of PDF for OPLL

Overall, addition of posterior instrumented fusion does not improve neurological recovery (Fig. 25.4) for OPLL patients in a meta-analysis of the latest version of OPLL guidelines edited by the Japanese Orthopaedics Association (JOA). However, PDF for patients with K-line (−) and/or with a canal occupying ratio of at least 60% or more tends to be effective ($p = 0.07$) (Fig. 25.4). By contrast, PDF significantly increases the incidence of postoperative segmental upper extremity motor palsy (so-called C5 palsy) (Fig. 25.4). Thus, PDF might be recommended not for all types of OPLL but for OPLL patients with K-line (−) and/or with a canal occupying ratio of at least 60% or more.

We previously reported a clinical case series and analyzed surgical outcome of PDF surgery for K-line (−) OPLL. The recovery rate of JOA score was approximately 40%, showing modest neurological recovery [19]. We compared the clinical outcome of laminoplasty, PDF, and ADF for K-line (−) OPLL. The JOA score recovery rate was approximately 60% in the ADF group, 40% in PDF group, and 20% in laminoplasty group. We found that PDF surgery produced a significantly better outcome than laminoplasty in the K-line (−) OPLL population. Therefore, laminoplasty should not be used for K-line (−) cervical OPLL [20]. ADF is a suitable surgical treatment for K-line (−) OPLL. However, adequate management of ADF-specific perioperative complications is needed. PDF is a possible alternative procedure for K-line (−) OPLL. Both ADF and PDF are applicable for K-line (−) OPLL according to indications set by each institute and decisions of individual surgeons. Our

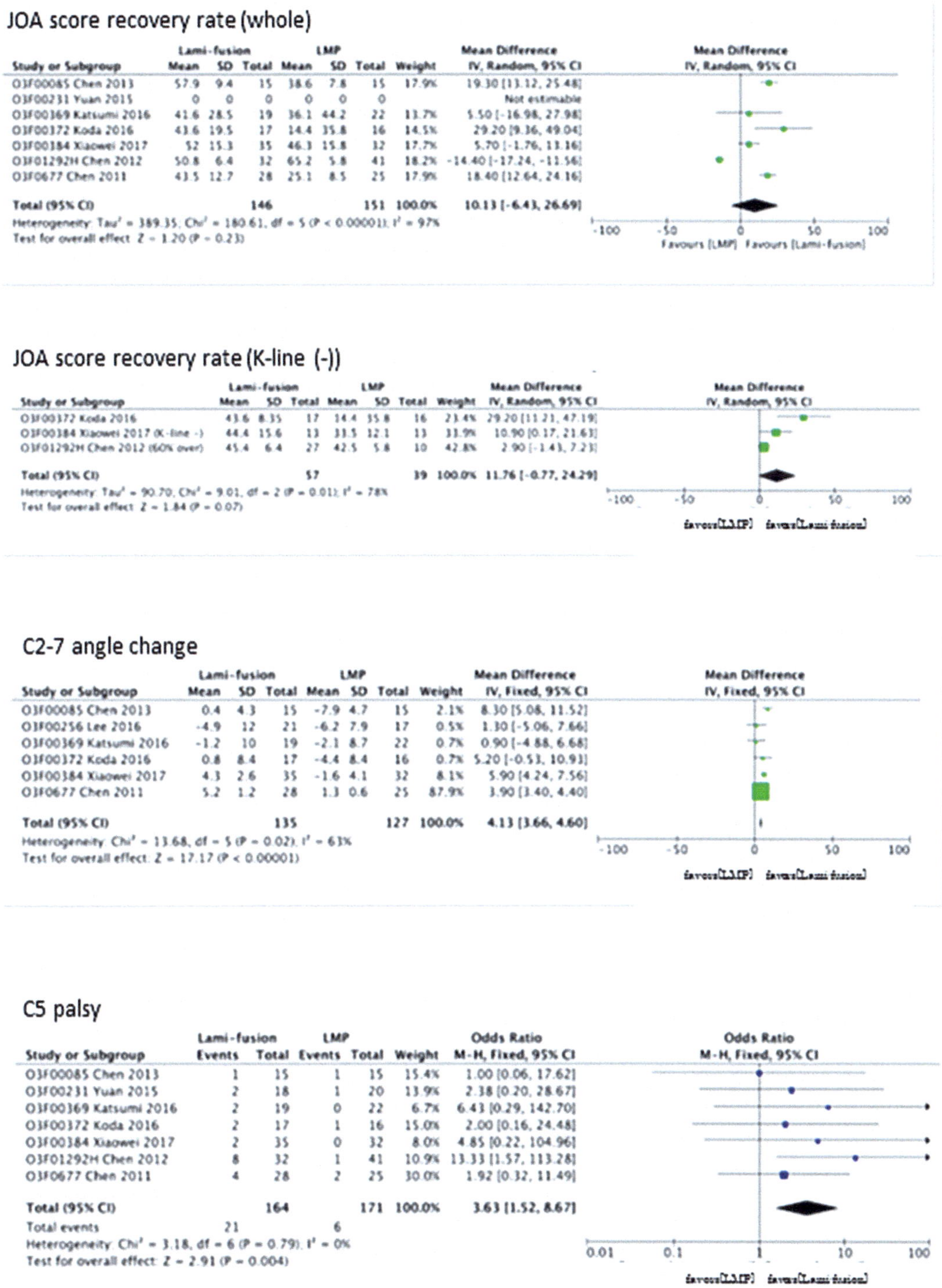

Fig. 25.4 Meta-analyses comparing laminoplasty and posterior decompression and fusion surgery

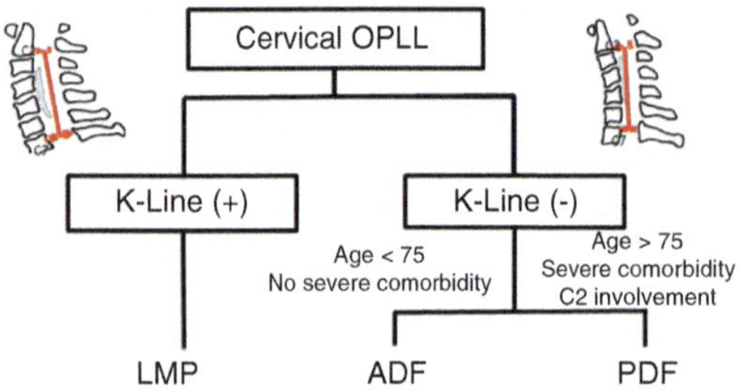

Fig. 25.5 Surgical decision-making for cervical OPLL based on K-line

current surgical choice between ADF and PDF is based on comorbidities, patient age, and location of the ossification foci. Anterior surgery should be avoided for patients having preoperative respiratory disorders and dysphagia, large ossification foci at the C2 level, and older patients (Fig. 25.5). Surgical complications specific to PDF surgery are neurovascular injury related to instrumentation and a higher incidence of proximal upper extremity palsy.

25.5 Future Perspectives

A recent study comparing ADF and PDF for OPLL found that there was no significant difference in clinical outcome between ADF and PDF in thick OPLL with lordotic alignment, whereas ADF showed a significantly better outcome than PDF in OPLL with kyphotic alignment [21]. Alignment might be a determinant of surgical procedures for patients with K-line (−) OPLL. Further exploration is needed to establish a standardized determination of surgical choices for K-line (−) OPLL.

Correction to lordosis theoretically promotes better spinal cord decompression by its bowstringing effects. Previously, we analyzed the factors that have a positive impact on better clinical outcome after PDF for K-line (−) type OPLL. Postoperative change of K-line from (−) to (+) was an independent factor for a better outcome. In other words, alignment correction to lordosis can result in better spinal cord decompression [22]. However, excessive correction of alignment can cause instrumentation failure and spinal cord/foraminal impingement. To date, there is no consensus about optimal alignment correction. Kurakawa reported that preoperative narrowing of intervertebral foramen is a predictive factor for postoperative C5 palsy and also reported the tolerable range of alignment correction according to the degree of preoperative foraminal stenosis [23]. Future investigation is needed to elucidate the tolerable alignment correction in patients with OPLL.

Recently, a correlation between spinal sagittal alignment and clinical symptoms has been highlighted [24]. Posterior cervical spine surgery potentially causes postoperative sagittal alignment change, possibly resulting in exacerbating neck pain and neurological symptoms. Whether addition of posterior instrumented fusion can prevent postoperative sagittal alignment deterioration after laminoplasty remains unclear. Our previous study revealed that the addition of posterior instrumentation can prevent postoperative kyphosis but cannot suppress deterioration of sagittal alignment [25]. The appropriate surgical procedure for preventing postoperative deterioration of sagittal alignment remains elusive.

25.6 Conclusions

Posterior decompression with fusion (PDF) surgery is an option for cervical OPLL. PDF might improve the clinical outcome of OPLL patients with K-line (−) and/or with a canal occupying ratio at least 60% or more. Care must be taken to avoid postoperative C5 palsy.

References

1. Smith ZA, Buchanan CC, Raphael D, et al. Ossification of the posterior longitudinal ligament: pathogenesis, management, and current surgical approaches. A review. Neurosurg Focus. 2011;30:E10. https://doi.org/10.3171/2011.1.FOCUS10256.
2. Matsumoto M, Chiba K, Toyama Y. Surgical treatment of ossification of the posterior longitudinal ligament and its outcomes: posterior surgery by laminoplasty. Spine (Phila Pa 1976). 2012;37:E303–8.
3. Ogawa Y, Toyama Y, Chiba K, et al. Long-term results of expansive open-door laminoplasty for ossification

of the posterior longitudinal ligament of the cervical spine. J Neurosurg Spine. 2004;1:168–74.
4. Mizuno J, Nakagawa H. Ossified posterior longitudinal ligament: management strategies and outcomes. Spine J. 2006;6(Suppl):282S–8S.
5. An HS, Al-Shihabi L, Kurd M. Surgical treatment for ossification of the posterior longitudinal ligament in the cervical spine. J Am Acad Orthop Surg. 2014;22:420–9.
6. Sodeyama T, Goto S, Mochizuki M, et al. Effect of decompression enlargement laminoplasty for posterior shifting of the spinal cord. Spine (Phila Pa 1976). 1999;24:1527–31.
7. Aita I, Hayashi K, Wadano Y, Yabuki T. Posterior movement and enlargement of the spinal cord after cervical laminoplasty. J Bone Joint Surg Br. 1998;80:33–7.
8. Iwasaki M, Okuda S, Miyauchi A, et al. Surgical strategy for cervical myelopathy due to ossification of the posterior longitudinal ligament: Part 1: Clinical results and limitations of laminoplasty. Spine (Phila Pa 1976). 2007;32:647–53.
9. Ogawa Y. Updates on ossification of posterior longitudinal ligament. Clinical results and problems of posterior decompression for OPLL of the cervical spine. Clin Calcium. 2009;19:1493–8.. [In Japanese]
10. Nishida N, Kanchiku T, Kato Y, et al. Biomechanical analysis of cervical myelopathy due to ossification of the posterior longitudinal ligament: effects of posterior decompression and kyphosis following decompression. Exp Ther Med. 2014;7:1095–9.
11. Fujiyoshi T, Yamazaki M, Kawabe J, et al. A new concept for making decisions regarding the surgical approach for cervical ossification of the posterior longitudinal ligament: the K-line. Spine (Phila Pa 1976). 2008;33:E990–3.
12. Liu H, Li Y, Chen Y, et al. Cervical curvature, spinal cord MRIT2 signal, and occupying ratio impact surgical approach selection in patients with ossification of the posterior longitudinal ligament. Eur Spine J. 2013;22:1480–8.
13. Yoshii T, Egawa S, Hirai T, Kaito T, Mori K, Koda M, Chikuda H, Hasegawa T, Imagama S, Yoshida M, Iwasaki M, Okawa A, Kawaguchi Y. A systematic review and meta-analysis comparing anterior decompression with fusion and posterior laminoplasty for cervical ossification of the posterior longitudinal ligament. J Orthop Sci. 2020;25(1):58–65. https://doi.org/10.1016/j.jos.2019.03.004.
14. Li H, Dai LY. A systematic review of complications in cervical spine surgery for ossification of the posterior longitudinal ligament. Spine J. 2011;11:1049–57.
15. Masaki Y, Yamazaki M, Okawa A, et al. An analysis of factors causing poor surgical outcome in patients with cervical myelopathy due to ossification of the posterior longitudinal ligament: anterior decompression with spinal fusion versus laminoplasty. J Spinal Disord Tech. 2007;20:7–13.
16. Azuma Y, Kato Y, Taguchi T. Etiology of cervical myelopathy induced by ossification of the posterior longitudinal ligament: determining the responsible level of OPLL myelopathy by correlating static compression and dynamic factors. J Spinal Disord Tech. 2010;23:166–9.
17. Nishida N, Kanchiku T, Kato Y, et al. Cervical ossification of the posterior longitudinal ligament: biomechanical analysis of the influence of static and dynamic factors. J Spinal Cord Med. 2015;38(5):593–8.
18. Maruo K, Moriyama T, Tachibana T, et al. The impact of dynamic factors on surgical outcomes after double-door laminoplasty for ossification of the posterior longitudinal ligament of the cervical spine. J Neurosurg Spine. 2014;21:938–43.
19. Saito J, Maki S, Kamiya K, Furuya T, Inada T, Ota M, Iijima Y, Takahashi K, Yamazaki M, Aramomi M, Mannoji C, Koda M. Outcome of posterior decompression with instrumented fusion surgery for K-line (−) cervical ossification of the longitudinal ligament. J Clin Neurosci. 2016;32:57–60.
20. Koda M, Mochizuki M, Konishi H, Aiba A, Kadota R, Inada T, Kamiya K, Ota M, Maki S, Takahashi K, Yamazaki M, Mannoji C, Furuya T. Comparison of clinical outcomes between laminoplasty, posterior decompression with instrumented fusion, and anterior decompression with fusion for K-line (−) cervical ossification of the posterior longitudinal ligament. Eur Spine J. 2016;25:2294–301.
21. Yoshii T, Sakai K, Hirai T, Yamada T, Inose H, Kato T, Enomoto M, Tomizawa S, Kawabata S, Arai Y, Okawa A. Anterior decompression with fusion versus posterior decompression with fusion for massive cervical ossification of the posterior longitudinal ligament with a ≥50% canal occupying ratio: a multicenter retrospective study. Spine J. 2016;16:1351–7.
22. Koda M, Furuya T, Saito J, Ijima Y, Kitamura M, Ohtori S, Orita S, Inage K, Abe T, Noguchi H, Funayama T, Kumagai H, Miura K, Nagashima K, Yamazaki M. Postoperative K-line conversion from negative to positive is independently associated with a better surgical outcome after posterior decompression with instrumented fusion for K-line negative cervical ossification of the posterior ligament. Eur Spine J. 2018;27:1393–400.
23. Kurakawa T, Miyamoto H, Kaneyama S, Sumi M, Uno K. C5 nerve palsy after posterior reconstruction surgery: predictive risk factors of the incidence and critical range of correction for kyphosis. Eur Spine J. 2016;25:2060–7.
24. Tang JA, Scheer JK, Smith JS, Deviren V, Bess S, Hart RA, Lafage V, Shaffrey CI, Schwab F, Ames CP, ISSG. The impact of standing regional cervical sagittal alignment on outcomes in posterior cervical fusion surgery. Neurosurgery. 2012;71:662–9.
25. Inada T, Furuya T, Ota M, Maki S, Ijima Y, Saito J, Kitamura M, Ohtori S, Orita S, Inage K, Yamazaki M, Koda M. Addition of instrumented fusion to laminoplasty cannot suppress postoperative sagittal balance exacerbation. J Clin Neurosci. 2017;45:214–7.

Anterior Cervical Decompression for Cervical OPLL: Technique, Complications, and Long-Term Results

26

Toshitaka Yoshii

Abstract

Anterior cervical decompression and fusion (ADF) is an effective treatment option for cervical ossification of the posterior longitudinal ligament (OPLL) because it provides direct decompression to the spinal cord and stabilizes the involved segments. The anterior floating method thins the ossification and disconnects it from the surrounding bony tissues, instead of resecting the OPLL. When the thinned OPLL appears to be like a board floating on water, decompression of the spinal cord is complete. For reconstruction, we normally use a fibular bone graft reinforced by an anterior plate. Alternative graft materials, such as allograft, prefabricated hydroxyapatite graft, and titanium cage, have been available, which decrease donor site morbidity. There are various perioperative complications related to ADF, including dysphagia, airway obstruction, cerebrospinal fluid leak, insufficient decompression, C5 palsy, and implant failure. Despite these perioperative complications, long-term surgical results of ADF for cervical OPLL are generally favorable.

Keywords

OPLL · Anterior · Floating · Complication
Long-term results

26.1 Surgical Technique

26.1.1 Positioning

The surgery is performed in the supine position under general anesthesia. A roll pillow is placed under the neck. Excessive extension of the cervical spine should be avoided to prevent neurological deterioration during surgery. The mandible is slightly rotated to the right to permit easy access to the cervical spine especially in high cervical cases. Spinal monitoring is routinely performed to prevent neurological complications. We typically measure compound muscle action potentials induced by brain stimulation to monitor the motor tract during surgery.

26.1.2 Procedure

A left-sided approach is usually used because of the more protected course of the recurrent laryngeal nerve in the tracheoesophageal groove. The skin incision level can be estimated from subcutaneous landmarks: The hyoid corresponds to C3, the thyroid cartilage to C4–5, and the cricoids to

T. Yoshii (✉)
Department of Orthopaedic Surgery, Tokyo Medical and Dental University, Tokyo, Japan
e-mail: yoshii.orth@tmd.ac.jp

A. Okawa et al. (eds.), *OPLL*, https://doi.org/10.1007/978-981-15-3855-1_26

C6. A transverse incision is made anterior to the appropriate interspace starting at the midline and extending laterally to the medial edge of sternocleidomastoid muscle (SCM). An oblique skin incision is preferable to use for 3-level fusion or more. The dissection is carried through the subcutaneous tissue to the platysma. The superficial cervical fascia is incised, and then the trachea, esophagus, and hyoid muscles are retracted medially to expose the prevertebral cervical fascia overlying the bodies of the cervical vertebrae. Bilateral longus colli muscles are retracted, and retractors are set up carefully on these edges to avoid injury to the esophagus, trachea, and carotid sheath. In OPLL cases, the anterior surface of the vertebral column is widely exposed (Fig. 26.1).

The disks should be sufficiently curetted between the bilateral uncovertebral joints to ensure accurate canal width. This also ensures maintenance of the correct midline of the vertebral column during surgery. The corpectomy is initiated by drilling bilateral holes in the uncovertebral joints and nibbling away at the vertebral body. Discectomy and corpectomy are performed in an alternating fashion. The width of corpectomy is carefully planned using preoperative CT images. Wide corpectomies are required in cases with wide OPLL in which we have to set the cutting line of the vertebrae close to the transverse foramen [1].

Upon reaching the posterior cortex, a careful and skillful air drill technique is required under a microscope. The ossification is thinned like a shape of the bottom of a ship until the soft tissue underneath the ossification is slightly visible (Fig. 26.2a). During the thinning process, the OPLL should be kept connected to the surrounding bone. When freeing the ossification from the surrounding bone tissues, the top and bottom ends of the ossification are released transversely and then the lateral side of OPLL is disconnected from the vertebral bodies and pedicles [2] (Fig. 26.3). When the thinned OPLL appears to be like a board floating on water, decompression of the entire spinal cord is complete. If the surrounding soft tissue is still hard, pedicles and uncovertebral joints are further removed to obtain a sufficient decompression (Fig. 26.2b). Early release of the OPLL from the vertebral bodies should be avoided as this may induce uneven decompression. In massive OPLL, thinning of OPLL is necessary for sufficient floating because

Fig. 26.1 Approach to the cervical spine

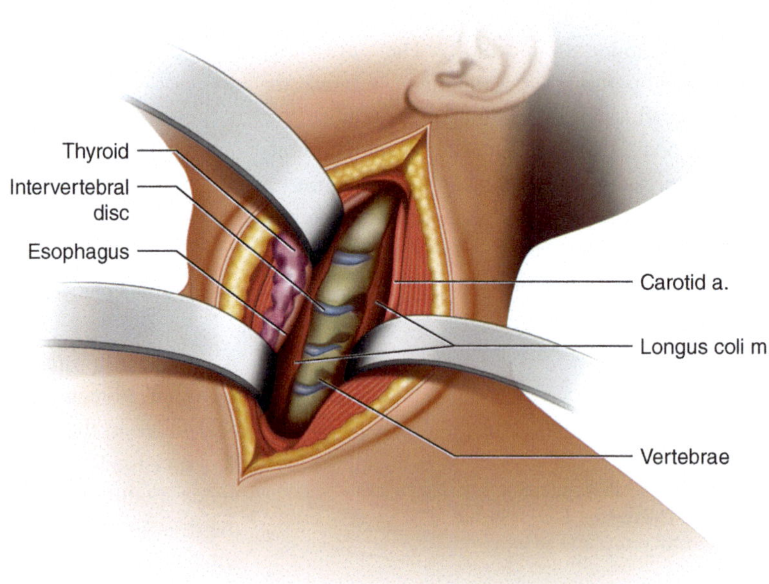

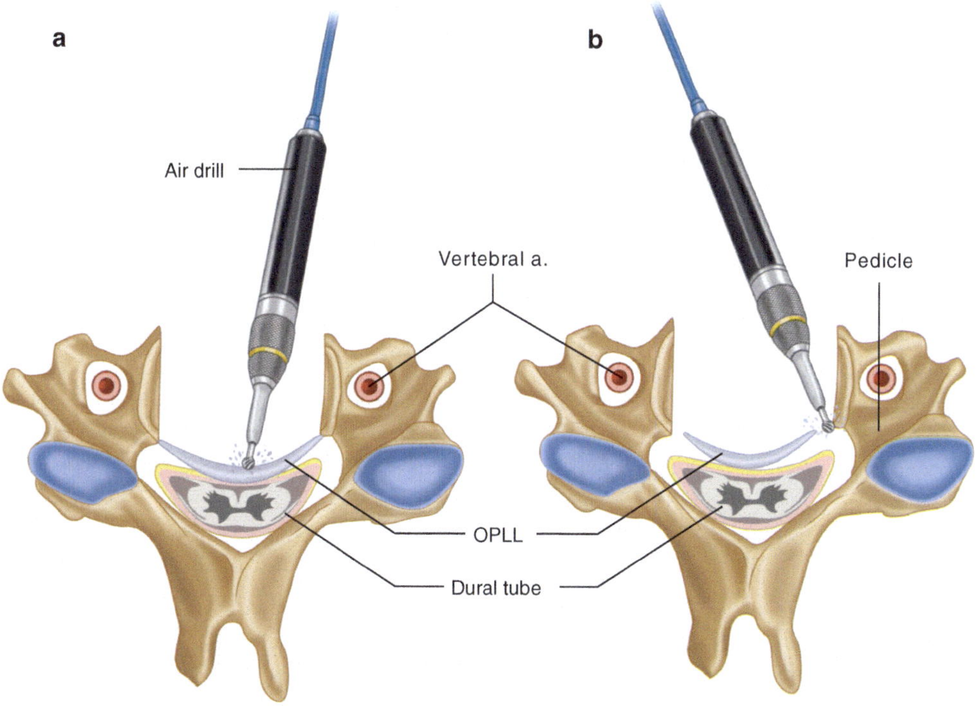

Fig. 26.2 Thinning the OPLL. The OPLL is thinned gradually while it is kept connected to the surrounding bone (*Left*). After the OPLL is thinned enough, the OPLL is disconnected from the surrounding bone (*Right*). If the conection of the OPLL to the surrounding tissue remains tight, wider margin around the OPLL shoud be taken by further removal of surrounding bone, pedicle, and uncovertebral joints

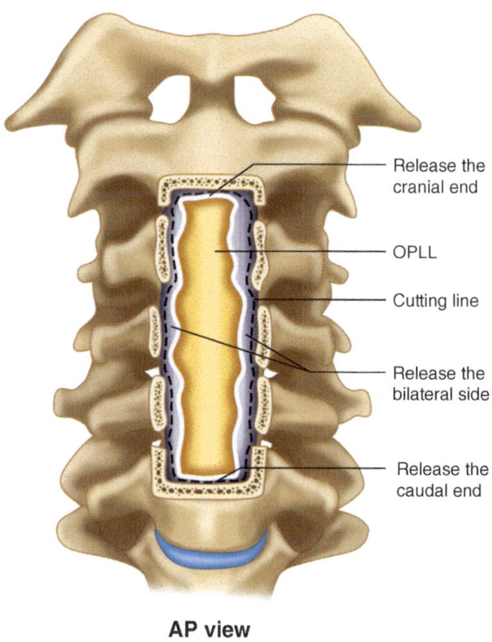

Fig. 26.3 Floating of the OPLL. The OPLL is disconnected from the surrounding bone. First, releasing at the cranial and caudal side is performed. Then, the OPLL is released bilaterally (more compressed side first)

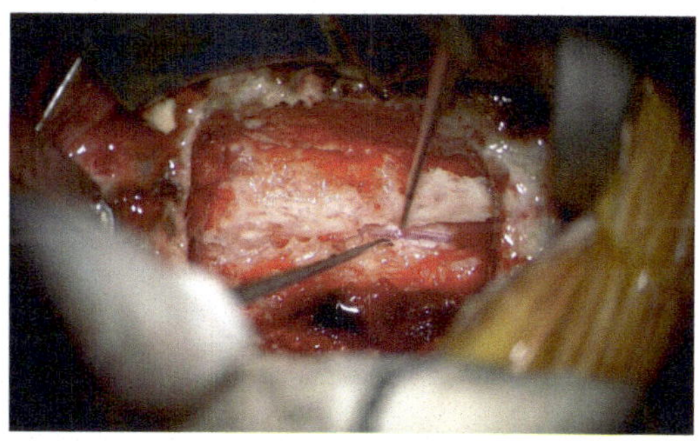

Fig. 26.4 Further splitting the OPLL after floating

an already mature, rocklike ossification does not float as easily as an immature small ossification. In addition, we sometimes need to split the OPLL transversely or longitudinally in order to float the OPLL completely (Fig. 26.4). Recently, high resolution reconstructed CT images can be obtained intraoperatively and are useful for the intraoperative evaluation of adequate decompression during the technically demanding anterior floating method [1]. In challenging OPLL cases, we usually evaluate the decompression during the surgery using the intraoperative CT (Fig. 26.5). The released ossification gradually migrates anteriorly over time to enlarge the vertebral canal, due to resorption of hematoma and pressure from the cerebrospinal fluid, up to 4–8 weeks postoperatively.

For reconstruction, autologous fibular/iliac bone, titanium cage, and artificial bone graft are available. Internal fixation using a plate stabilizes the cervical spine immediately after the operation, making a postoperative care easy. Additionally, it can prevent postoperative graft dislodging and spine deformity before fusion is complete. We prefer using synthetic hydroxyapatite graft for cases in which we need two continuous corpectomies or less [3]. Philadelphia neck collar is generally applied for 3 months after surgery. Hybrid procedures of corpectomy and anterior discectomy with fusion (ACDF) can also be applied for multilevel OPLL if we can preserve a vertebra within the decompression levels. The hybrid procedure provides better stability and less chance of graft dislodgement/subsidence (Fig. 26.6).

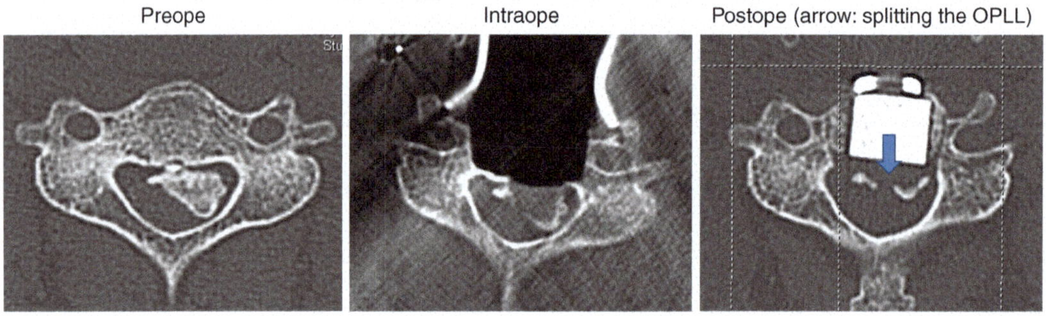

Fig. 26.5 Preoperative (left), intraoperative (middle), and postoperative (right) CT images of patients who received anterior decompression with floating method. The OPLL was split at the middle (arrow) after floating to achieve complete decompression

Fig. 26.6 (**a**) Fibula bone graft. (**b**) Hybrid graft using synthetic hydroxyapatite

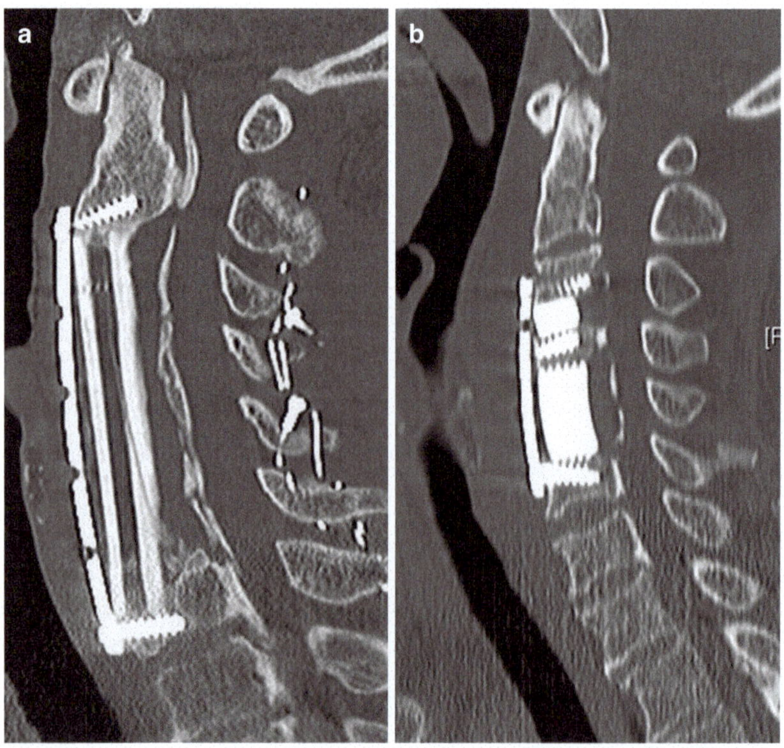

26.2 Complications

The overall complication rates were higher in ADF when compared with posterior laminoplasty. According to recent meta-analysis, the overall complication rate was 21.4% in the ADF group, whereas the rate was 12.9% in laminoplasty (odds ratio: 2.19) [4].

Common complications related to the anterior approach are recurrent laryngeal nerve palsy and dysphagia. The mechanism includes direct injury, traction, edema, or tethering of the recurrent laryngeal nerve against the endotracheal tube. Recurrent laryngeal nerve injury can be minimized using gentle tissue retraction [5]. Dysphagia is associated with retropharyngeal tissue edema from esophageal retraction or from plate prominence. The incidence of dysphagia in anterior cervical surgery is reported to be as high as 50% postoperatively, but this generally decreases over time [6]. Postoperative dysphagia occurs more frequently in women and in cases of multilevel anterior fusion. The use of lower profile plates may decrease the risk for dysphagia.

Vertebral artery injury can occur from excessive lateral dissections or from an abnormal course of the vertebral artery [7]. The width of the corpectomy should be carefully planned before surgery using the preoperative CT and MRI images. The uncovertebral joint and bottom of the transverse process are reliable anatomical landmarks for the lateral border of the vertebral body. Airway destruction due to the development of retropharyngeal tissue swelling and/or hematoma are also common and potentially catastrophic complications. In case of acute respiratory distress, emergent reintubation/tracheostomy should be considered.

The incidence of dural tears and CSF fistulas after cervical corpectomy for all pathologies has been reported to be between 0 and 8% [8]. However, the incidence of a CSF leak after anterior cervical OPLL resection is reported to be much higher (between 6.7 and 31.8%) [8]. Floating method can reduce the incidence of CSF leak or fistula to be 5.1% [2]. In our experience, even in cases with a dural tear or dural defect, CSF leak can be managed without lumbar drainage by placing polyglycolic acid sheet on the floating OPLL followed by spraying of fibrin glue.

Graft-related complications are also common in cases with multiple corpectomies. One of the risk factors for graft dislodgement/ migration after cervical corpectomies is the number of segments involved in the surgery. It is reported that the odds ratio for having a displaced graft with each additional level was 1.65 [9]. Cervical alignment also influences the incidence of graft complications. Hyperlordosis of the spine also negatively influences the incidence of graft complications because of the inappropriate fitting of the graft to the host bone [10]. In our experience, a graft that is too long causes anterior slipping of the graft or a vertebral body fracture. The length of the graft should be carefully determined such that the decompressed cervical column is extended slightly by mild manual power or by a Casper distractor.

C5 palsy is a well-recognized complication that can occur with either anterior or posterior cervical surgery. The incidence of C-5 nerve palsy after anterior cervical decompression has been reported to occur in 1.6–12.1% of patients [8], whereas the incidence of C5 palsy after ADF for OPLL is reported to be higher (9.5–13.3%) [2, 11]. In ADF, various factors can cause C5 palsy such as direct injury during the surgery, postoperative alignment change due to subsidence of the graft, insufficient decompression, and foraminal stenosis.

26.3 Long-Term Results

Long-term surgical results of ADF for cervical OPLL are favorable. Sakai et al. have reported that the JOA recovery rate at postoperative 2 years was 64.8%, which was well maintained at 5 years postoperatively (71.4%) [12]. Matsuoka et al. have also reported that the JOA recovery rate at 1 year is 61.2%, which was well maintained at 10 years after surgery (66.5%) [2]. After anterior surgery, progression of OPLL rarely occurs, especially at the operated segments. The alignment of cervical spine is preserved for long once it is fused. Therefore, deterioration of neurological symptoms is not frequently observed during long-term follow-up if the initial decompression was adequately performed [2].

References

1. Yoshii T, Hirai T, Yamada T, Inose H, Kato T, Sakai K, Enomoto M, Kawabata S, Arai Y, Okawa A. Intraoperative evaluation using mobile computed tomography in anterior cervical decompression with floating method for massive ossification of the posterior longitudinal ligament. J Orthop Surg Res. 2017;12(1):12.
2. Matsuoka T, Yamaura I, Kurosa Y, Nakai O, Shindo S, Shinomiya K. Long-term results of the anterior floating method for cervical myelopathy caused by ossification of the posterior longitudinal ligament. Spine (Phila Pa 1976). 2001;26(3):241–8.
3. Yoshii T, Hirai T, Sakai K, Sotome S, Enomoto M, Yamada T, Inose H, Kato T, Kawabata S, Okawa A. Anterior cervical corpectomy and fusion using a synthetic hydroxyapatite graft for ossification of the posterior longitudinal ligament. Orthopedics. 2017;40(2):e334–e9.
4. Yoshii T, Egawa S, Hirai T, Kaito T, Mori K, Koda M, Chikuda H, Hasegawa T, Imagama S, Yoshida M, Iwasaki M, Okawa A, Kawaguchi Y. A systematic review and meta-analysis comparing anterior decompression with fusion and posterior laminoplasty for cervical ossification of the posterior longitudinal ligament. J Orthop Sci. 2020;25(1):58–65.
5. Apfelbaum RI, Kriskovich MD, Haller JR. On the incidence, cause, and prevention of recurrent laryngeal nerve palsies during anterior cervical spine surgery. Spine (Phila Pa 1976). 2000;25(22):2906–12.
6. Bazaz R, Lee MJ, Yoo JU. Incidence of dysphagia after anterior cervical spine surgery: a prospective study. Spine (Phila Pa 1976) [Clinical Trial Research Support, Non-U.S. Gov't]. 2002;27(22):2453–8.
7. Smith MD, Emery SE, Dudley A, Murray KJ, Leventhal M. Vertebral artery injury during anterior decompression of the cervical spine. A retrospective review of ten patients. J Bone Joint Surg Br. 1993;75(3):410–5.
8. Cardoso MJ, Koski TR, Ganju A, Liu JC. Approach-related complications after decompression for cervical ossification of the posterior longitudinal ligament. Neurosurg Focus [Review]. 2011;30(3):E12.
9. Wang JC, Hart RA, Emery SE, Bohlman HH. Graft migration or displacement after multilevel cervical corpectomy and strut grafting. Spine (Phila Pa 1976). 2003;28(10):1016–21; discussion 21–2.
10. Okawa A, Sakai K, Hirai T, Kato T, Tomizawa S, Enomoto M, Kawabata S, Takahashi M, Shinomiya K. Risk factors for early reconstruction failure of multilevel cervical corpectomy with dynamic plate fixation. Spine (Phila Pa 1976). 2011;36(9):E582–7.
11. Kimura A, Seichi A, Hoshino Y, Yamazaki M, Mochizuki M, Aiba A, Kato T, Uchida K, Miyamoto K, Nakahara S, Taniguchi S, Neo M, Taguchi T, Endo K, Watanabe M, Takahashi M, Kaito T, Chikuda H, Fujimori T, Ito T, Ono A, Abumi K, Yamada K, Nakagawa Y, Toyama Y. Perioperative complications of anterior cervical decompression with fusion in patients with ossification of the posterior longitudinal ligament: a retrospective, multi-institutional study. J Orthop Sci. [Multicenter Study Research Support, Non-U.S. Gov't]. 2012;17(6):667–72.
12. Sakai K, Okawa A, Takahashi M, Arai Y, Kawabata S, Enomoto M, Kato T, Hirai T, Shinomiya K. Five-year follow-up evaluation of surgical treatment for cervical myelopathy caused by ossification of the posterior longitudinal ligament: a prospective comparative study of anterior decompression and fusion with floating method versus laminoplasty. Spine (Phila Pa 1976). 2012;37(5):367–76.

27 Surgical Indications and Choice of Surgical Procedure for Thoracic OPLL

Kei Ando, Kazuyoshi Kobayashi, Hiroaki Nakashima, Masayoshi Morozumi, Masaaki Machino, Naoki Ishiguro, and Shiro Imagama

Abstract

The surgical indication for T-OPLL can be classified into three groups: first, myelopathy caused by T-OPLL requires surgical intervention; second, the discontinuous type across the disc space between the rostral and caudal ossification regions requires special care without myelopathy, and immediate surgical intervention if myelopathy develops; and third, the continuous type without myelopathy at the initial visit can be observed with confidence.

Surgical treatment can be divided into two categories based on the type of decompression. The first is direct removal of the T-OPLL through an anterior or posterior approach, and the second is indirect posterior decompression of the spinal cord without directly touching the OPLL. In a recent multicenter study, posterior decompression and fusion with instrumentation were performed in most cases (74%), and the rate of surgery with instrumentation of 88% reflects the current major trend toward posterior instrumented fusion surgery for T-OPLL. However, the most common postoperative complication may be aggravation of motor weakness in the lower extremities (32.2%, $n = 37$). A second surgery of OPLL resection could be performed in cases with no improvement or aggravation of symptoms within 3 weeks after posterior decompression and fusion surgery.

Keywords

Thoracic ossification of posterior longitudinal ligament · Surgical indications · Discontinuous type · Surgical procedures · Direct removal · Indirect posterior decompression · Instrumentation

27.1 Introduction

In a radiologic study conducted by Mori et al., the prevalence of thoracic ossification of the posterior longitudinal ligament (T-OPLL) was 1.9% in 3013 subjects on computed tomography (CT), which was significantly lower than that of 1.9–4.3% for OPLL of the cervical vertebrae [1]. In a study of the natural history of untreated OPLL, Matsunaga et al. found that 17% of patients with OPLL without signs of myelopathy progressed to development of myelopathy [2]. However, T-OPLL has not been widely examined in this respect because of its low prevalence and the small number of cases treated conservatively due to the vulnerable spinal cord at a thoracic lesion.

K. Ando · K. Kobayashi · H. Nakashima
M. Morozumi · M. Machino · N. Ishiguro
S. Imagama (✉)
Department of Orthopaedic Surgery, Nagoya University Graduate School of Medicine, Nagoya, Aichi, Japan
e-mail: imagama@med.nagoya-u.ac.jp

A. Okawa et al. (eds.), *OPLL*, https://doi.org/10.1007/978-981-15-3855-1_27

However, an understanding of the pathological mechanism of development of myelopathy in T-OPLL is important for monitoring of conservative treatment and for establishment of the indication for surgery. Here, we discuss this indication and surgical methods for T-OPLL.

27.2 Surgical Indication

T-OPLL generally requires surgical intervention because of its progressive nature and poor response to conservative therapy [3, 4]. There have been some studies of the natural course of cervical myelopathy in OPLL, but little is known about thoracic myelopathy [2, 5]. Dynamic factors may play an important role in progression of myelopathy due to OPLL in addition to static compression. The range of motion (ROM) of the cervical spine with OPLL, as seen in radiography, affects onset and aggravation of myelopathy [2]. Patients with mild stenosis (<60%) who also have myelopathy have a more extensive ROM (75.6°) compared to those without myelopathy (36.5°) [2].

The thoracic spine has a lower ROM during flexion and extension compared with the cervical and lumbar spine because the ROM of the thoracic spine is restricted by the rib cage. Morita et al. [6] investigated dynamic alignment and ROM of the thoracic spine at the segmental level using multidetector-row CT and found total kyphotic angles (T1/L1) of 40.2 ± 11.4° and 8.5 ± 12.8° in flexion and extension, respectively. The apex of the kyphotic angle was at T6/7 in flexion, total ROM (T1/L1) was 31.7 ± 11.3°, segmental ROM decreased from T1/2 to T4/5, but increased gradually from T4/5 to T12/L1, maximum ROM was at T12/L1 (4.2 ± 2.1°), and minimum ROM was at T4/5 (0.9 ± 3.0°) [6]. Ando et al. compared cases that did and did not undergo surgery [7]. Radiologically, conservatively treated patients had a lower discontinuous (across the disc space between the rostral and caudal ossification regions) rate on sagittal CT (Fig. 27.1) and a higher rate of a high intensity area on MRI although there were no differences between the two groups in T-OPLL level, number of T-OPLLs, and canal diameter ratio of OPLL [7]. The discontinuous region (Fig. 27.2) refers to micromotion at the intervertebral level, and micromotion may lead to OPLL progression, even within essentially immobile thoracic spine segments. It was also suggested that this micromotion secondary to segmental discontinuity of OPLL might cause deterioration of the vulnerable spinal cord [7].

These reports suggest that the surgical indication can be classified into three groups: first, myelopathy caused by T-OPLL requires surgical intervention; second, the discontinuous type across the disc space between the rostral and caudal ossification regions requires special care without myelopathy and immediate surgical intervention if myelopathy develops; and third, the continuous type without myelopathy at the initial visit can be observed with confidence (Fig. 27.3).

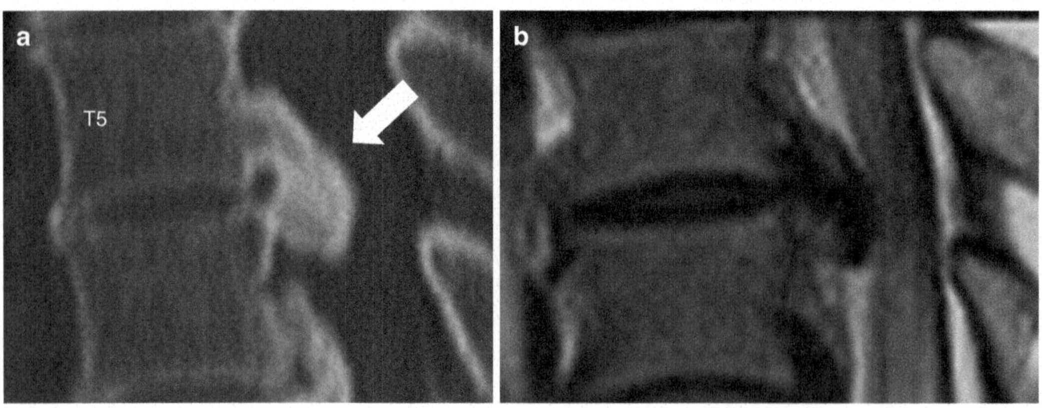

Fig. 27.1 (**a**) Sagittal CT image of beak-type continuous OPLL at T5–6. (**b**) MRI showing severe canal stenosis at several OPLL locations without a high intensity area

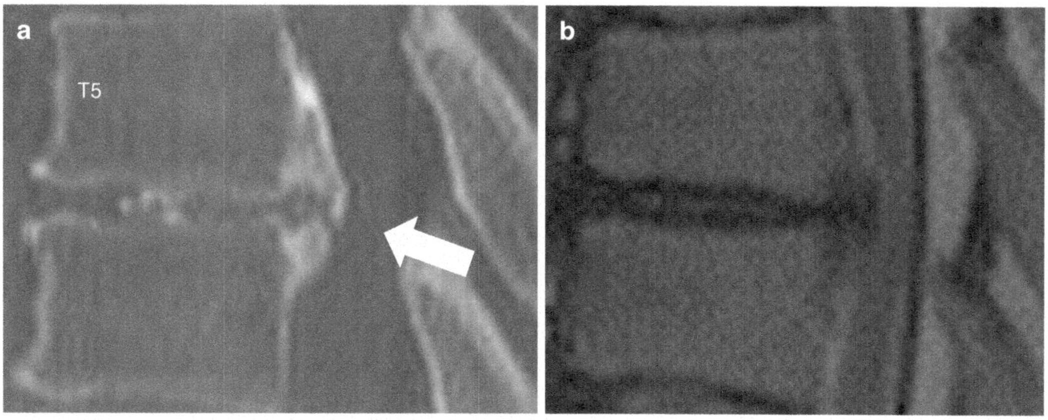

Fig. 27.2 (**a**) Sagittal CT image of beak-type OPLL at T5-6 with discontinuity between the rostral and caudal ossification regions. (**b**) MRI showing intramedullary signal intensity change at the same location as the OPLL

Fig. 27.3 A case of beak-type continuous OPLL at T4-6 with mild leg numbness without palsy. (**a**) CT image. (**b**) MRI revealed severe canal stenosis at several OPLL locations without a high intensity area. At final follow-up after 3 years, the neurological status was unchanged, and OPLL had not extended or expanded [7]

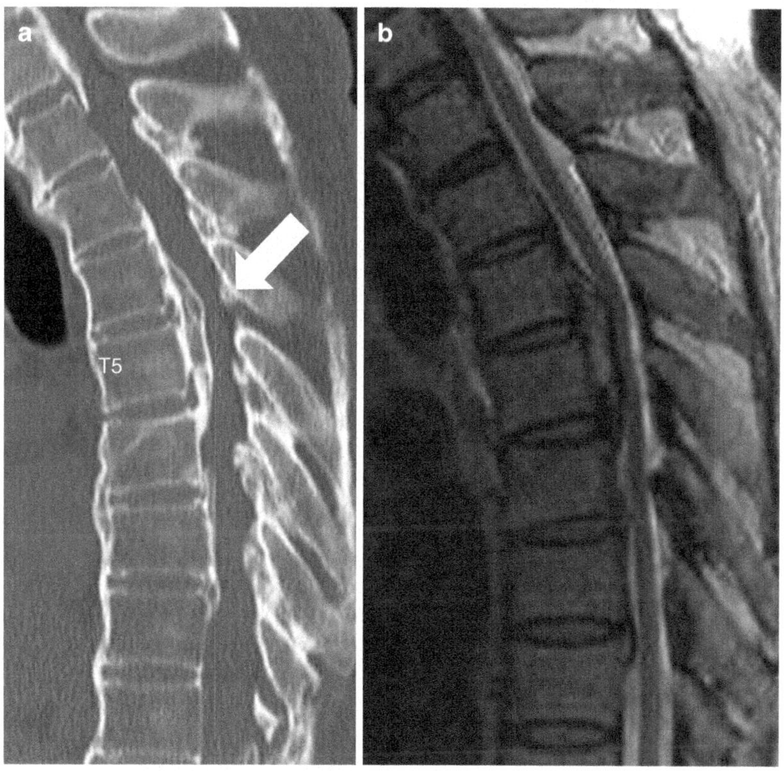

27.3 Choice of Surgical Procedures

Surgical treatment can be divided into two categories based on the type of decompression. The first is direct removal of the T-OPLL through an anterior or posterior approach [8–10] (Figs. 27.4 and 27.7), and the second is indirect posterior decompression of the spinal cord without directly touching the OPLL [3, 11, 12] (Figs. 27.5 and 27.6).

In 2008, a research group for ossification of the spinal ligament sponsored by the Japanese

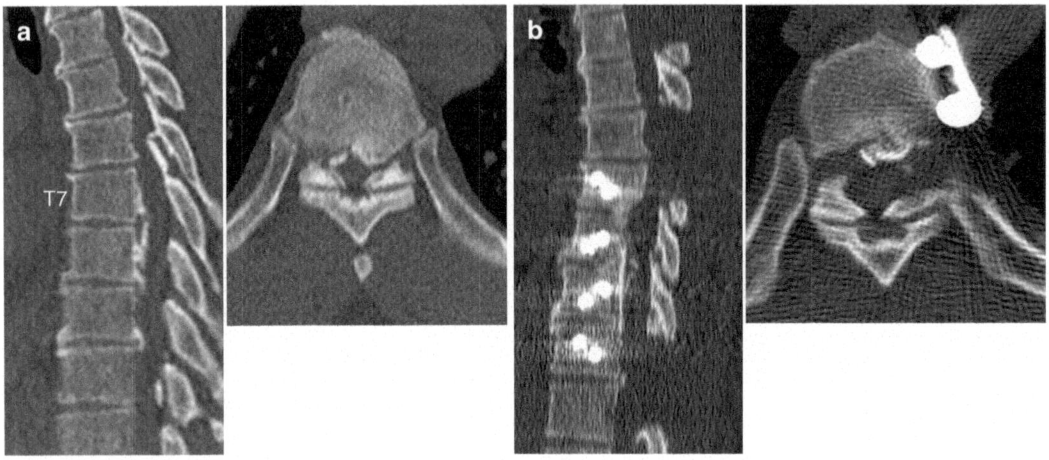

Fig. 27.4 A case of mixed-type OPLL at T7-10 with progressive myelopathy. (**a**) Preoperative sagittal CT images showed discontinuity between the rostral and caudal ossification regions. (**b**) Sagittal CT images after T7-10 anterior decompression and fusion with instrumentation

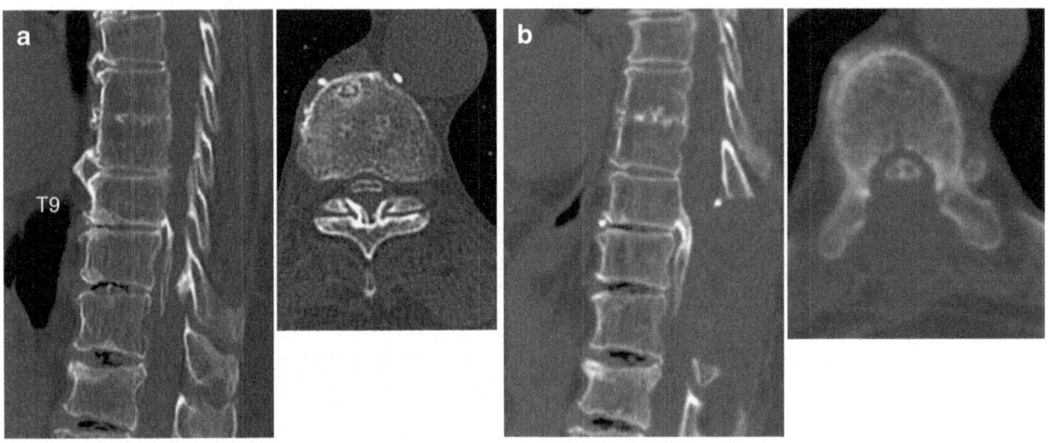

Fig. 27.5 A case of continuous-type OPLL at T9-11 and T10/11 ossification of the ligamentum flavum (OLF) with progressive myelopathy. (**a**) Preoperative sagittal CT images showed discontinuity between the OPLL and T11 vertebra without kyphosis of this region. (**b**) Sagittal CT images after T9-11 laminectomy

Ministry of Health, Labor and Welfare (MHLW) and with members from major Japanese institutions that treat spinal diseases conducted a multi-institutional retrospective survey of patients who underwent surgery for T-OPLL [13]. The surgical procedures were laminectomy (n = 36 patients), laminoplasty (n = 51), anterior decompression and fusion via an anterior extrapleural or transpleural approach (n = 25), anterior decompression via a posterior approach (n = 29), circumferential decompression and fusion via a combined anterior and posterior approach (n = 8), and anterior decompression and fusion via a sternal splitting approach (n = 5). Augmentation by spinal instrumentation (n = 52, 33%), posterior instrumentation (n = 50), and anterior instrumentation (n = 2) were also conducted [13].

In 2018, a prospective nationwide multicenter study of T-OPLL surgeries was conducted using data from the Japanese Multicenter Research Organization for Ossification of the Spinal Ligament (JOSL), instituted by the MHLW [14]. In this report, the surgical procedures were laminectomy (n = 6, 5.2%), posterior fusion without

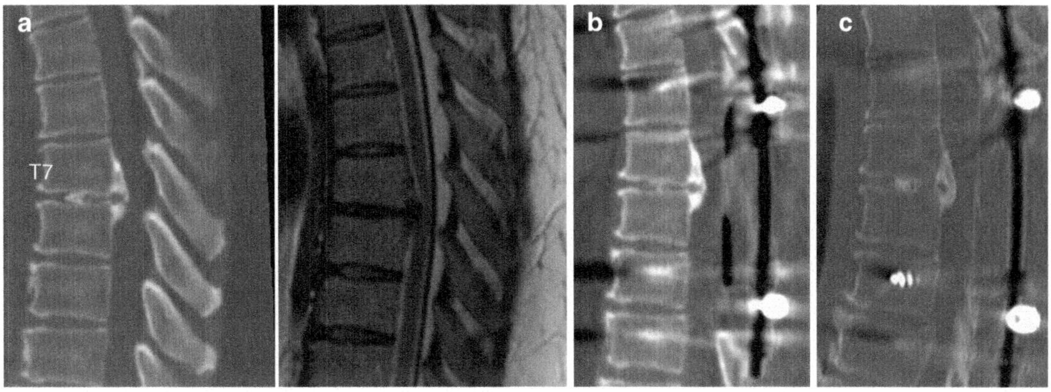

Fig. 27.6 A case of beak-type OPLL at T7/8 with progressive myelopathy. (**a**) Preoperative sagittal CT and MRI showed discontinuity between the rostral and caudal ossification regions. (**b**) CT after T5-10 posterior decompression and fusion with instrumentation. (**c**) CT at follow-up after 6 months, at which time neurological status had recovered and OPLL was continuous

laminectomy (*n* = 4, 3.5%), anterior resection via an anterior approach (*n* = 8, 7%), anterior resection via a posterior approach (*n* = 12, 10.4%), and posterior decompression and fusion with instrumentation with or without concomitant dekyphosis (*n* = 85, 74%). Decompression only was used in six cases (5.2%). The rate of surgery with instrumentation was 88% (101 cases) [14]. Thus, instrumentation surgeries for T-OPLL have increased considerably in 10 years.

Instrumentation is not necessary for upper and lower thoracic lesions because the spinal curvature is usually lordotic or only slightly kyphotic at the cervicothoracic junction, and dorsal shift and decompression of the spinal cord can be achieved by posterior decompression alone [13]. However, use of instrumentation is recommended for a middle thoracic OPLL, which is the most frequently affected level, to prevent intra- and postoperative paralysis by the change of kyphotic alignment [3, 15]. Regarding the choice of surgical procedure, Matsuyama et al. reported that anterior decompression surgery via an anterior approach is technically demanding and is associated with a risk of intrathoracic complications although it allows effective decompression. Anterior decompression via a posterior approach is an effective procedure but is also technically demanding and has the risk of kyphotic progression. Expansive laminoplasty is a relatively safe procedure with clinical outcomes comparable to those of anterior decompression. However, cases of postoperative neurologic deterioration do occasionally occur [3].

In the recent multicenter study [14], posterior decompression and fusion with instrumentation and with or without concomitant dekyphosis were performed in most cases (74%, Fig. 27.6), and the rate of surgery with instrumentation of 88% reflects the current major trend toward posterior instrumented fusion surgery for T-OPLL [14]. However, the most common postoperative complication may be aggravation of motor weakness in the lower extremities (32.2%, *n* = 37) [14]. In the 37 cases with this complication, 27 (73.0%) recovered after rehabilitation in bed or systemic corticosteroid infusion without additional surgery, but 9 (24.3%) required additional surgery, including extension of posterior fusion (*n* = 4), T-OPLL resection from a posterior approach (*n* = 2), hematoma removal and irrigation (*n* = 2), and additional laminectomy following T-OPLL resection from an anterior approach (*n* = 1) [14]. Imagama et al. suggested that a second surgery of OPLL resection (Fig. 27.7) should be performed in cases with no improvement or aggravation of symptoms within 3 weeks after posterior decompression and fusion surgery [9].

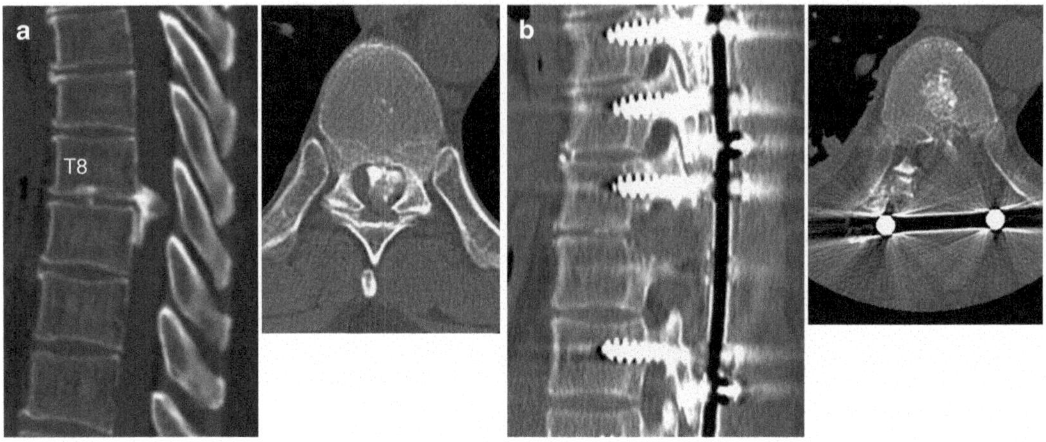

Fig. 27.7 A case of beak-type OPLL at T8/9 with progressive myelopathy. (**a**) Preoperative CT. The patient underwent T6-11 posterior decompression and fusion with instrumentation, but there was no improvement of symptoms by 3 weeks after surgery. (**b**) CT after resection of beak-type T-OPLL from a posterior approach (RASPA) [10]

References

1. Mori K, et al. Prevalence, distribution, and morphology of thoracic ossification of the posterior longitudinal ligament in Japanese: results of CT-based cross-sectional study. Spine (Phila Pa 1976). 2014;39(5):394–9.
2. Matsunaga S, et al. Clinical course of patients with ossification of the posterior longitudinal ligament: a minimum 10-year cohort study. J Neurosurg. 2004;100(3 Suppl Spine):245–8.
3. Matsuyama Y, et al. Surgical outcome of ossification of the posterior longitudinal ligament (OPLL) of the thoracic spine: implication of the type of ossification and surgical options. J Spinal Disord Tech. 2005;18(6):492–7; discussion 498.
4. Yonenobu K, et al. Lateral rhachotomy for thoracic spinal lesions. Spine (Phila Pa 1976). 1990;15(11):1121–5.
5. Matsunaga S, Sakou T. Ossification of the posterior longitudinal ligament of the cervical spine: etiology and natural history. Spine (Phila Pa 1976). 2012;37(5):E309–14.
6. Morita D, et al. Range of motion of thoracic spine in sagittal plane. Eur Spine J. 2014;23(3):673–8.
7. Ando K, et al. Comparative study of surgical treatment and nonsurgical follow up for thoracic ossification of the posterior longitudinal ligament: radiological and clinical evaluation. Spine (Phila Pa 1976). 2017;42(6):407–10.
8. Fujimura Y, et al. Long-term follow-up study of anterior decompression and fusion for thoracic myelopathy resulting from ossification of the posterior longitudinal ligament. Spine (Phila Pa 1976). 1997;22(3):305–11.
9. Imagama S, et al. Risk factors for ineffectiveness of posterior decompression and dekyphotic corrective fusion with instrumentation for beak-type thoracic ossification of the posterior longitudinal ligament: a single institute study. Neurosurgery. 2017;80(5):800–8.
10. Imagama S, et al. Resection of beak-type thoracic ossification of the posterior longitudinal ligament from a posterior approach under intraoperative neurophysiological monitoring for paralysis after posterior decompression and fusion surgery. Global Spine J. 2016;6(8):812–21.
11. Matsuyama Y, et al. Indirect posterior decompression with corrective fusion for ossification of the posterior longitudinal ligament of the thoracic spine: is it possible to predict the surgical results? Eur Spine J. 2009;18(7):943–8.
12. Yamazaki M, et al. Posterior decompression with instrumented fusion for thoracic myelopathy caused by ossification of the posterior longitudinal ligament. Eur Spine J. 2010;19(5):691–8.
13. Matsumoto M, et al. Surgical results and related factors for ossification of posterior longitudinal ligament of the thoracic spine: a multi-institutional retrospective study. Spine (Phila Pa 1976). 2008;33(9):1034–41.
14. Imagama S, et al. Perioperative complications after surgery for thoracic ossification of posterior longitudinal ligament: a Nationwide multicenter prospective study. Spine (Phila Pa 1976). 2018;43(23):E1389–97.
15. Yamazaki M, et al. Transient paraparesis after laminectomy for thoracic myelopathy due to ossification of the posterior longitudinal ligament: a case report. Spine (Phila Pa 1976). 2005;30(12):E343–6.

Posterior Decompression and Fusion for Thoracic OPLL: Surgical Techniques, Outcomes, Timing, and Complications

28

Shiro Imagama, Kei Ando, Kazuyoshi Kobayashi, Hiroaki Nakashima, and Naoki Ishiguro

Abstract

Thoracic OPLL (T-OPLL) has an operative indication in most cases due to preoperative severe myelopathy. However, poor surgical outcomes and postoperative complications are major problems, and there is no consensus on surgical timing and operative procedures. A recent nationwide multicenter prospective study of T-OPLL surgery in Japan indicated a complication rate of 51.3%, including a rate of 32.2% for postoperative motor palsy, but the positive 1-year surgical outcome (JOA score recovery rate) of 55% was better than those in previous multicenter retrospective studies in Japan and in a recent systematic review. Therefore, surgical outcomes are improving but are still not satisfactory in all T-OPLL cases, and establishment of optimal surgical procedures and methods for reducing complications are required. In our department, posterior decompression and dekyphotic corrective fusion with instrumentation are performed because it achieves good surgical outcomes (JOA score recovery rate: 68%), can be applied for many T-OPLL cases, and can include rescue procedures to prevent spinal cord damage based on intraoperative neurophysiological monitoring. This procedure is a good surgical option, but some cases need T-OPLL resection from a posterior approach (RASPA). Therefore, we use two-stage surgery of posterior decompression and dekyphotic corrective fusion with instrumentation followed by RASPA if there is no improvement or aggravation occurs at about 3 weeks after the first surgery. A study in our department revealed that a positive preoperative prone and supine position test, non-ambulatory status, and severe radiographic spinal cord compression on MRI are significantly related to a poor surgical outcome, and we recommend earlier surgery for patients with these factors.

Keywords

Thoracic ossification of the posterior longitudinal ligament (T-OPLL) · Nationwide multicenter prospective study · Perioperative complication · Postoperative motor palsy
Good surgical outcome · Two-stage T-OPLL resection

S. Imagama (✉) · K. Ando · K. Kobayashi
H. Nakashima · N. Ishiguro
Department of Orthopaedic Surgery,
Nagoya University Graduate School of Medicine,
Nagoya, Aichi, Japan
e-mail: imagama@med.nagoya-u.ac.jp

A. Okawa et al. (eds.), *OPLL*, https://doi.org/10.1007/978-981-15-3855-1_28

28.1 Introduction

Thoracic OPLL (T-OPLL) is a rare but difficult-to-treat disease due to the lack of effective conservative therapy, preoperative severe myelopathy, and poor surgical outcomes with postoperative complications [1–3]. There is no consensus on surgical timing and ideal operative procedures though many surgical procedures have been described [4–9]. In Japan, posterior decompression and fusion surgery has recently been reported to give a favorable outcome [10–12], and this has led us to perform posterior decompression and dekyphotic instrumented fusion surgery, especially for beak type T-OPLL (Fig. 28.1). In this chapter, we discuss the complication rate in a multicenter prospective study [13], surgical techniques and timing, and factors associated with good surgical outcomes at our hospital [14–19].

28.2 Improved Surgical Outcomes, But High Complication Rates, in a Multicenter Prospective Study

The first nationwide prospective multicenter study for evaluation of perioperative complications in surgery for T-OPLL was conducted from 2011 to 2016 by the Japanese Multicenter Research Organization for Ossification of the Spinal Ligament (JOSL) with the assistance of the Japanese Ministry of Health, Labour and Welfare (MHLW) and the Japan Agency for Medical Research and Development (AMED) [13]. A total of 115 cases (males: 55, females: 60, average age 53.1 years, mean body mass index (BMI) 30.4 kg/m^2) were included in the study. Surgical procedures, preoperative radiographic findings, pre- and postoperative thoracic myelop-

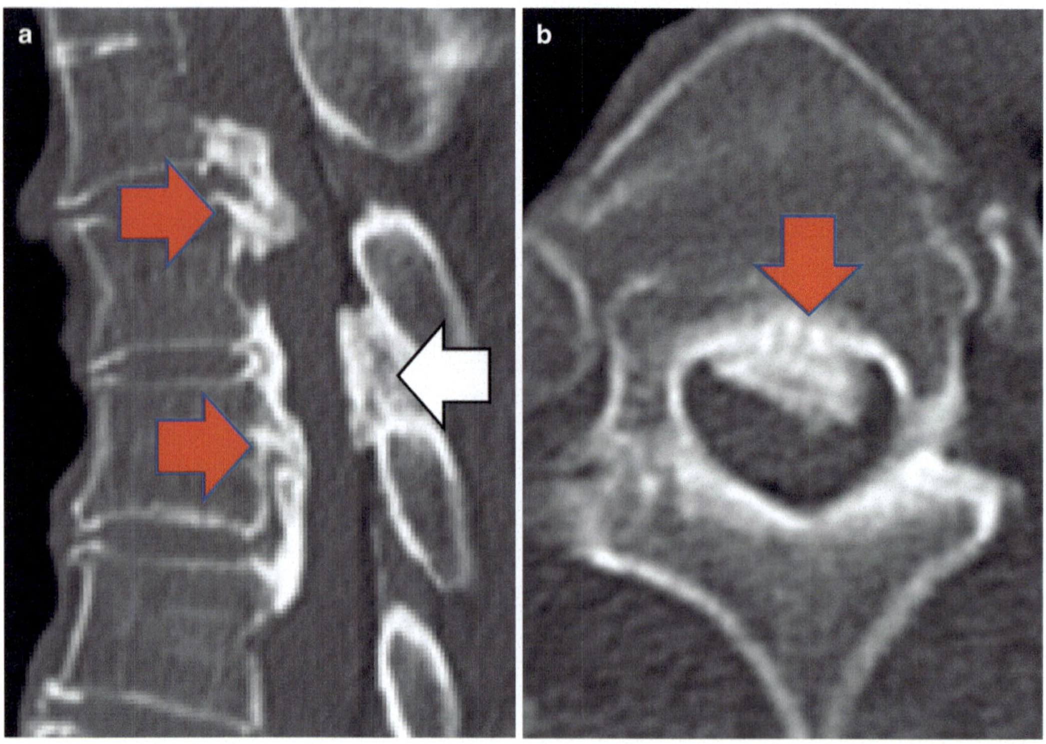

Fig. 28.1 Beak type T-OPLL on CT images. (**a**) Sagittal plane and (**b**) axial plane. Red arrows indicate T-OPLL. White arrows indicate T-OLF

athy (Japanese Orthopaedic Association (JOA) score), prone and supine position test (PST) status, intraoperative ultrasonography, and intraoperative neurophysiological monitoring (IONM) were investigated in these patients.

Posterior decompression and fusion with instrumentation with or without dekyphosis was performed in 85 of the 115 cases (74%). T-OPLL resection from a posterior approach, T-OPLL resection from an anterior approach, laminectomy only, and posterior fusion without laminectomy were performed in 10.4%, 7.0%, 5.2%, and 3.5%, respectively. The rate of instrumentation surgery of 88% reflects the current major trend toward posterior instrumented fusion surgery for T-OPLL.

The complication rate was 51.3% in all cases, including 32.2% with postoperative motor palsy (Fig. 28.2). This complication rate is higher than those of 40.8% in a 2011 JOSL retrospective multicenter study of fusion surgery for T-OPLL [2], and 39.4% in a 2017 systematic review of 15 retrospective articles on complications in T-OPLL surgery [3]. Postoperative neurological deficit occurred at rates of 11.7% in a 2008 JOSL retrospective multicenter study of all types of T-OPLL surgery [1], 26.3% in the 2011 JOSL study [2], and 13.9% in the 2017 review [3]. Thus, the prospective data in the 2011–2016 study may provide a better understanding of perioperative complications, which is needed for obtaining informed consent from patients, evidence-based decision making, and establishment of prophylactic procedures.

The 2011–2016 prospective study included dorsal column symptoms of the spinal cord and urinary tract infections as minor complications but also revealed major complications of two cases of pulmonary infarction and one of cerebral infarction (Table 28.1). This indicates the importance of prevention of such major general complications as well as surgical site complications. Significant factors related to perioperative complications included a larger number of T-OPLL levels, lower preoperative JOA score, higher preoperative positive PST rate, longer operative time, and a lower rate of intraoperative spinal cord floating in ultrasonography along with a tendency for an effect of a history of thoracic surgery (Table 28.2). Postoperative motor palsy was

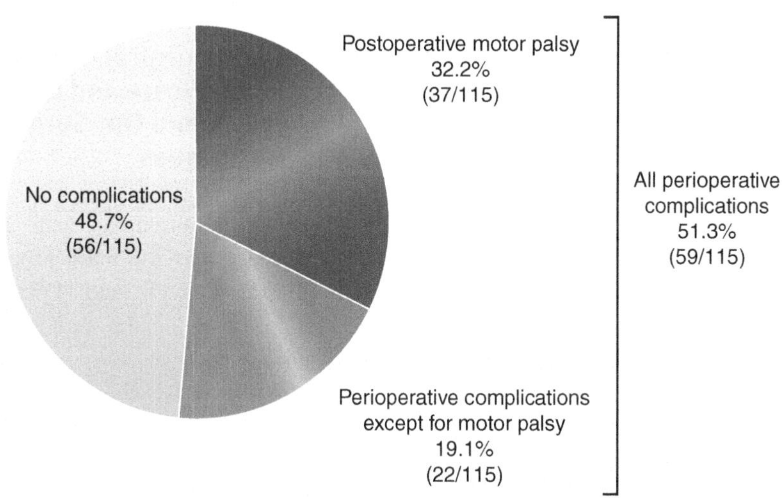

Fig. 28.2 Perioperative complications. The overall perioperative complication rate was 51.3%, including 32.2% for postoperative motor palsy. *Source*: Imagama S, et al. Perioperative Complications After Surgery for Thoracic Ossification of Posterior Longitudinal Ligament: A Nationwide Multicenter Prospective Study. Spine (Phila Pa 1976). 2018 Dec 1;43(23):E1389–E1397. doi: 10.1097/BRS.0000000000002703, journal URL: https://journals.lww.com/spinejournal/fulltext/2018/12010/Perioperative_Complications_After_Surgery_for.6.aspx

Table 28.1 Perioperative complications in 115 cases

Complication	Number
Intraoperative (16 complications)	
Dural tear	16
Postoperative (72 complications)	
Motor palsy in the lower extremities	37[a]
Liquorrhea	10
Deep wound infection	5
Hematoma at surgical site	3
Vertebral fracture	3
Pleural effusion due to liquorrhea	3
Pulmonary infarction	2
Cerebral infarction	1
Atelectasis	1
Sepsis	1
Superficial wound infection	1
Urinary tract infection	1
Horner sign	1
Dorsal column symptom of spinal cord	1
Numbness in upper extremity due to intraoperative prone position	1

Imagama S, et al. Perioperative Complications After Surgery for Thoracic Ossification of Posterior Longitudinal Ligament: A Nationwide Multicenter Prospective Study. Spine (Phila Pa 1976). 2018 Dec 1;43(23):E1389–E1397. doi: 10.1097/BRS.0000000000002703, journal URL: https://journals.lww.com/spinejournal/fulltext/2018/12010/Perioperative_Complications_After_Surgery_for.6.aspx

[a]Includes five cases of motor palsy on day 1 to day 12 after surgery. The number is all complications in 59 cases with complications. Paralyzed cases include transient palsy

significantly related to comorbid ossification of the ligamentum flavum (OLF), estimated blood loss (EBL), and deterioration of IONM in addition to the factors for all complications listed above (Table 28.3). In an analysis of comorbidities and complications, diabetes mellitus was a significant risk factor for postoperative deep surgical site infection. Identification of these risk factors may allow development of preventive methods to reduce perioperative complications and postoperative palsy.

Another finding in the 2011–2016 study was that motor palsy fully recovered with a mean recovery period of 2.7 months, except for one case of postoperative cerebral palsy. However, spinal cord regeneration therapy is not fully established, and some cases may still have high risk of permanent postoperative motor palsy. A high number of T-OPLL levels, lower preoperative JOA score, and greater EBL were significantly associated with a long recovery period for postoperative motor palsy. Thus, a large number of T-OPLL levels, low preoperative JOA score, and a preoperative positive PST may suggest a need for earlier surgery to prevent postoperative complications. A less invasive procedure, better decompression of the spinal cord, and stable IONM during surgery are also likely to be associated with fewer complications.

Despite the higher complication rate, surgical outcomes based on the positive 1-year JOA score recovery rate of 55% were better than those of 36.8% in the 2008 study [1], 45.4% in the 2011 study [2], and 50.4% in the 2017 review [3] in which surgical outcomes were based on longer postoperative follow-up. We believe that this better outcome is due to appropriate selection of the surgical procedure based on improved knowledge of T-OPLL, innovation in instrumentation, and better and safer procedures using IONM. However, the surgical outcome is still not satisfactory in all T-OPLL patients, and there is still a need to establish optimal surgical procedures, timing, and preventive methods to reduce postoperative complications.

28.3 Good Surgical Outcome in JOA Score and Quality of Life and Our Surgical Techniques

Posterior decompression and instrumented fusion surgery was the main procedure in the 2011–2016 nationwide study [13], and we prospectively perform posterior decompression and dekyphotic corrective fusion with instrumentation for beak type T-OPLL (Table 28.4, left column). Our procedure involves dekyphosis for the thoracic lesion after laminectomy, which enables additional indirect spinal cord decompression without T-OPLL resection after laminectomy by decreasing thoracic kyphosis [10, 17, 18]. The gradual improvement in JOA score was expected for at least 1 year after this surgery (Fig. 28.3), and quality of life with the SF-36 (Japanese ver. 2.0) at 1 year after surgery was also improved (Fig. 28.4). This procedure

Table 28.2 Comparison of patients with and without perioperative complications

Item	Complications (*n* = 59)	No complications (*n* = 56)	*P*
Age (year)	52.1 ± 14.1	54.1 ± 15.3	0.46
Gender (male %)	40.7% (24/59)	55.4% (31/56)	0.14
Body mass index (kg/m²)	30.7 ± 7.45	30.2 ± 6.1	0.71
Comorbidity (%)	57.6% (34/59)	57.1% (32/56)	0.88
History of thoracic surgery (+) (%)	20.3% (12/59)	7.1% (4/56)	0.055
Number of T-OPLL levels	**3.3 ± 2.5**	**2.1 ± 1.4**	**0.022**
Ossification of the ligamentum flavum (+) (%)	45.8% (27/59)	33.9% (19/56)	0.17
Preoperative JOA score	**4.0 ± 2.5**	**5.0 ± 2.0**	**0.018**
Preoperative positive PST (%)	**32.2% (19/59)**	**12.5% (7/56)**	**0.028**
Operative time (min)	**469.9 ± 198.2**	**364.8 ± 166.1**	**0.0060**
Estimated blood loss (mL)	1098.5 ± 1330.4	733.6 ± 855.6	0.11
Intraoperative spinal cord floating (+) in ultrasonography (%)	**53.7% (29/54)**	**83.7% (41/49)**	**0.020**

JOA Japanese Orthopaedic Association, *PST* prone and supine position test, *T-OPLL* thoracic ossification of the posterior longitudinal ligament
Data are shown as mean ± standard deviation
The figure in parentheses is the number of patients. The total number of patients is 115 for all comparisons except for intraoperative spinal cord floating (+) in ultrasonography (*n* = 103)
Bold values indicate significant difference
Source: Imagama S, et al. Perioperative Complications After Surgery for Thoracic Ossification of Posterior Longitudinal Ligament: A Nationwide Multicenter Prospective Study. Spine (Phila Pa 1976). 2018 Dec 1;43(23):E1389–E1397. doi: 10.1097/BRS.0000000000002703, journal URL: https://journals.lww.com/spinejournal/fulltext/2018/12010/Perioperative_Complications_After_Surgery_for.6.aspx

Table 28.3 Comparison of patients with and without postoperative palsy

Item	Palsy (*n* = 37)	No Palsy (*n* = 78)	*P*
Pre- and intraoperative findings (n = 115)			
Age, year	52.9 ± 1 5.8	53.2 ± 14.3	0.92
Gender (male %)	37.8% (14/37)	52.6% (41/78)	0.16
Body mass index, kg/m²	32.0 ± 8.2	29.7 ± 5.9	0.093
Comorbidity (%)	59.5% (22/37)	56.4% (44/78)	0.84
History of thoracic surgery (+) (%)	16.2% (6/37)	11.5% (9/78)	0.55
Number of T-OPLL levels	**3.7 ± 2.5**	**2.2 ± 1.6**	**0.0025**
Ossification of the ligamentum flavum (+) (%)	**59.5% (22/37)**	**30.8% (24/78)**	**0.035**
Preoperative JOA score	**3.7 ± 2.3**	**4.9 ± 2.2**	**0.0092**
Preoperative positive PST (%)	**48.6% (18/37)**	**10.3% (8/78)**	**0.0009**
Operative time, min	**481.5 ± 210.0**	**385.3 ± 171.6**	**0.0020**
Estimated blood loss, mL	**1253.5 ± 1572.1**	**751.9 ± 801.4**	**0.042**
Intraoperative spinal cord finding in ultrasonography (n = 103)			
Spinal cord floating (+) (%)	**48.6% (17/35)**	**77.9% (53/68)**	**0.031**
Intraoperative neurophvsiologica monitoring (IONM) (n = 100)			
Deterioration of IONM during surgery (%)	**84.4% (27/32)**	**27.9% (19/68)**	**<0.0001**
No restoration of aggravated amplitude (%)	**85.2% (23/27)**	**10.59% (2/19)**	**<0.0001**
No deterioration of IONM at end of surgery (%)	**28.1% (9/32)**	**97.1% (66/68)**	**<0.0001**

JOA Japanese Orthopaedic Association, *PST* prone and supine position test, *T-OPLL* thoracic ossification of the posterior longitudinal ligament
Data are shown as mean ± standard deviation
The figure in parentheses is the number of patients
Bold values indicate significant difference
Source: Imagama S, et al. Perioperative Complications After Surgery for Thoracic Ossification of Posterior Longitudinal Ligament: A Nationwide Multicenter Prospective Study. Spine (Phila Pa 1976). 2018 Dec 1;43(23):E1389–E1397. doi: 10.1097/BRS.0000000000002703, journal URL: https://journals.lww.com/spinejournal/fulltext/2018/12010/Perioperative_Complications_After_Surgery_for.6.aspx

Table 28.4 Surgical tips for posterior decompression and dekyphotic corrective fusion with instrumentation

Surgical procedure		Surgical tips (summary)
1	Position change from supine to prone	Perform gently because this position change may induce spinal cord injury
2	Exposure of laminae	Perform the procedure as quickly as possible
3	Pedicle screw insertion	Full segmental pedicle screws are advantageous and should be inserted very gently
4	Temporary unilateral rod fixation with in situ alignment	"In situ temporary rod fixation" No dekyphosis procedure is done before laminectomy
5	Posterior decompression with laminectomy using an air drill	Rough en-bloc laminectomy procedures should not be performed because of a high risk for intraoperative spinal cord damage (avoid "seesaw movement")
6	Ultrasonography (first time)	Check a fully decompressed spinal cord so as to make the lateral side of the dura mater visible for subsequent safe dekyphosis
7	Dekyphosis with bilateral rods	Cantilever maneuver and compression with pedicle screws made of a bilateral cobalt-chromium alloy rods of ≥6 mm in diameter (estimated dekyphosis of 10 degrees)
8	Ultrasonography (second time)	Additional dekyphosis procedure after Ponte osteotomy can be selected for insufficient indirect spinal cord decompression in second ultrasonography
9	Irrigation and skin closure	Thick drainage tubes after irrigation with sufficient saline, and the intrawound administration of vancomycin may be helpful to prevent surgical site infection

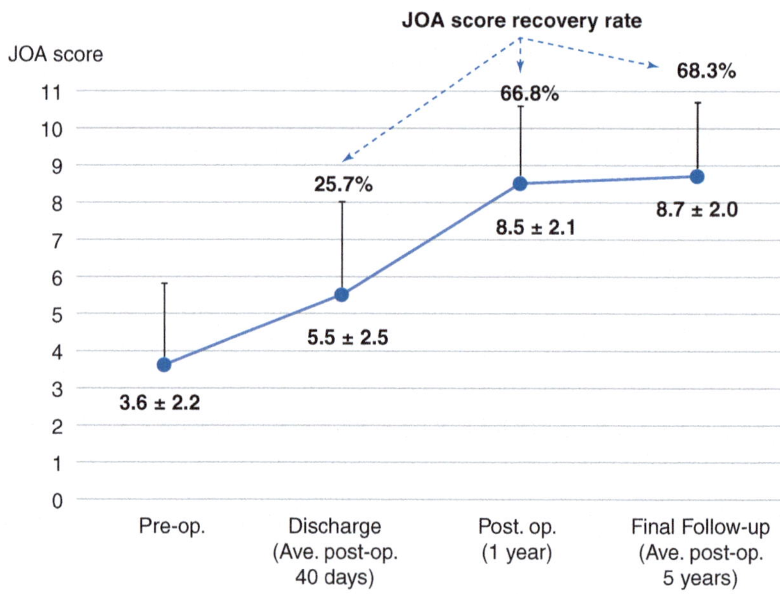

Fig. 28.3 Gradual improvement in JOA score after posterior decompression and dekyphotic corrective fusion with instrumentation

achieves excellent surgical outcomes (JOA score recovery rate of 68%) at the follow-up period of a minimum of 2 years and an average of 5 years [18] and is a good option for posterior surgery.

28.3.1 Surgical Tips (Table 28.4)

There are many tips that assist with obtaining a good surgical outcome. In the operating room, the change from a supine to prone position should be

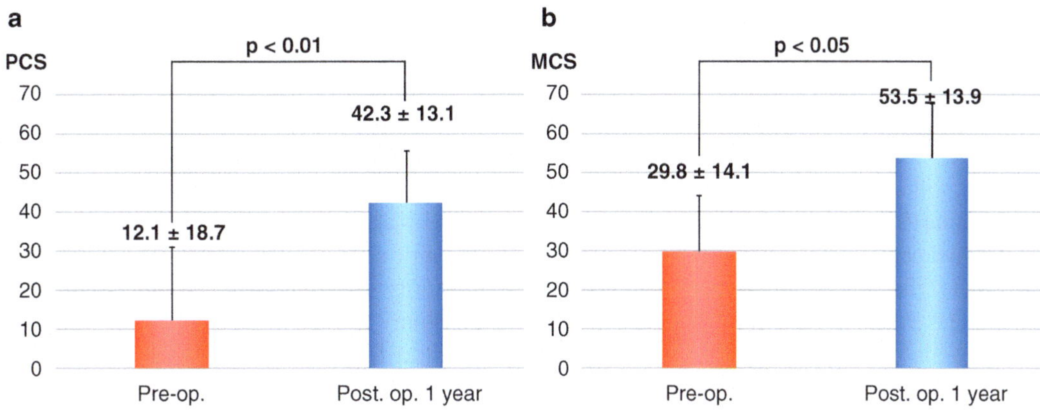

Fig. 28.4 Improvement of QOL with the two summary measures of the SF-36 at 1 year after surgery. (**a**) PCS (the physical component summary), (**b**) MCS (the mental component summary)

performed gently because this position change may induce spinal cord injury in patients with T-OPLL. The prone position itself is often harmful for a severely compressed spinal cord, and thus, decompression and fusion procedures should be performed as quickly as possible. After exposure of laminae, full segmental pedicle screws, which are beneficial to prevent postoperative motor paralysis due to rod bending, should be inserted at all pedicles in the fusion area [19]. Then these are fixed in situ by a unilateral rod to prevent paralysis due to spinal cord damage after the alignment change during performance of laminectomy with an air drill. At this time, since the spinal cord has not been decompressed, pedicle screws should be inserted very gently, with a focus on in situ temporary rod fixation. If any spinal alignment change occurs in fixing the unilateral temporary rod, it easily induces spinal cord injury. No dekyphosis procedure is done before laminectomy. After in situ temporary rod fixation, posterior decompression and removal of thin laminae with an air drill should be performed. En bloc laminectomy should not be performed in patients with T-OPLL associated with dural adhesion and ossification for avoiding the spinal cord compression due to "seesaw movement" when en bloc lamina was removed. The laminae were thinned to like a paper using the drill and then removed from the dura using a small raspatorium so that we can avoid the spinal cord compression by laminae under IONM. In a case with extensive OLF, the laminae were first removed at the area without OLF at the cranial and rostral site and the dura mater was exposed. As for patients with OLF with a large OPLL at the same level, it is safer for prevention of paralysis to approach from the caudal, distal and lateral sides of the spinal cord with partial or total removal of the facet joint if needed. Throughout the surgery, rough procedures can easily cause postoperative deterioration or motor paralysis. All laminectomy should be performed with a fully decompressed spinal cord so as to make the lateral side of the dura mater visible for subsequent safe dekyphosis. The extent of spinal cord decompression and movement should be checked with intraoperative ultrasonography. Acceptable spinal cord decompression in beak type T-OPLL is judged as observation of spinal cord floating in the spinal central canal, but most cases do not have sufficient decompression at this time point. Next, slowly dekyphosis procedure (estimated dekyphosis of 10 degrees) is performed using cantilever force and compression with pedicle screws made of a bilateral cobalt-chromium alloy rods of ≥6 mm in diameter, after which a second ultrasonography check is performed. If indirect spinal cord decompression is insufficient in ultrasonography, a second dekyphosis procedure after Ponte osteotomy is effective for achieving more spinal cord decompression in cases without massive ossification of the anterior longitudinal ligaments. After confirming sufficient spinal cord decompression in ultrasonography, decortication and local bone graft are performed, followed by soft tissue closure with thick drainage tubes after irrigation with sufficient saline to prevent surgical site infection (SSI). In our department, vancomycin (VCM) hydrochloride powder (1 g for adult) was applied to the wound after approval by the Institutional Review Board of our university, and the intrawound administration of VCM is thought to be effective to prevent SSI in cases with high risks of infection [20].

28.3.2 Rescue Procedures Based on IONM Deterioration (Table 28.5)

IONM is also essential to achieve a good surgical outcome. Deterioration of IONM is common in T-OPLL surgery, reflecting the vulnerable thoracic spinal cord, and so we prepare rescue procedures for each surgical procedure at the time of IONM deterioration to prevent permanent spinal cord paralysis (Table 28.5). In a case with a positive preoperative PST, IONM is checked in the supine position and at the time of the change from a supine to prone position. When IONM deteriorates in the position change, the appropriateness of the prone position should be checked, including checking the cervical spinal alignment. If IONM is aggravated at pedicle screw insertion, insertion of pedicle screws should be skipped to give priority to spinal cord decompression with laminectomy after unilateral temporary rod fixation with a few pedicle screws. The remaining screws can be inserted after laminectomy to prepare for the dekyphosis procedure. The most critical procedure that is likely to have IONM deterioration is decompression with an air drill, reflecting spinal cord damage by compression, vibration, and heat of the air drill. If this occurs, the surgical procedure should be stopped, the surgical site should be filled with warm saline, and blood pressure and body temperature should be raised to reduce the spinal cord damage. When the IONM amplitude recovers, laminectomy can be restarted. If IONM deteriorates after completed posterior decompression, indirect decompression by dekyphosis should be quickly performed.

Table 28.5 Surgical procedures for posterior decompression and dekyphotic corrective fusion with instrumentation and rescue procedures after IONM deterioration

Surgical procedure		Rescue procedure after IONM deterioration
1	Position change from supine to prone	Check the position, including cervical spinal alignment (IONM wave derivations are recommended at supine position before position change)
2	Exposure of laminae	Perform the procedure as quickly as possible to complete the decompression and fusion in a short time
3	Pedicle screw insertion	Skip insertion of pedicle screws and give priority to spinal cord decompression with laminectomy after bilateral temporary rod fixation with a few pedicle screws
4	Temporary unilateral rod fixation with in situ alignment	Recheck in situ fixation of temporary rod (confirm that there is no dekyphosis)
5	Posterior decompression with laminectomy using an air drill	Stop the surgical procedure, fill the surgical site with warm saline, and raise blood pressure and body temperature
6	Ultrasonography (first time)	Recheck insufficient laminectomy that may have induced spinal cord damage
7	Dekyphosis with bilateral rods	
8	Ultrasonography (second time)	Additional dekyphosis with or without Ponte osteotomy
9	Irrigation and skin closure	NA

IONM deterioration is defined as a decrease of amplitude of ≥70% from the control. The definition of IONM deterioration in T-OPLL surgery requires further investigation
NA not available

The important point is to avoid neglecting IONM findings and proceeding with surgery since this may cause permanent spinal cord injury. The recent prospective multicenter study about the alert timing and rescue procedures with IONM for high-risk spinal surgery concluded that appropriate intervention immediately after the IONM alert might prevent neurological deterioration even in high-risk spinal pathologies including T-OPLL, though the rescue ratios for T-OPLL was relatively low (40%) [21]. Therefore, we should perform a less invasive surgical procedure to prevent intraoperative spinal cord damage as well as IONM which will be also advantageous in T-OPLL surgery.

28.3.3 RASPA as Second Surgery (and a Suggested Indication for RASPA as First Surgery)

Posterior decompression and dekyphotic corrective fusion with instrumentation surgery can give good surgical outcomes using the above surgical tips and IONM findings. However, some cases need additional T-OPLL resection surgery, and we inform patients of the possible need for a two-stage strategy of posterior decompression and dekyphotic corrective fusion with instrumentation as the first surgery, and T-OPLL resection (Resection at an Anterior site of the Spinal cord from a Posterior Approach (RASPA)) as the second surgery if there is no improvement or there is aggravation at about 3 weeks after the first surgery [16, 17].

We have described RASPA in detail in the literature (Fig. 28.5) [16, 17]. Briefly, the RASPA procedure as the second surgery is as follows. After a unilateral rod and a few pedicle screws are removed at the level of OPLL resection, resection of the transverse process and pedicle is performed with spinal root sacrifice at the OPLL resection level. Posterior partial osteotomy of the vertebra and OPLL resection are performed with an air drill from the posterolateral direction with the instrument leaned laterally as much as possible to permit resection of the OPLL of the anterior spinal cord without causing spinal cord damage. We do not retract or rotate the vulnerable thoracic spinal cord to avoid spinal cord damage with frequent checking of IONM during surgery. If these surgical devices are obstructed by a posterior rib, partial resection of the rib (costotransversectomy) should be helpful. The same procedure is performed on the contralateral side according to OPLL extension after resetting of the temporary rod. As a residual thin OPLL may help to avoid CSF leakage and a thin OPLL does not usually prevent spinal cord decompression, spinal cord floating without total resection of the OPLL is usually sufficient. Spinal cord decompression can be confirmed with ultrasonography, and use of an intraoperative CT-based navigation system is helpful to check the amount of residual T-OPLL. After removal of the OPLL, additional dekyphosis with a bilateral rod can be performed in cases with T-OPLL at another site. This gives indirect decompression at another OPLL level that does not need OPLL resection, and spinal cord shortening is achieved after dekyphosis and a compression maneuver that may increase the blood supply to the spinal cord.

In our study, 4 of 70 cases (5.7%) needed two-stage T-OPLL resection (one case with an anterior approach and 3 with RASPA), but their mean JOA score recovery rate of 59% after two-stage surgery was good, and not significantly different from those for single posterior decompression and dekyphotic corrective fusion with instrumentation [17]. The three patients treated with RASPA as the second surgery could walk unaided or with one cane and had an average JOA score recovery rate of 80.5%. Therefore, we recommend this two-stage strategy of posterior decompression and dekyphotic corrective fusion with instrumentation and RASPA for cases without recovery or with aggravation, especially for beak type T-OPLL.

We believe that complete decompression of the spinal cord is ideal and advantageous for postoperative spinal cord recovery, but T-OPLL resection often induces massive blood loss and is an invasive surgery for the general condition and the spinal cord, particularly in cases with multiple T-OPLLs combined with OLF. In such cases, we select RASPA as the first surgery for short (one or two) segments of beak type T-OPLL in relatively young patients, given the surgical invasiveness of T-OPLL resection, but there are relatively few of these mild T-OPLL cases.

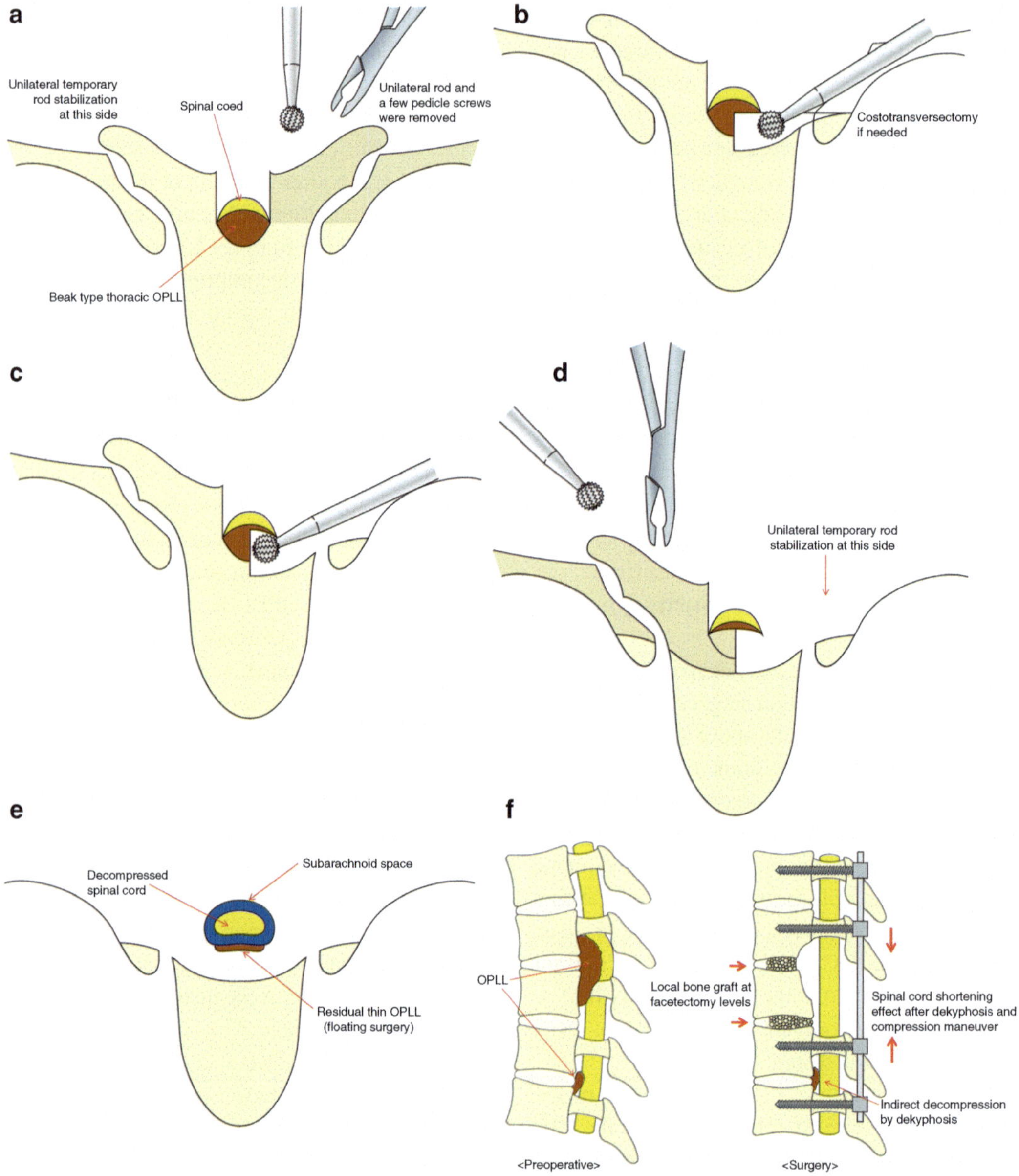

Fig. 28.5 Surgical procedures in RASPA surgery. (**a**) Unilateral rod and a few pedicle screws were removed. Resection of the transverse process and pedicle with spinal root sacrifice at the OPLL resection level. (**b**) Posterior partial osteotomy of vertebra and OPLL resection with an air drill from the posterolateral direction, with costotransversectomy if needed. (**c**) We do not retract or rotate the vulnerable thoracic spinal cord to avoid spinal cord injury. Surgical devices should be leaned laterally as much as possible. IOM should be checked frequently during surgery. (**d**) Same procedure on the contralateral side according to OPLL extension after resetting the temporary rod. (**e**) Spinal cord decompression was achieved with confirmation of the subarachnoid space in intraoperative ultrasonography. (**f**) After removal of the OPLL, additional dekyphosis and compression maneuver with a bilateral rod is performed, which gives indirect decompression at other OPLL levels with spinal cord compression and spinal cord shortening. Local bone graft is performed at the OPLL resection level because discectomy is usually straightforward. *Source*: Resection of beak-type thoracic ossification of the posterior longitudinal ligament from a posterior approach under intraoperative neurophysiological monitoring for paralysis after posterior decompression and fusion surgery. Imagama S, Ando K, Ito Z, Kobayashi K, Hida T, Ito K, Ishikawa Y, Tsushima M, Matsumoto A, Tanaka S, Morozumi M, Machino M, Ota K, Nakashima H, Wakao N, Nishida Y, Matsuyama Y, Ishiguro N. Global Spine J. 2016 Dec;6(8):812-821. Epub 2016 Feb 24

28.4 Factors and Optimal Surgical Timing for Good Surgical Outcomes

In a previous study, we examined factors for a good surgical outcome in posterior decompression and dekyphotic corrective fusion with instrumentation for T-OPLL prospectively in 71 cases [18]. These cases were divided into good or poor outcomes based on a JOA score recovery rate of ≥50% and <50%, respectively, in a mean follow-up period of 5 years with a minimum of 2 years. Preoperatively, the group with a good outcome (76%) had significantly lower rates of non-ambulatory status and positive PST; of T-OPLL, OLF, and a high intensity area (HIA) at the same level on MRI, of thoracic spinal cord misalignment (OPLL-SKAD), and of spinal canal stenosis on MRI. Perioperatively, this group had lower estimated blood loss (EBL) and higher rates of intraoperative spinal cord floating and absence of deterioration of IONM. Postoperatively, lower rates of postoperative complications were significantly related to a good outcome as expected. In a multivariate logistic regression analysis based on these findings, a negative PST (odds ratio [OR]: 17.0), preoperative ambulatory status (OR: 6.1), absence of T-OPLL, OLF, and HIA at the same level (OR: 5.8), intraoperative spinal cord floating (OR: 5.0), and lower EBL (OR: 1.0) were identified as significant independent factors associated with a good surgical outcome.

As described above, the 2011–2016 nationwide prospective multicenter study of perioperative complications and recovery from postoperative palsy showed that a large number of T-OPLL levels, low preoperative JOA score, and a positive preoperative PST suggest the need for earlier surgical timing to prevent complications [13]. Our prospective study of surgical outcomes suggests that a positive preoperative PST, preoperative non-ambulatory status, radiographic severe spinal canal stenosis, and spinal cord damage (T-OPLL, OLF, and HIA at the same level on MRI T2-weighted images) may also indicate a need for early surgical intervention [18]. The appropriate timing of surgery requires evaluation in a randomized controlled trial, but such a trial is difficult to conduct ethically, given the potential disadvantages to patients. Thus, the above factors associated with perioperative complications in the 2011–2016 nationwide study and those linked to the surgical outcome in our study may currently be the most effective basis for determining the appropriate surgical timing for treatment of T-OPLL (Table 28.6).

Table 28.6 Factors and optimal surgical timing for good surgical outcomes

Goal	The factors for earlier surgical timing
For preventing the perioperative complications	Large number of T-OPLL levels
	Low preoperative JOA score
	Positive preoperative PST
For good surgical outcome	Positive preoperative PST
	Preoperative non-ambulatory
	Presence of T-OPLL, OLF, and HIA at the same level on preoperative MRI

Note: Surgery before positive PST and non-ambulatory with severe preoperative symptoms will be more advantageous for symptomatic T-OPLL patients

Acknowledgements The authors thank all members of the Investigation Committee on the Ossification of the Spinal Ligaments of the Japanese Ministry of Public Health and Welfare for their assistance throughout the nationwide multicenter prospective study of T-OPLL surgery.

Conflicts of interest and source of funding: The nationwide multicenter prospective study of T-OPLL surgery was supported by a Japanese Health Labor Sciences Research Grant (Grant number 040), and Japan Agency for Medical Research and Development (AMED, Grant number JP15ek0109136).

References

1. Matsumoto M, Chiba K, Toyama Y, Takeshita K, Seichi A, Nakamura K, et al. Surgical results and related factors for ossification of posterior longitudinal ligament of the thoracic spine: a multi-institutional retrospective study. Spine (Phila Pa 1976). 2008;33(9):1034–41.
2. Matsumoto M, Toyama Y, Chikuda H, Takeshita K, Kato T, Shindo S, et al. Outcomes of fusion surgery for ossification of the posterior longitudinal ligament of the thoracic spine: a multicenter retrospective survey: clinical article. J Neurosurg Spine. 2011;15(4):380–5.

3. Xu N, Yu M, Liu X, Sun C, Chen Z, Liu Z. A systematic review of complications in thoracic spine surgery for ossification of the posterior longitudinal ligament. Eur Spine J. 2017;26(7):1803–9.
4. Aizawa T, Sato T, Sasaki H, Matsumoto F, Morozumi N, Kusakabe T, et al. Results of surgical treatment for thoracic myelopathy: minimum 2-year follow-up study in 132 patients. J Neurosurg Spine. 2007;7(1):13–20.
5. Kato S, Murakami H, Demura S, Yoshioka K, Hayashi H, Tsuchiya H. Novel surgical technique for ossification of posterior longitudinal ligament in the thoracic spine. J Neurosurg Spine. 2012;17(6):525–9.
6. Kawahara N, Tomita K, Murakami H, Hato T, Demura S, Sekino Y, et al. Circumspinal decompression with dekyphosis stabilization for thoracic myelopathy due to ossification of the posterior longitudinal ligament. Spine (Phila Pa 1976). 2008;33(1):39–46.
7. Takahata M, Ito M, Abumi K, Kotani Y, Sudo H, Minami A. Clinical results and complications of circumferential spinal cord decompression through a single posterior approach for thoracic myelopathy caused by ossification of posterior longitudinal ligament. Spine (Phila Pa 1976). 2008;33(11):1199–208.
8. Tokuhashi Y, Matsuzaki H, Oda H, Uei H. Effectiveness of posterior decompression for patients with ossification of the posterior longitudinal ligament in the thoracic spine: usefulness of the ossification-kyphosis angle on MRI. Spine (Phila Pa 1976). 2006;31(1):E26–30.
9. Yamazaki M, Okawa A, Koda M, Goto S, Minami S, Moriya H. Transient paraparesis after laminectomy for thoracic myelopathy due to ossification of the posterior longitudinal ligament: a case report. Spine (Phila Pa 1976). 2005;30(12):E343–6.
10. Matsuyama Y, Sakai Y, Katayama Y, Imagama S, Ito Z, Wakao N, et al. Indirect posterior decompression with corrective fusion for ossification of the posterior longitudinal ligament of the thoracic spine: is it possible to predict the surgical results? Eur Spine J. 2009;18(7):943–8.
11. Yamazaki M, Mochizuki M, Ikeda Y, Sodeyama T, Okawa A, Koda M, et al. Clinical results of surgery for thoracic myelopathy caused by ossification of the posterior longitudinal ligament: operative indication of posterior decompression with instrumented fusion. Spine (Phila Pa 1976). 2006;31(13):1452–60.
12. Yamazaki M, Okawa A, Fujiyoshi T, Furuya T, Koda M. Posterior decompression with instrumented fusion for thoracic myelopathy caused by ossification of the posterior longitudinal ligament. Eur Spine J. 2010;19(5):691–8.
13. Imagama S, Ando K, Takeuchi K, Kato S, Murakami H, Aizawa T, et al. Perioperative complications after surgery for thoracic ossification of posterior longitudinal ligament: a Nationwide multicenter prospective study. Spine (Phila Pa 1976). 2018;43(23):E1389–E97.
14. Ando K, Imagama S, Ito Z, Kobayashi K, Ukai J, Muramoto A, et al. Ponte osteotomy during Dekyphosis for indirect posterior decompression with ossification of the posterior longitudinal ligament of the thoracic spine. Clin Spine Surg. 2017;30(4):E358–E62.
15. Ando K, Imagama S, Kobayashi K, Hida T, Ito K, Tsushima M, et al. Comparative study of surgical treatment and nonsurgical follow up for thoracic ossification of the posterior longitudinal ligament: radiological and clinical evaluation. Spine (Phila Pa 1976). 2017;42(6):407–10.
16. Imagama S, Ando K, Ito Z, Kobayashi K, Hida T, Ito K, et al. Resection of beak-type thoracic ossification of the posterior longitudinal ligament from a posterior approach under intraoperative neurophysiological monitoring for paralysis after posterior decompression and fusion surgery. Global Spine J. 2016;6(8):812–21.
17. Imagama S, Ando K, Ito Z, Kobayashi K, Hida T, Ito K, et al. Risk factors for ineffectiveness of posterior decompression and Dekyphotic corrective fusion with instrumentation for beak-type thoracic ossification of the posterior longitudinal ligament: a single institute study. Neurosurgery. 2017;80(5):800–8.
18. Imagama S, Ando K, Kobayashi K, Hida T, Ito K, Tsushima M, et al. Factors for a good surgical outcome in posterior decompression and Dekyphotic corrective fusion with instrumentation for thoracic ossification of the posterior longitudinal ligament: prospective single-center study. Oper Neurosurg (Hagerstown). 2017;13(6):661–9.
19. Imagama S, Ando K, Kobayashi K, Hida T, Ito K, Tsushima M, et al. Atypical vertebral column fracture at the middle of fused area after instrumented posterior decompression and fusion surgery for beak type thoracic ossification of the posterior longitudinal ligament. J Orthop Sci. 2018;23(6):1100–4.
20. Hida T, Ando K, Kobayashi K, Ito K, Tsushima M, Matsumoto A, et al. Intrawound vancomycin powder as the prophylaxis of surgical site infection after invasive spine surgery with a high risk of infection. Nagoya J Med Sci. 2017;79(4):545–50.
21. Yoshida G, Ando M, Imagama S, Kawabata S, Yamada K, Kanchiku T, et al. Alert timing and corresponding intervention with intraoperative spinal cord monitoring for high-risk spinal surgery. Spine (Phila Pa 1976). 2019;44(8):E470–E9.

Anterior Decompression and Fusion for Thoracic OPLL: Transthoracic and Transsternal Approaches

29

Shigeo Shindo, Koichi Mizuno, Kazuyuki Otani, Kazuo Kusano, and Osamu Nakai

Abstract

Ossification of the poster longitudinal ligament (OPLL) lessens the sagittal diameter of the canal and compresses the spinal cord anteriorly. Anterior decompression directly relieves the spinal cord, as well as restores the spinal cord to its original position. Anterior decompression for OPLL is a rational operative method. In the case of the thoracic spine, the approach method differs depending on the spinal level. The manubrium splitting approach is indicated for cases of OPLL located from cervical to T3. Transpleural approach is indicated below T2 level to thoraco-lumbar level. For 55 cases, we performed anterior decompression for thoracic OPLL, and noted the surgical approach, surgical result. The JOA (Japanese Orthopedic Association) scores were investigated. We modified the scoring system for cervical myelopathy established by the JOA by excluding items involving the upper extremities. Surgical approaches were transpleural approach in 47 cases and manubrium splitting approach in 8 cases. The mean recovery rate was 42.7% for manubrium splitting approach and 53.8% with transpleural approach. The frequency of laryngeal nerve palsy was over 50% with manubrium splitting approach. Leakage of cerebrospinal fluid in the thoracic cavity was seen frequently with the transpleural approach; however, it healed spontaneously without additional treatment. Although the anterior approach is associated with some problems (such as surgical invasiveness and postoperative complications), this surgical method resulted in positive outcomes, indicating that it is a useful technique.

Keywords

Ossification of the posterior longitudinal ligament (OPLL) · Thoracic myelopathy Transthoracic approach · Transpleural approach · Transsternal approach · Sternal splitting approach · Manubrium splitting approach · Anterior decompression and fusion · Anterior floating method

S. Shindo (✉) · K. Mizuno · K. Otani · K. Kusano
O. Nakai
Department of Orthopedic Surgery,
Kudanzaka Hospital, Tokyo, Japan
e-mail: sindou_s@kudanzaka.com

29.1 Introduction

Ossification of the poster longitudinal ligament (OPLL) lessens the sagittal diameter of the cervical canal and compresses the spinal cord anteriorly. Anterior decompression for OPLL is a rational operative method [1]. Anterior decompression directly relieves the cervical spinal cord, as well as restores the spinal cord to its original

A. Okawa et al. (eds.), *OPLL*, https://doi.org/10.1007/978-981-15-3855-1_29

position—especially the alignment of the thoracic spine is kyphotic. Compression is likely to remain in posterior decompression. Anterior decompression and fixation are necessary [2–4].

29.2 Approaches

In the case of the thoracic spine, the approach method differs depending on the spinal level (i.e., sternal splitting approach and the transpleural < extrapleural > approach). There are several types of sternal splitting [5–8]. In our department, the Manubrium splitting approach was selected.

29.3 Surgical Technique

29.3.1 Manubrium Splitting Approach [9]

The manubrium splitting approach is indicated for cases of OPLL located from cervical to T3. Above T1/2, it may be reachable by the approach without adding sternal splitting, but sternal splitting is often required to approach T3.

The patient is placed in the supine position. The cervical spine is in a neutral position. The skin incision is an oblique incision along the medial edge of the sternocleidomastoid muscle, reaching the midline of the manubrium end, while the suprasternal is a dogleg shaped incision in the midline longitudinal incision. Basically, it approaches from the left side. There is an exceptional existence on the right side (the so-called non-recurrent laryngeal nerve), in which case there is the possibility of nerve damage [10, 11].

The superficial cervical fascia is cut longitudinally, followed by blunt dissection between the hyoid muscle group and the sternocleid muscle, and retraction of the esophagus and trachea to the middle (while the carotid sheath to lateral reaches the vertebral body). If the lower thyroid artery crosses the operative area, it will be ligated and cut off. Detachment of the sternothyroid muscle and the sternocleid muscle (which are attached to the sternum) is then achieved.

This is followed by detachment of the periosteum (front of the sternum) to a sternal angle using raspatrium. After manual exfoliation of the ventral side of the sternum, a spatula is inserted under the sternum for the purpose of protecting the mediastinum tissue, and the manubrium is longitudinally split with a bone saw. Next the cartilaginous junction between manubrium and corpus sterni is cut with an osteotome. Opening the longitudinal split with a spreader reveals the adipose tissue below the sternum. Large blood vessels exist inside this adipose tissue (Fig. 29.1). The brachiocephalic trunk is retracted inferiorly, and corpectomy and anterior floating method are performed [1]. A graft from the fibula or iliac bone is inserted into the decompression space, and the vertebral bodies are fixed using a plate. A titanium cable is used to fasten the longitudinally split and the cartilaginous junction. The hyoid muscle group detached from the manubrium is re-sutured and the wound is closed.

29.3.2 Transthoracic Approach (Transpleural Approach and Extrapleural Approach) [12–18]

This approach is indicated below the T2 level to the thoraco-lumbar level.

The patient is placed in the lateral decubitus position placing a triangular mat to protect the down-facing upper limb and abduct or flex the upper-facing involved limb. A skin incision is made along the line of the rib that corresponded to the thoracic vertebra one or two levels above the involved vertebra. But in the upper thoracic vertebra, the incision is at the same level or one lower. The latissimus dorsi muscle and the seratus anterior muscle are then opened in the direc-

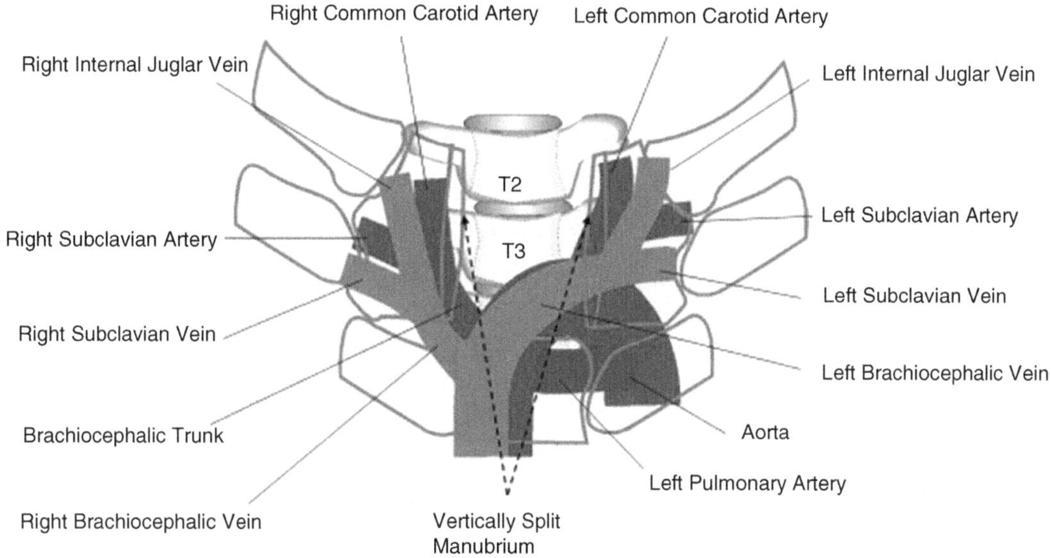

Fig. 29.1 When the manubrium is vertically split and opened, fat tissue appears, and the brachiocephalic vein is present inside the fat tissue. Upper edge of brachiocephalic vein is T3 vertebra body

tion of the skin incision to reach the rib. The rib is exfoliated under the periosteum using a raspatrium. Next the rib is cut off and used for a bone graft. In the case of the transpleural approach, the pleura is incised to enter the pleural cavity, and pleura of vertebra side is longitudinally cut and exfoliated from the vertebral body to expose the lateral vertebral body and the rib head. In the case of the extrapleural approach, the parietal pleura is carefully exfoliated from the chest wall with a gauze ball (or manually) to reach the vertebral body. The segmental vessels on the involved vertebrae are ligated and detached from the vertebral body. In the left approach the lung and the aorta are retracted anteriorly. The sympathetic trunk running longitudinally on the side of the vertebral body is retracted posteriorly. The head of the ribs is then excised to identify the pedicle, posterior end of the disk, and the intervertebral foramen. The posterior half of the vertebral body in a box shape is next resected using an osteotome, and the posterior wall of the vertebral body is thinned using an osteotome or a high-speed drill. After the OPLL was exposed, it was thinned, released from the pedicles, and cut transversely on the cranial and caudal sides, allowing it to move forward (Fig. 29.2). The resected rib is then inserted into the space where the decompression was performed, and the spine is fixed with an instrument. An expiration tube is set into the thoracic cavity, after which the intercostal muscle is closed, along with the latissimus dorsi muscle and the seratus anterior muscle and skin.

29.4 Material

Cases of anterior decompression surgery performed from 1990 in our hospital are the subjects of this study (except for cases in which the main lesion was cervical OPLL). We treated a total of 55 cases (29 males and 26 females). Age at time of surgery was

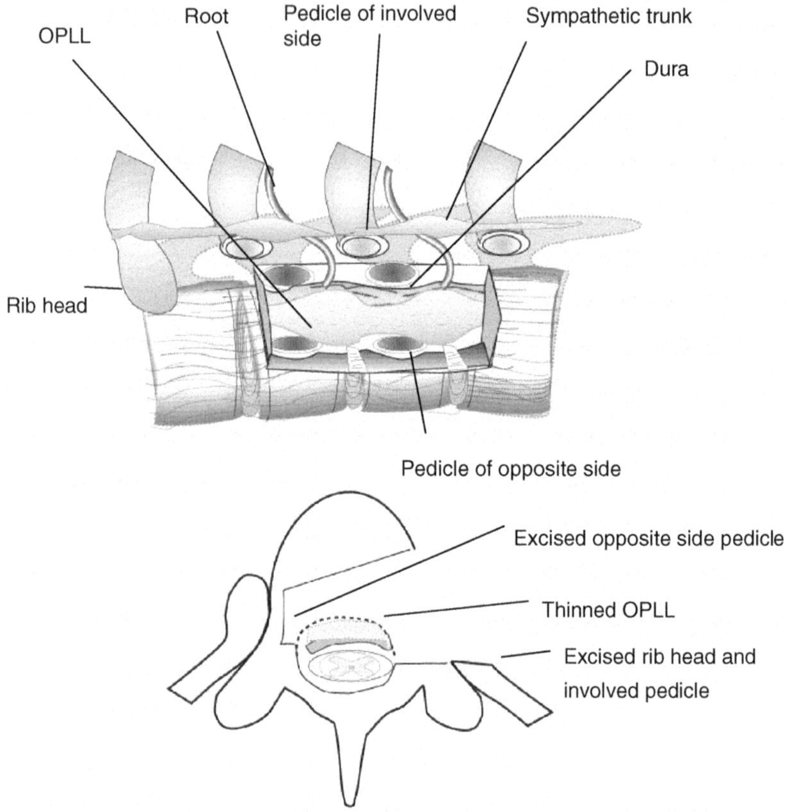

Fig. 29.2 After excision of the posterior part of the vertebral body, the spinal canal is exposed with rib heads and the pedicles dissection, and the configuration of OPLL is grasped; after thinning the anterior side of the OPLL, the opposite side pedicle is dissected, and the OPLL on the cranio-caudal side is cut; then the OPLL is released and floated

27–80, with a mean age of 52.1. Patients were followed up with for at least 1 year. The observation period was 1-year-and-2-months to 24 years, with a mean observation period of 8 years and 1 month. The Manubrium splitting approach is indicated for cases of OPLL located between Th1 to Th3, whereas the transpleural approach is indicated for cases below T2. In the munubrium splitting approach subtotal corpectomy and anterior decompression floating method are performed. Fibula graft is used and fixed using a plate. In the transthoracic approach iliac or rib graft is used in one level decompression. In multilevel decompression, a rib or fibula graft is applied. Recently, we have used instrumentation as an alternative.

29.5 Method

For 55 cases, we performed anterior decompression for thoracic OPLL, and noted the surgical approach, surgical time, number of decompression segments, amount of bleeding, and complications. In addition, the JOA (Japanese Orthopedic Association) scores were investigated. We modified the scoring system for cervical myelopathy established by the JOA by excluding items involving the upper extremities. The modified system has a normal score of 11 points (JOA score) (Table 29.1). The patient's recovery rates were calculated from the preoperative and postoperative JOA scores.

29.6 Result

Surgical approaches were transthoracic approach in 47 cases and manubrium splitting approach in 8 cases.

29.6.1 Manubrium Splitting Approach

The number of decompression segments was one case in 2 levels decompression, four cases in 3 levels, and one case in 4 levels. The involving caudal end vertebra is 1 case at T2 and 7 cases at T3. The surgical time was 3 h and 28 min to 12 h and 11 min, with a mean of 6 h and 36 min. The amount of bleeding was 440–3670 mL, with a mean of 1705 mL. the JOA score had improved from the preoperative mean points of 4.4 to post-operative mean points of 6.4, at final evaluation. The mean recovery rate was 42.7%.

Table 29.1 Evaluation of thoracic myelopathy (Japanese Orthopedic Association score)

Function point score	
Lower extremity motor function	
Unable to stand up and walk	0
Unable to walk without a cane or other support on level surface	1
Walks independently on level surface, but needs support on stairs	2
Capable of fast walking but is clumsy	3
Normal	4
Sensory function	
1. Lower extremity	0
Apparent sensory loss	1
Minimal sensory loss	2
Normal	
2. Trunk	
Apparent sensory loss	0
Minimal sensory loss	1
Normal	2
Bladder function	
Urinary retention and/or incontinence	0
Sense of retention and/or dribbling and/or thin stream	1
Urinary retardation and/or pollakiuria	2
Normal	3
Total for normal patient	11

Recovery rate = (postoperative score − preoperative score)/(11 − preoperative score) × 100%

29.6.2 Transpleural Approach

The number of decompression segments was 27 cases in one level decompression, 8 cases in 2 levels, 8 cases in 3 levels, and 4 cases in 4 levels. Decompression segments ranged across all thoracic levels, showing middle thoracic domination. The surgical time was 3 h and 25 min to 14 h and 15 min, with a mean of 6 h and 31 min. The amount of bleeding was 200–12,625 mL, with a mean of 2019 mL. As the surgical time was longer, a large amount of bleeding was seen, as expected (Table 29.2). The JOA score was preoperatively 4.1 and at the final follow-up was 7.8. The recovery rate was 53.8%.

Postoperatively, scores gradually improve and reach maximum score at one or 2 years after operation, and then decline in the long term with age and recurrence of myelopathy caused by thoracic OPLL at another level, ossification of yellow ligament, and cervical OPLL (Table 29.3).

Table 29.2 Involving vertebra level and surgical time, amount of bleeding

Segments	Surgical time	Amount of bleeding
1 levels (27 cases)	Ave. 5:40 (3:25–7:34)	Ave. 1452 mL (290–3230 mL)
2 levels (8 cases)	Ave. 6:32 (4:02–10:34)	Ave. 2171 mL (200–5100 mL)
3 levels (8 cases)	Ave. 8:50 (4:32–14:35)	Ave. 4036 mL (500–12,625 mL)
4 levels (4 cases)	Ave. 7:56 (7:18–8:51)	Ave. 1501 mL (1000–2370 mL)

Table 29.3 Average JOA scores and recovery rate

	Preoperative score	Maximum recovery score	Maximum recovery rate (%)	Postoperative score	Final recovery rate (%)
Manubrium splitting	4.4	8.2	60.2	6.4	42.7
Transpleural	4.1	8.0	56.9	7.8	53.7

29.7 Complications

Pseudo-meningocele and Hornel signs and hoarseness, swallowing dysfunction caused by paralysis of recurrence of the laryngeal nerve were a complication with the manubrium splitting approach. The frequency of laryngeal nerve palsy was over 50%. However, all recovered within a month or two.

Pooling of cerebrospinal fluid in the thoracic cavity was seen frequently with the transpleural approach; however, it healed spontaneously without additional treatment. But in two cases it was treated by spinal drainage. One case required fistula repair. Recently, NIPPV (noninvasive positive pressure ventilation) has been applied for patients with cerebrospinal fluid fistula [19–21]. Injury of the sympathetic nerve trunk on the upper thoracic caused dysfunction of perspiration in 6 cases. Two cases showed no sign of recovery [22, 23]. Three cases had neurological deterioration. The palsy recovered within several weeks after the operation,

29.8 Case Presentation

Case 1: 50-year-old man: C6-T3 anterior decompression and fusion using a plate through manubrium splitting approach were performed. His JOA score improved preoperatively 2 points to 11 points postoperatively (Fig. 29.3).

Case 2: 32-years-old female: T4–8 anterior decompression and fusion through extrapleural approach was performed. She couldn't stand on admission. After operation, she was able to walk using a cane. Her JOA score improved 1 point to 4.5 points (Fig. 29.4).

29.9 Discussion

Anterior decompression is necessary for thoracic OPLL because the alignment of the thoracic spine is kyphotic. Anterior decompression via anterior approach is a rational surgical method for thoracic OPLL to be able to operate under direct visualization of OPLL, and to restore the spinal cord to its correct physiological position. The surgical result was good. Anterior decompression via manubrium splitting approach is restricted to OPLL located above T3. The number of spinal segments to be decompressed is limited to five segments for graft length and fusion stability. But the latter problem may be solved with spinal instrumentation. Although the anterior approach is associated with some problems, such as surgical invasiveness (long surgical time, large amount of bleeding), postoperative complication, and the progress of skill to perform the procedure will improve these problems.

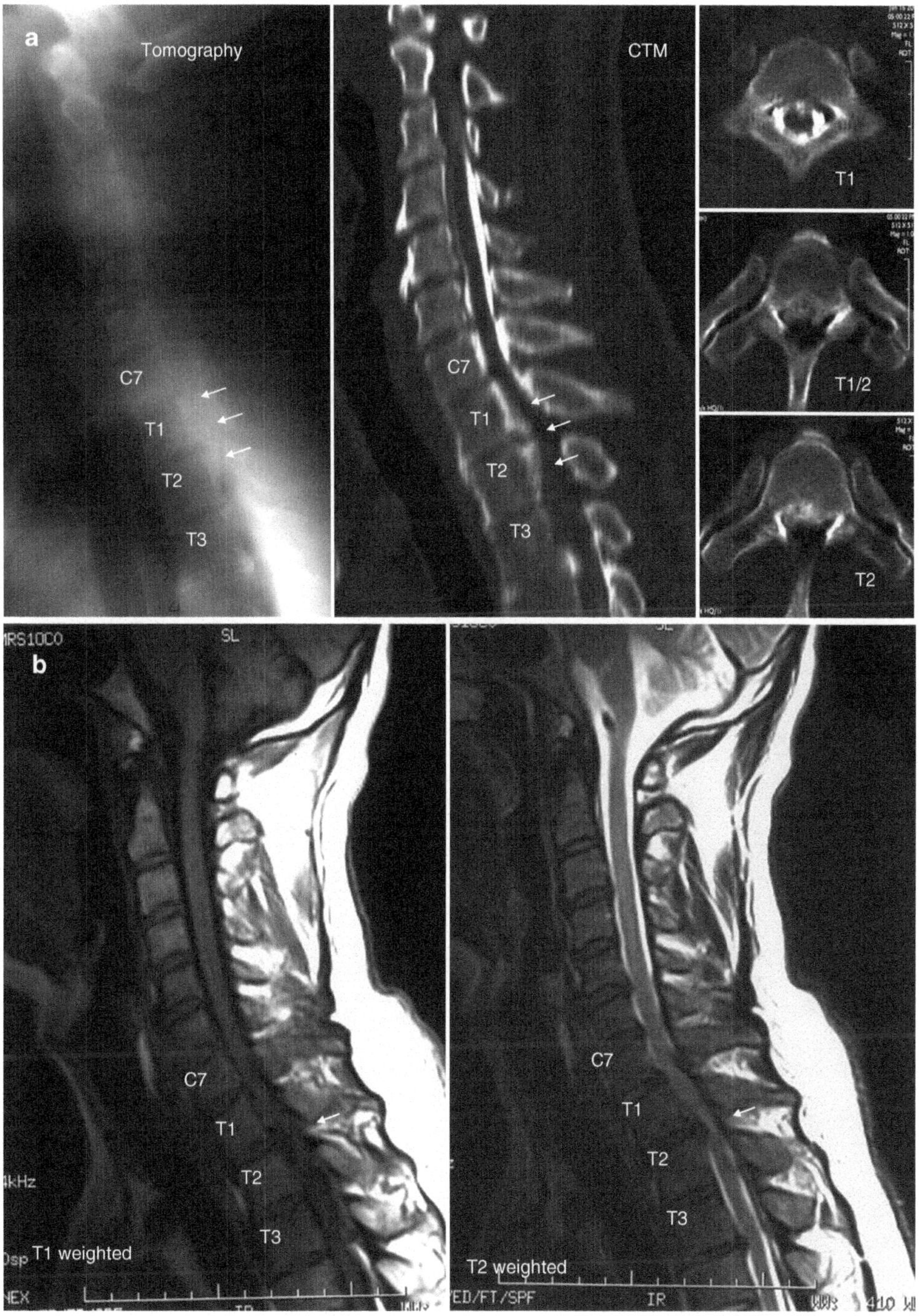

Fig. 29.3 (**a**) Preoperative tomography and reconstructed CT, CT myelography. OPLL is present from T1 to T2, and narrowing the spinal canal. (**b**) Preoperative MRI. Spinal cord was compressed by OPLL at the level of T1–T2. T2 weighted MRI shows a high intensity signal in the cord at the T1–T2 level. (**c**) Postoperative X-ray, tomography, CT, and MRI show good decompression. Spinal compression was alleviated and spinal cord moved anterior

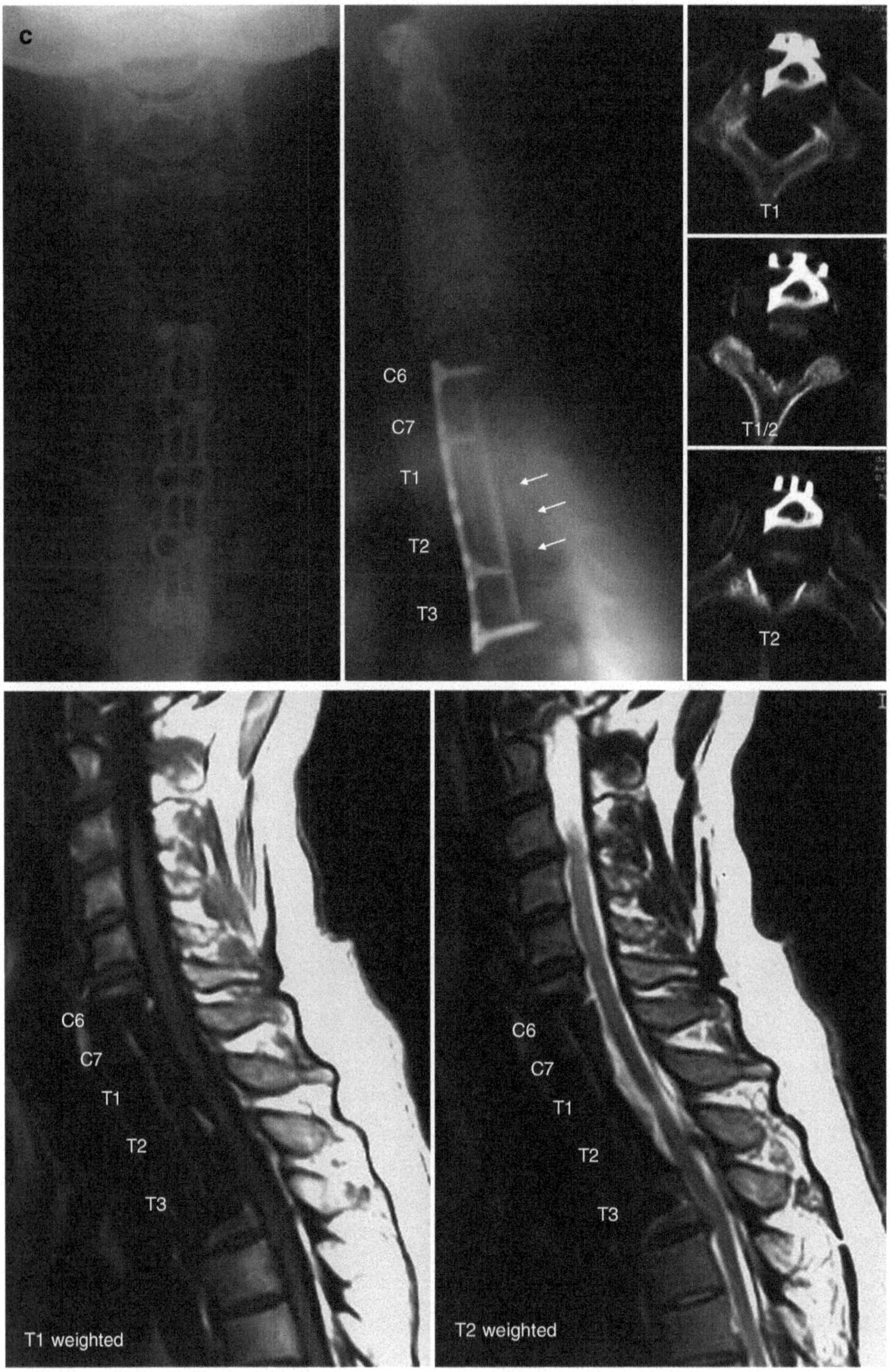

Fig. 29.3 (continued)

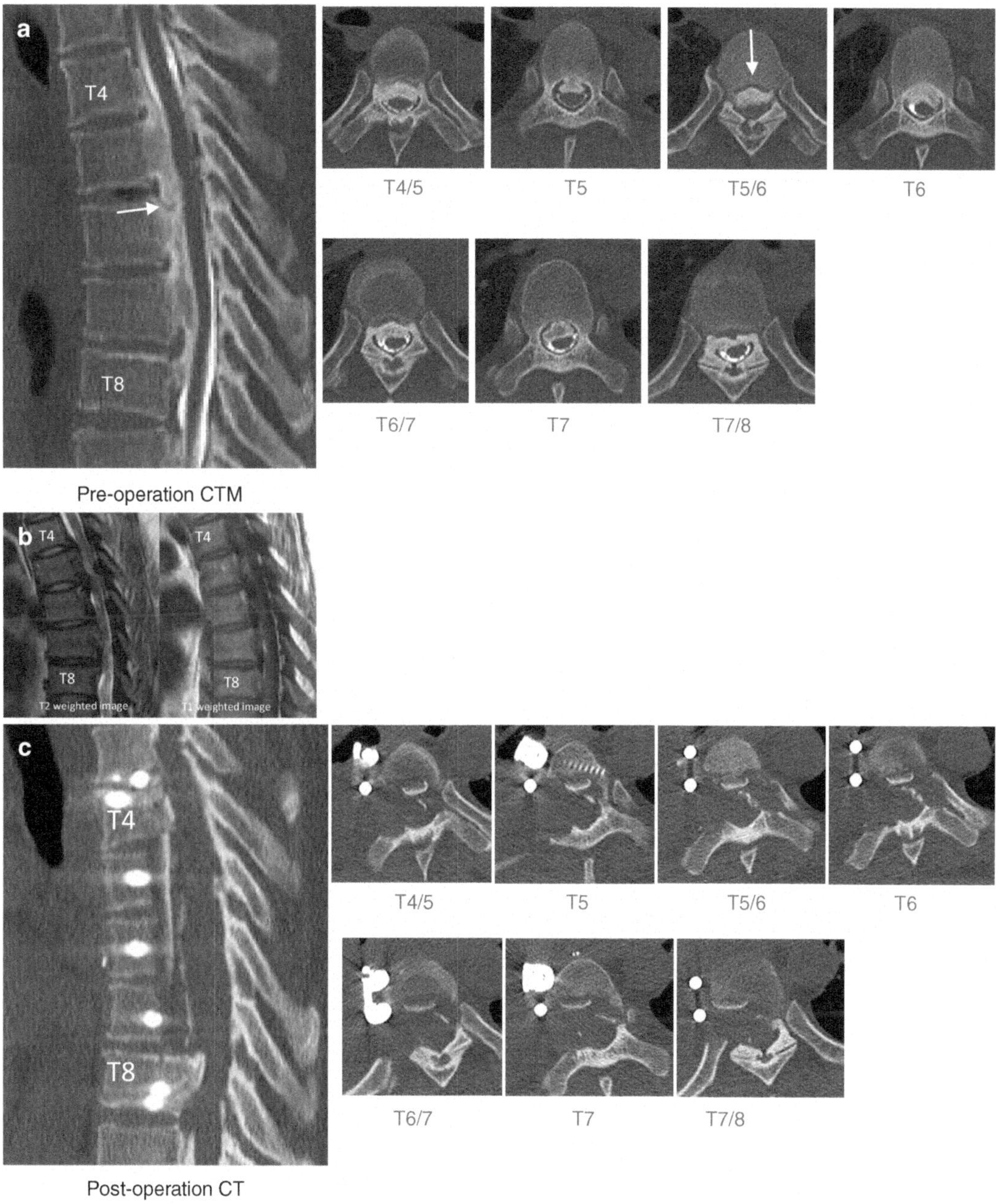

Fig. 29.4 (**a**) There is a huge continuous type OPLL at the level of T4–T8. (**b**) Spinal cord was compressed by OPLL at the level of T4-T8. (**c**) Postoperatively, the OPLL has moved forward and the spinal canal is expanding

29.10 Conclusion

We presented the outcomes and complications of thoracic OPLL patients treated with anterior decompression and fusion via manubrium splitting approach or transpleural approach. Although the anterior approach is associated with some problems (such as surgical invasiveness, and postoperative complications), this surgical method resulted in positive outcomes, indicating that it is a useful technique.

References

1. Yamaura I, Kurosa Y, Matsuoka T, et al. Anterior floating method for cervical myelopathy caused by ossification of the posterior longitudinal ligament. Clin Orthop. 1999;359:27–34.
2. Matsumoto M, Chiba K, Toyama Y, et al. Surgical results and related factors for ossification of posterior longitudinal ligament of the thoracic spine: a multi-institutional retrospective study. Spine (Phila Pa 1976). 2008;33:1034–41.
3. Matsumoto M, Toyama Y, Chikuda H, et al. Outcomes of fusion surgery for ossification of the posterior longitudinal ligament of the thoracic spine: a multicenter retrospective survey: clinical article. J Neurosurg Spine. 2011;15:380–5.
4. Imagama S, Ando K, Takeuchi K, et al. Perioperative complications after surgery for thoracic ossification of posterior longitudinal ligament a nationwide multicenter prospective study. Spine. 2018;43(23):E1389–97.
5. Cauchoix J, Binet JP. Anterior surgical approaches to the spine. Ann R Coll Surg Engl. 1957;21:237–43.
6. Kurtz LT, Pursel SE, Herkowitz HN. Modified anterior approach to the cervicothoracic junction. Spine. 1991;16:S542–7.
7. Knoller SM, Brethner L. Surgical treatment of the spine at the cervicothoracic junction:an illustrated review of a modified sternotomy approach with the description of tricks and pitfalls. Arch Orthop Trauma Surg. 2002;122:365–8.
8. Tamura M, Saito M, Machida M, Shibasaki K. A trans-sternoclavicular approach for the anterior decompression and fusion of the upper thoracic spine. Technical note. J Neurosurg Spine. 2005;2:226–9.
9. Fujimura Y, Nishi Y, Nakamura M, Toyama Y, Suzuki N. Anterior decompression and fusion for ossification of the posterior longitudinal ligament of the upper thoracic spine causing myelopathy using manubrium splitting. Spinal Cord. 1996;34:387–93.
10. Henry JF, Audiffret J, Denizot A. The nonrecurrent inferior laryngeal nerve: review of 33 cases, including two on the left side. Surgery. 1988;104:977–84.
11. Stewart GR, Mountain JC, Colcock BP. Non-recurrent laryngeal nerve. Br J Surg. 1972;59:379–81.
12. Fujimura Y, Nishi Y, Nakamura M, et al. Anterior decompression and fusion for ossification of the posterior longitudinal ligament of the upper thoracic spine causing myelopathy: using the manubrium splitting approach. Spinal Cord. 1996;34:387–93.
13. Hanai K, Ogikubo O, Miyashita T. Anterior decompression for myelopathy resulting from thoracic ossification of the posterior longitudinal ligament. Spine. 2002;27:1070–6.
14. Fujimura Y, Nishi Y, Nakamura M, et al. Myelopathy secondary to ossification of the posterior longitudinal ligament of the thoracic spine treated by anterior decompression and bony fusion. Spinal Cord. 1997;35:777–84.
15. Fujimura Y, Nishi Y, Nakamura M, et al. Long-term follow-up study of anterior decompression and fusion for thoracic myelopathy resulting from ossification of the posterior longitudinal ligament. Spine. 1997;22:305–11.
16. Kurosa Y, Yamaura I, Nakai O, Shinomiya K. Selecting a surgical method for thoracic myelopathy caused by ossification of the posterior longitudinal ligament. Spine. 1996;21:1458–66.
17. Ohtani K, Nakai S, Fujimura Y, et al. Anterior surgical decompression for thoracic myelopathy as a result of ossification of the posterior longitudinal ligament. Clin Orthop. 1982;166:82–8.
18. Yonenobu K, Korkusuz F, Hosono N, Ebara S, Ono K. Lateral rhachotomy for thoracic spinal lesions. Spine. 1990;15:1121–5.
19. Schlag HR, Muquit S, Hristov TB, et al. Subarachnoidal pleural fistula after resection of intradural thoracic disc herniation and multimodal treatment with noninvasive positive pressure ventilation (NPPV). Eur Spine J. 2016;25(1):155–9.
20. Kurata Y, Yoshimoto M, Takebayashi T, et al. Subarachnoid-pleural fistula treated with noninvasive positive pressure ventilation: a two-case report and literature review. Spine. 2010;35(18):E908–11.
21. Ido K, Shimizu K, Nakamura T. Management of cerebrospinal fluid leakage complicating anterior procedures through thoracotomy: report of three cases. Neurosurg Rev. 2002;25:174–6.
22. Adson AW, Craig WM, Brown GE. Essentialyperhidrosis cured by sympathetic gang-Lionectomy and trunk resection. Arch Surg. 1935;31:794–8.
23. Sahina M, Mathias CJ, Katagiri A, et al. Sudomotor and cardiovascular dysfunction in patients with early untreated Parkinson's disease. J Parkinsons Dis. 2014;4:385–93.

Circumferential Decompression Through Posterior Approach for Thoracic OPLL: Technique and Complications

30

Satoshi Kato

Abstract

In patients with thoracic myelopathy resulting from OPLL in the thoracic spine with a kyphotic curve, anterior spinal cord decompression via OPLL removal or floating is logical and the most effective method for relieving pressure on the spinal cord. Anterior (circumferential) spinal cord decompression through a posterior approach was first reported by Ohtsuka et al. in 1983 and has been used by several surgeons. The disadvantage of this procedure is that anterior decompression and resection of OPLL using an air-drill is mostly performed with a blind procedure. Since 2011, we have employed a surgical technique via a posterolateral approach that allows the surgeon to perform anterior spinal cord decompression more safely and effectively than the conventional procedures. This maneuver includes laminectomies and total resection of the transverse processes and pedicles, which allows space creation bilateral to the dural sac and the targeted OPLL for subsequent anterior decompression. The thoracic nerves at the levels of anterior decompression were ligated bilaterally and lifted to improve the view of the OPLL and the anterolateral aspect of the dural sac. In this procedure, surgeons can perform anterior decompression with adequate recognition of the positions of the OPLL and the whole dural sac at every point in time. Patients with a localized spinal cord compression by a beak-type OPLL with a ≥50% canal occupying ratio in the kyphotic thoracic spine is indicated for anterior decompression via a posterolateral approach. However, the procedure should not be applied for thoracic OPLL with multi-level spinal compressions.

Keywords

Anterior decompression · Complication
Ossification of the posterior longitudinal ligament (OPLL) · Posterior approach
Technique · Thoracic spine

Abbreviations

ADF	Anterior decompression and fusion
OPLL	Ossification of the longitudinal ligament
PDF	Posterior decompression and fusion

S. Kato (✉)
Department of Orthopaedic Surgery, Graduate School of Medical Sciences, Kanazawa University, Kanazawa, Japan

A. Okawa et al. (eds.), *OPLL*, https://doi.org/10.1007/978-981-15-3855-1_30

30.1 Histories and Recent Innovation of Circumferential Decompression Through Posterior Approach for Thoracic OPLL

Ossification of the posterior longitudinal ligament (OPLL) in the thoracic spine is a rare but clinically significant spinal disorder that causes progressive thoracic myelopathy and responds poorly to conservative therapy. Surgery is the only effective treatment option. However, the surgical outcome for thoracic OPLL compares unfavorably with that for cervical OPLL [1]. This is due to anatomic factors and the pathophysiology of T-OPLL: (1) the thoracic spine is naturally kyphotic, and posterior decompression is less effective since backward movement of the spinal cord is restricted; (2) the spinal cord is more vulnerable at the site of compression because of its relative avascularity [2]; and (3) the ossified ligament adheres strongly to the ventral aspect of the dural sac; this increases the difficulty in direct removal of the OPLL and increases the risk of spinal cord injury during decompression maneuvers.

Spine surgeons have faced significant challenges in determining the most effective surgical procedure and preventing surgical complications [1, 3, 4]. In patients with thoracic myelopathy resulting from OPLL in the thoracic spine with a kyphotic curve, anterior spinal cord decompression via OPLL removal or floating is logical and the most effective method for relieving pressure on the spinal cord [5–8]. However, anterior decompression is technically demanding and associated with significant surgical complications, including postoperative neurologic degradation [5–8]. Although anterior decompression is recommended owing to the anatomical features of thoracic OPLL, posterior decompression and instrumented fusion are widely applied for the treatment of this disease [1, 3]. Most spine surgeons perform posterior decompression surgery as the primary treatment, regardless of the size and type of OPLL, and spinal alignment at the affected level [9, 10, 11].

Anterior spinal cord decompression surgeries and resection of thoracic OPLL using the anterior [5, 6], posterior [7, 12], and posterior–anterior combined approaches [8, 13] were reported. However, only a limited number of surgeons have employed these surgeries. Anterior (circumferential) spinal cord decompression through a posterior approach was first reported by Ohtsuka et al. in 1983 [12]. After a wide laminectomy, the medial portions of the facet joints, pedicles, and pars interarticularis were removed bilaterally using an air-drill to make space between the lateral side of the dural sac and pedicles for manipulating the targeted OPLL via a posterior approach. Some surgeons performed additional resection of the posterior surface of the transverse process and total facetectomy [14]. Then, anterior spinal cord decompression was performed posteriorly. The posterior portions of the vertebral bodies were excavated using an air-drill from the bilateral sides of the dural sac to lower the ossified ligament into the vertebral body (OPLL floating). Hirabayashi et al. reported that special attention was required at the time of separation of the most cranial and caudal ends of the OPLL from the vertebral body because this was a completely blind procedure [14]. Abumi and his colleagues used the same technique in circumferential spinal cord decompression for thoracic OPLL [7, 15]. Tsuzuki and his colleagues reported staged surgery via a posterior single approach [16, 17]. The primary surgery is expansive laminoplasty from the cervical level to the thoracic level to separate the spinal cord from the thoracic OPLL posteriorly to the extent possible. If improvement cannot effectively be obtained after the primary surgery, anterior spinal cord decompression via a posterior approach is carried out about 1 month later. The disadvantage of anterior spinal cord decompression via a posterior approach is that anterior decompression and resection of OPLL using an air-drill is mostly performed with a blind procedure. Moreover, in this procedure, it is often difficult to control the bleeding from the epidural venous plexus and vessels accompanying the nerve roots. A clear operative field with controlled bleeding is mandatory in safe and feasible anterior spinal cord decompression via a posterior approach. Therefore, the surgical maneuver in the conventional procedure has a potential risk of spinal cord injury, which causes a limited application in the clinical treatment even among specialized spine surgeons.

Since 2011, we have employed a surgical technique to remove or float the OPLL in the thoracic spine via a posterolateral approach that allows the surgeon to perform anterior decompression for thoracic OPLL more safely and effectively than the conventional procedures [18]. The features of this surgical technique were derived from the surgical maneuver in total en bloc spondylectomy for spinal tumors [19, 20]. We reported favorable clinical results and a considerable indication of the surgical procedure for thoracic OPLL [18, 21, 22]. It is especially useful for cases of beak-type OPLL, the most complicated type to treat surgically [9, 23, 24]. In the latter part of this chapter, we present the technique and potential complications of circumferential spinal cord decompression via a posterolateral approach.

30.2 Techniques and Indication of Circumferential Decompression Through Posterolateral Approach for Thoracic OPLL

With the patient in the prone position, we performed total resection of the posterior elements at the anterior decompression levels. This maneuver includes laminectomies and total resection of the transverse processes and pedicles, which allows space creation bilateral to the dural sac and the targeted OPLL for subsequent anterior decompression (Fig. 30.1). The thoracic nerves at the levels of anterior decompression were ligated bilaterally and lifted to improve the view of the OPLL and the anterolateral aspect of the dural sac (Fig. 30.2a). Lifting the nerve roots facilitates control of bleeding from the varix in the canal and vessels in the intervertebral foramen (Fig. 30.2b). It does not create the risk of spinal cord rotation because the anterior aspect of the dural sac adheres to the OPLL. After these maneuvers afforded adequate working space and

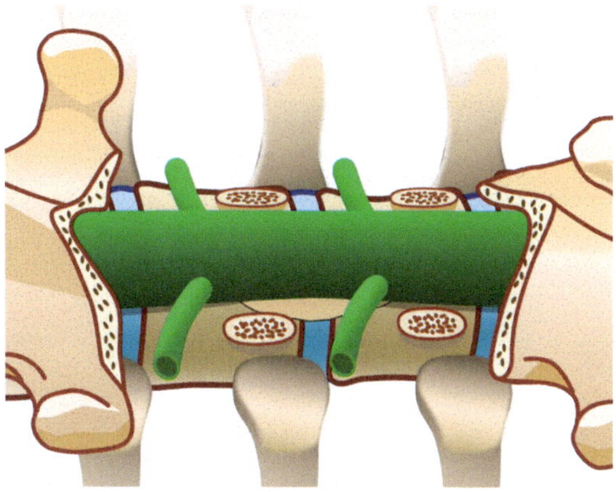

Fig. 30.1 Total resection of the posterior elements allows space creation bilateral to the dural sac and the targeted OPLL for subsequent anterior decompression

good visualization of the operative field with controlled bleeding, anterior decompression was performed postero-laterally (Fig. 30.3). This is similar in terms of approach and visualization to methods used when treating the epidural tumor from the vertebral body, the dural sac, and the nerve roots to remove the tumor including negative margins in total en bloc spondylectomy for spinal tumors [19, 20]. In every step of anterior decompression using this approach, surgeons can have visual contact with both the OPLL and dural sac. As same as the conventional procedure, the surgeons were allowed to leave the OPLL floating, and OPLL removal was not required (Fig. 30.4a, b). Gradual migration of the floated plaques provided additional spinal cord decompression during the postoperative course [21]. A larger and smoother excavation of the vertebral body with a sufficient cutting margin for the OPLL floating can be obtained in this procedure because more space was created on the bilateral sides of the dural sac with resection of the pedicles and lifting of the ligated nerve roots (Fig. 30.4a, b; [21, 22]). It is a key to make an effective migration of the floating plaques. Before anterior decompression, we perform posterior instrumentation at the spinal level, including that at least 2 levels above and 2 levels below the anterior decompression. Posterolateral fusion using local bone chips of the resected laminae and transverse processes was conducted after spi-

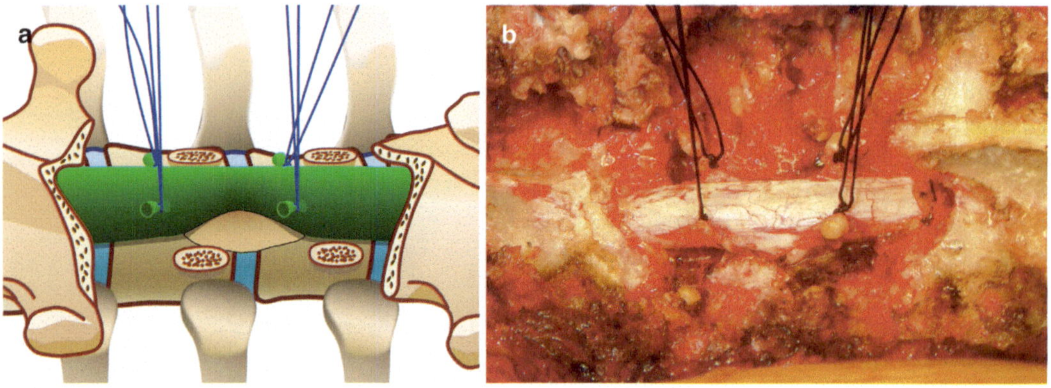

Fig. 30.2 Lifting of the ligated nerve roots at the levels of anterior decompression improves the view of the OPLL and the anterolateral aspect of the dural sac. It facilitates control of bleeding from the varix in the canal and vessels in the intervertebral foramen. (**a**) Illustration of intraoperative view (**b**) Intraoperative photograph. (Figures 30.2a, b, and 30.4b are modified and reprinted with permission from Kato S, Murakami H, Demura S, Yoshioka K, Hayashi H, Yokogawa N, Fang X, Tsuchiya H (2015) Gradual spinal cord decompression through migration of floated plaques after anterior decompression via a posterolateral approach for OPLL in the thoracic spine. J Neurosurg Spine 23 (4):479–483)

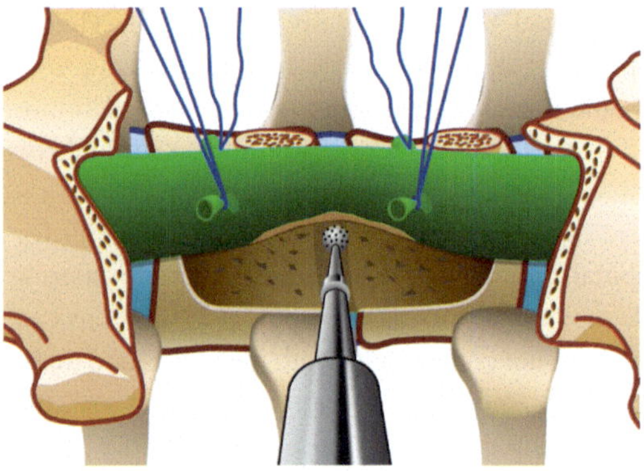

Fig. 30.3 In this procedure, surgeons can perform anterior decompression with adequate recognition of the positions of the OPLL and the whole dural sac

nal cord decompression. In the patients who had OPLL floating, kyphosis correction with posterior instrumentation was applied after the OPLL floating because we observed with ultrasonography that the spinal cord compression was relieved but still retained by the floated OPLL. We used intraoperative spinal cord monitoring during the surgery in all the patients.

A main advantage of this procedure is that it provides more space on the bilateral sides of the dural sac for maneuvering during anterior decompression relative to the conventional posterior approach [7, 12] (Fig. 30.5). Additionally, this space, combined with lifting of the ligated thoracic nerves, allows surgeons to directly visualize the targeted OPLL and the anterolateral aspect of the dural sac. In this procedure, surgeons can perform anterior decompression with adequate recognition of the positions of the OPLL and the whole dural sac at every point in time, and this facilitates the anterior decompression procedure. This is a major advantage of the procedure that cannot be obtained with the conventional anterior or posterior approaches. We therefore consider that our surgical technique based on a posterolateral approach is relatively safe and feasible for anterior decompression of thoracic OPLL. Imagama et al. reported a similar surgical procedure and its favorable outcome [25].

This surgical procedure via a posterolateral approach has other advantages. This surgical approach has all the advantages related to the conventional posterior approach [26]; (1) a clear, shallow, and wide surgical field can be obtained and freely extended toward craniocaudal direction, (2) less surgical stress and easier control of CSF leakage without thoracotomy, and (3) removal of the ossification of ligamentum flavum which frequently accompanies thoracic OPLL. The procedure allows easier correction of kyphosis with posterior instrumen-

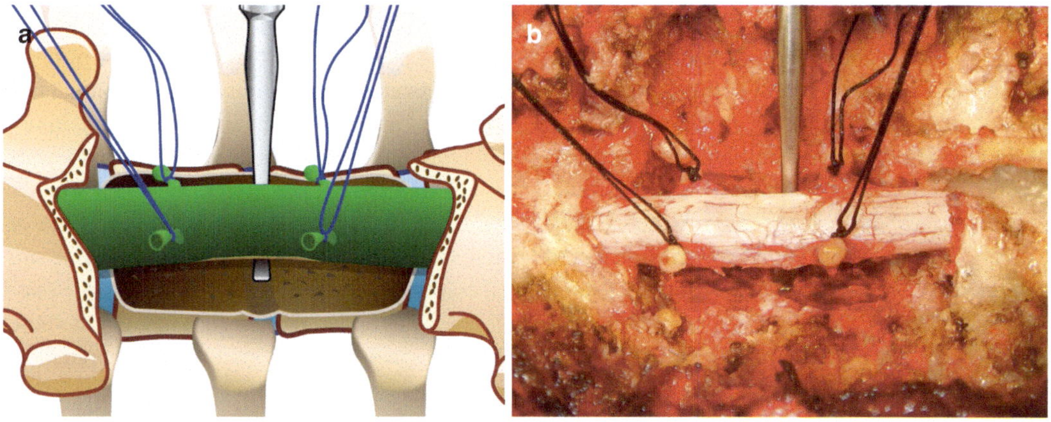

Fig. 30.4 After anterior decompression (floating of OPLL), a surgical spatula can be easily inserted into the ventral side of the dural sac, and the tip of the spatula can be observed from the opposite side. (**a**) Illustration of intraoperative view. (**b**) Intraoperative photograph

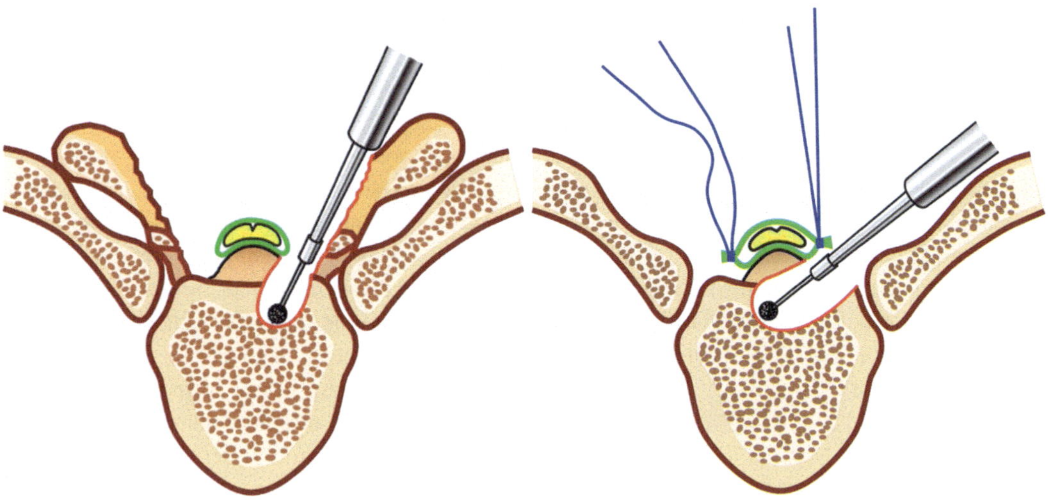

Fig. 30.5 Axial image of a conventional posterior approach (left) and our posterolateral approach (right). (Figures 30.3, 30.4a, and 30.5 are modified and reprinted with permission from Kato S, Murakami H, Demura S, Yoshioka K, Yokogawa N, Shimizu T, Oku N, Tsuchiya H (2020). Indication for anterior spinal cord decompression via a posterolateral approach for the treatment of ossification of the posterior longitudinal ligament in the thoracic spine: A prospective cohort study. Eur Spine J 29 (1):113–121)

tation than the conventional posterior approach because the thoracic spine at the decompression levels becomes more flexible by removal of the transverse processes and pedicles. The correction of kyphosis is the maneuver to reduce the compressive pressure of the OPLL on the spinal cord [13, 27]. It is especially useful if complete removal of the OPLL cannot be achieved and the floated plaque still compresses the spinal cord.

In the literature on OPLL in the cervical spine, for patients with a more severely compromised spinal canal, especially a canal occupying ratio >50% [28, 29] or 60% [30], data suggests that the results of anterior decompression and fusion (ADF) were better than those of laminoplasty or posterior decompression and fusion (PDF). Koda et al. examined the clinical outcomes of patients with K-line (−) OPLL who underwent surgical treatments consisting of laminoplasty, PDF, and

ADF [31]. They demonstrated that the recovery rate of Japan Orthopaedic Association score was significantly higher in the ADF group than those in the laminoplasty and PDF groups. The results of these studies demonstrate that even for a certain portion of patients with OPLL in the lordotic cervical spine, anterior decompression is indicated owing to severely compromised spinal cord compression by a large OPLL from the ventral side and/or local kyphotic alignment. Based on the results of these studies on cervical OPLL and the development of a safe and feasible anterior decompression for thoracic OPLL via the posterolateral approach, patients with a localized spinal cord compression by a large OPLL with a ≥50% canal occupying ratio in the kyphotic thoracic spine (e.g., large beak-type OPLL) has been indicated for anterior decompression in our institute since 2012 [22]. Imagama et al. reported their case series with beak-type thoracic OPLL treated with PDF and risk factors for ineffectiveness of the surgery and concluded that the OPLL canal occupying ratio, OPLL length in the sagittal plane on computed tomography, and spinal cord kyphotic angle difference from upper instrumented vertebra to the lowest instrumented vertebra were risk factors associated with ineffectiveness of PDF and revision surgery of anterior decompression [9].

30.3 Potential Complications of Anterior Decompression Through Posterolateral Approach for Thoracic OPLL

In the procedure, a risk of ischemic spinal cord injury was presented because thoracic nerve roots were ligated at the anterior decompression levels. There were no significant changes detected on spinal cord monitoring in the patients after ligation of the thoracic nerve roots in a maximum of two consecutive levels bilaterally in our patients. On the basis of the results of the total spondylectomy for spine tumors, Murakami et al. reported that surgeons are allowed to sacrifice up to three pairs of thoracic nerve roots even including the level of the artery of Adamkiewicz without ischemic neurologic deterioration [32]. In animal studies, Kato et al. reported that ligation of bilateral segmental arteries four or more consecutive levels has a risk of ischemic spinal cord injury including the level of the artery of Adamkiewicz [33]. Fujimaki et al. reported in animal studies that ligation of bilateral segmental arteries five or more consecutive levels has a risk of ischemic spinal cord injury in the levels equivalent to the middle thoracic spine in human [34]. From these points of view, the ligation of thoracic nerve roots for anterior decompression described here can be indicated for T-OPLL within three consecutive levels. Unnecessary nerve root ligations should be avoided in the procedure. In some patients, ligation of unilateral nerve roots can be preserved owing to asymmetric or eccentrical location of the OPLL. Considering risk prevention, a localized spinal cord compression by a large beak-type OPLL, which is known as the most complicated for surgery [23, 24], is a good indication for the surgical procedure. However, the procedure should not be applied for thoracic OPLL with multi-level spinal compressions. Takahata et al. reported a greater range of circumferential spinal cord decompression (five or more vertebral levels) via a posterior approach carried a high risk of unfavorable surgical outcome [7].

Another concern is that lifting of the ligated nerve roots leads to spinal cord rotation which causes spinal cord injury. Actually in the procedure of anterior spinal cord decompression, the maneuver does not create the risk of spinal cord rotation because the anterior aspect of the dural sac strongly adheres to the OPLL. However, the surgeons should be aware of the situation that the spinal cord is easily rotated by lifting the nerve roots after the OPLL removal or floating.

Thirteen patients underwent a circumferential spinal cord decompression via a posterolateral approach in our institute between April 2011 and May 2018. Transient neurological deterioration and dural tear were observed in one or two patients. Dural tear and cerebrospinal fluid leakage often happen in thoracic OPLL surgery, especially in anterior spinal cord decompression. Posterior-based surgery has an advantage in controlling cerebrospinal fluid leakage compared to anterior-based surgery with thoracotomy. We have not experienced any other complications including surgical site infection and instrumentation failure.

References

1. Matsumoto M, Chiba K, Toyama Y, Takeshita K, Seichi A, Nakamura K, Arimizu J, Fujibayashi S, Hirabayashi S, Hirano T, Iwasaki M, Kaneoka K, Kawaguchi Y, Ijiri K, Maeda T, Matsuyama Y, Mikami Y, Murakami H, Nagashima H, Nagata K, Nakahara S, Nohara Y, Oka S, Sakamoto K, Saruhashi Y, Sasao Y, Shimizu K, Taguchi T, Takahashi M, Tanaka Y, Tani T, Tokuhashi Y, Uchida K, Yamamoto K, Yamazaki M, Yokoyama T, Yoshida M, Nishiwaki Y. Surgical results and related factor for ossification of posterior longitudinal ligament of the thoracic spine. A multi-institutional retrospective study. Spine (Phila Pa 1976). 2008;33(9):1034–41.
2. Lazorthes G, Gouaze A, Zadeh JO, Santini JJ, Lazorthes Y, Burdin P. Arterial vascularization of the spinal cord. Recent studies of the anastmotic susstitution pathways. J Neurosurg. 1971;35(3):253–62.
3. Imagama S, Ando K, Takeuchi K, Kato S, Murakami H, Aizawa T, Ozawa H, Hasegawa T, Matsuyama Y, Koda M, Yamazaki M, Chikuda H, Shindo S, Nakagawa Y, Kimura A, Takeshita K, Wada K, Katoh H, Watanabe M, Yamada K, Furuya T, Tsuji T, Fujibayashi S, Mori K, Kawaguchi Y, Watanabe K, Matsumoto M, Yoshii T, Okawa A. Perioperative complications after surgery for thoracic ossification of posterior longitudinal ligament—nationwide multicenter prospective study. Spine (Phila Pa 1976). 2018;43(23):E1389–97.
4. Matsumoto M, Toyama Y, Chikuda H, Takeshita K, Kato T, Shindo S, Abumi K, Takahata M, Nohara Y, Taneichi H, Tomita K, Kawahara N, Imagama S, Matsuyama Y, Yamazaki M, Okawa A. Outcomes of fusion surgery for ossification of the posterior longitudinal ligament of the thoracic spine: a multicenter retrospective survey: clinical article. J Neurosurg Spine. 2011;15(4):380–5.
5. Fujimura Y, Nishi Y, Nakamura M, Watanabe M, Matsumoto M. Myelopathy secondary to ossification of the posterior longitudinal ligament of the thoracic spine treated by anterior decompression and bony fusion. Spinal Cord. 1997;35(11):777–84.
6. Min JH, Jang JS, Lee SH. Clinical results of ossification of the posterior longitudinal ligament (OPLL) of the thoracic spine treated by anterior decompression. J Spinal Disord Tech. 2008;21(2):116–9.
7. Takahata M, Ito M, Abumi K, Kotani Y, Sudo H, Minami A. Clinical results and complications of circumferential spinal cord decompression through a single posterior approach for thoracic myelopathy caused by ossification of posterior longitudinal ligament. Spine (Phila Pa 1976). 2008;33(11):1199–208.
8. Tomita K, Kawahara N, Baba H, Kikuchi Y, Nishimura H. Circumspinal decompression for thoracic myelopathy due to combined ossification of the posterior longitudinal ligament and ligamentum flavum. Spine (Phila Pa 1976). 1990;15(11):1114–20.
9. Imagama S, Ando K, Ito Z, Kobayashi K, Hida T, Ito K, Tsushima M, Ishikawa Y, Matsumoto A, Morozumi M, Tanaka S, Machino M, Ota K, Nakashima H, Wakao N, Nishida Y, Matsuyama Y, Ishiguro N. Risk factors for ineffectiveness of posterior decompression and dekyphotic corrective fusion with instrumentation for beak-type thoracic ossification of the posterior longitudinal ligament: a single institute study. Neurosurgery. 2017;80(5):800–8.
10. Koda M, Furuya T, Okawa A, Inada T, Kamiya K, Ota M, Maki S, Takahashi K, Yamazaki M, Aramomi M, Ikeda O, Mannoji C. Mid- to long-term outcomes of posterior decompression with instrumented fusion for thoracic ossification of the posterior longitudinal ligament. J Clin Neurosci. 2016a;27:87–90.
11. Yamazaki M, Okawa A, Fujiyoshi T, Furuya T, Koda M. Posterior decompression with instrumented fusion for thoracic myelopathy caused by ossification of the posterior longitudinal ligament. Eur Spine J. 2010;19(5):691–8.
12. Ohtsuka K, Terayama K, Tsuchiya T, Wada K, Furukawa K, Ohkubo M. A surgical procedure of the anterior decompression of the thoracic spinal cord through the posterior approach [in Japanese]. Seikei Saigai Geka (Orthoped Surg Traumatol). 1983;26(8):1083–1090.
13. Kawahara N, Tomita K, Murakami H, Hato T, Demura S, Sekino Y, Nasu W, Fujimaki Y. Circumspinal decompression with dekyphosis stabilization for thoracic myelopathy due to ossification of the posterior longitudinal ligament. Spine (Phila Pa 1976). 2008;33(1):39–46.
14. Hirabayashi S, Kitagawa T, Iwahori T, Yamamoto I, Yamada K, Matsushita T. Surgical technique and clinical results of circumferential decompression surgery via posterior approach alone for thoracic ossification of the posterior longitudinal ligament (OPLL). J Spine Res. 2015;6(5):886–91.
15. Abumi K, Suda K. Surgical strategy for thoracic OPLL [in Japanese]. Seikei Saigai Geka (Orthoped Surg Traumatol). 2002;45(6):615–621.
16. Hirabayashi S, Matsushita T, Tsuzuki N. Surgical treatment for ossification of the ligaments at the thoracic spine especially for OPLL [in Japanese]. Sekitsuisekizui (Spine & Spinal Cord). 2009;22(2):171–178.
17. Tsuzuki N, Hirabayashi S, Abe R, Saiki K. Staged spinal cord decompression through posterior longitudinal ligament. Spine (Phila Pa 1976). 2001;26(14):1623–30.
18. Kato S, Murakami H, Demura S, Yoshioka K, Hayashi H, Tsuchiya H. Novel surgical technique for ossification of posterior longitudinal ligament in the thoracic spine. J Neurosurg Spine. 2012;17(6):525–9.

19. Kawahara N, Tomita K, Murakami H, Demura S. Total en bloc spondylectomy for spinal tumors: surgical techniques and related basic background. Orthop Clin North Am. 2009;40(1):47–63.
20. Tomita K, Kawahara N, Baba H, Tsuchiya H, Nagata S, Toribatake Y. Total en bloc spondylectomy for solitary spinal metastases. Int Orthop. 1994;18(5):291–8.
21. Kato S, Murakami H, Demura S, Yoshioka K, Hayashi H, Yokogawa N, Fang X, Tsuchiya H. Gradual spinal cord decompression through migration of floated plaques after anterior decompression via a posterolateral approach for OPLL in the thoracic spine. J Neurosurg Spine. 2015;23(4):479–83.
22. Kato S, Murakami H, Demura S, Yoshioka K, Yokogawa N, Shimizu T, Oku N, Tsuchiya H. Indication for anterior spinal cord decompression via a posterolateral approach for the treatment of ossification of the posterior longitudinal ligament in the thoracic spine: a prospective cohort study. Eur Spine J. 2020;29(1):113–21.
23. Matsuyama Y, Yoshihara H, Tsuji T, Sakai Y, Yukawa Y, Nakamura H, Ito K, Ishiguro N. Surgical outcome of ossification of the posterior longitudinal ligament (OPLL) of the thoracic spine: implication of the type of ossification and surgical options. J Spinal Disord Tech. 2005;18(6):492–7; discussion 498.
24. Tokuhashi Y, Matsuzaki H, Oda H, Uei H. Effectiveness of posterior decompression for patients with ossification of posterior longitudinal ligament in the thoracic spine: usefulness of the ossification-kyphosis angle on MRI. Spine (Phila Pa 1976). 2006;31(1):E26–30.
25. Imagama S, Ando K, Ito Z, Kobayashi K, Hida T, Ito K, Ishikawa Y, Tsushima M, Matsumoto A, Tanaka S, Morozumi M, Machino M, Ota K, Nakashima H, Wakao N, Nishida Y, Matsuyama Y, Ishiguro N. Resection of beak-type thoracic ossification of the posterior longitudinal ligament from a posterior approach under intraoperative neurophysiological monitoring for paralysis after posterior decompression and fusion surgery. Global Spine J. 2016;6(8):812–21.
26. Hirabayashi S, Kitagawa T, Yamamoto I, Yamada K, Kawano H. Surgical treatment for ossification of the posterior longitudinal ligament (OPLL) at the thoracic spine: usefulness of the posterior approach. Spine Surg Relat Res. 2018;2(3):169–76.
27. Ando K, Imagama S, Ito Z, Kobayashi K, Ukai J, Muramoto A, Shinjo R, Matsumoto T, Nakashima H, Matsuyama Y, Ishiguro N. Ponte osteotomy during dekyphosis for indirect posterior decompression with ossification of the posterior longitudinal ligament of the thoracic spine. Clin Spine Surg. 2017;30(4):E358–62.
28. Sakai K, Okawa A, Takahashi M, Arai Y, Kawabata S, Enomoto M, Kato T, Hirai T, Shinomiya K. Five-year follow-up evaluation of surgical treatment for cervical myelopathy caused by ossification of the posterior longitudinal ligament: a prospective comparative study of anterior decompression and fusion with floating method versus laminoplasty. Spine (Phila Pa 1976). 2012;37(5):367–76.
29. Yoshii T, Sakai K, Hirai T, Yamada T, Inose H, Kato T, Enomoto M, Tomizawa S, Kawabata S, Arai Y, Okawa A. Anterior decompression with fusion versus posterior decompression with fusion for massive cervical ossification of the posterior longitudinal ligament with a >/=50% canal occupying ratio: a multicenter retrospective study. Spine J. 2016;16(11):1351–7.
30. Iwasaki M, Okuda S, Miyauchi A, Sakaura H, Mukai Y, Yonenobu K, Yoshikawa H. Surgical strategy for cervical myelopathy due to ossification of the posterior longitudinal ligament: part 2: advantages of anterior decompression and fusion over laminoplasty. Spine (Phila Pa 1976). 2007;32(6):654–60.
31. Koda M, Mochizuki M, Konishi H, Aiba A, Kadota R, Inada T, Kamiya K, Ota M, Maki S, Takahashi K, Yamazaki M, Mannoji C, Furuya T. Comparison of clinical outcomes between laminoplasty, posterior decompression with instrumented fusion, and anterior decompression with fusion for K-line (−) cervical ossification of the posterior longitudinal ligament. Eur Spine J. 2016b;25(7):2294–301.
32. Murakami H, Kawahara N, Tomita K, Demura S, Kato S, Yoshioka K. Does interruption of the artery of Adamkiewicz during total en bloc spondylectomy affect neurologic function? Spine (Phila Pa 1976). 2010;35(22):E1187–92.
33. Kato S, Kawahara N, Tomita K, Murakami H, Demura S, Fujimaki Y. Effects on spinal cord blood flow and neurologic function secondary to interruption of bilateral segmental arteries which supply the artery of Adamkiewicz: an experimental study using a dog model. Spine (Phila Pa 1976). 2008;33(14):1533–41.
34. Fujimaki Y, Kawahara N, Tomita K, Murakami H, Ueda Y. How many ligations of bilateral segmental arteries cause ischemic spinal cord dysfunction? An experimental study using a dog model. Spine (Phila Pa 1976). 2006;31(21):E781–9.

Surgery for Ossification of the Ligamentum Flavum: Posterior Decompression with or Without Fusion

31

Takashi Kaito

Abstract

Ossification of the ligamentum flavum (OLF) is a major cause of thoracic myelopathy. Surgical treatment is indicated when conservative treatment loses efficacy and symptoms of myelopathy appear. Either of the two surgical techniques are usually employed based on the observed ossification type after resection or division and thinning of the laminae. They include the double open-door and en bloc resection techniques, which are indicated in cases without and with bony fusion in the midline, respectively. The surgical outcomes are generally good. However, the presence of dural ossification has a negative impact on treatment outcomes and is related to a higher risk of surgical complications. The preoperative diagnosis of dural ossification is of considerable value, as it prepares surgeons for possible complications.

Keywords

Ossification · Ligamentum flavum
Myelopathy · Surgery · Dural ossification
Complications · Thoracic spine

T. Kaito (✉)
Department of Orthopaedic Surgery, Osaka University Graduate School of Medicine, Osaka, Japan
e-mail: takashikaito@ort.med.osaka-u.ac.jp

31.1 Introduction

Ossification of the ligamentum flavum (OLF) is one of the major causes of thoracic myelopathy, occurring in 42.4% of cases. It usually occurs at the lower thoracic spine (T10-12), followed by the upper thoracic spine. On plain radiographs, the incidence has been reported to be 3.8–26% [1–3]. However, recent studies using CT have demonstrated a higher incidence of 36% [4]. Although the definite etiology of OLF has not been elucidated, the high incidence of concurrent ossification of the posterior longitudinal ligament suggests the involvement of genetic and metabolic factors [5]. Mechanical factors have also been implicated [6]. The hypertrophied and ossified ligamentum flavum may cause compression of the spinal cord and nerve roots, which may lead to various neurological symptoms in accordance with the spinal levels of compression. In cases where conservative treatment is ineffective, surgical decompression is indicated when the symptoms of myelopathy appear. In this chapter, we will discuss about the preoperative evaluation, surgical techniques, and surgery-related complications of OLF.

31.2 Radiographic Classification of OLF

The ligamentum flavum independently connects bilateral superior articular processes to the cranial ventral laminae. Therefore, ossification

A. Okawa et al. (eds.), *OPLL*, https://doi.org/10.1007/978-981-15-3855-1_31

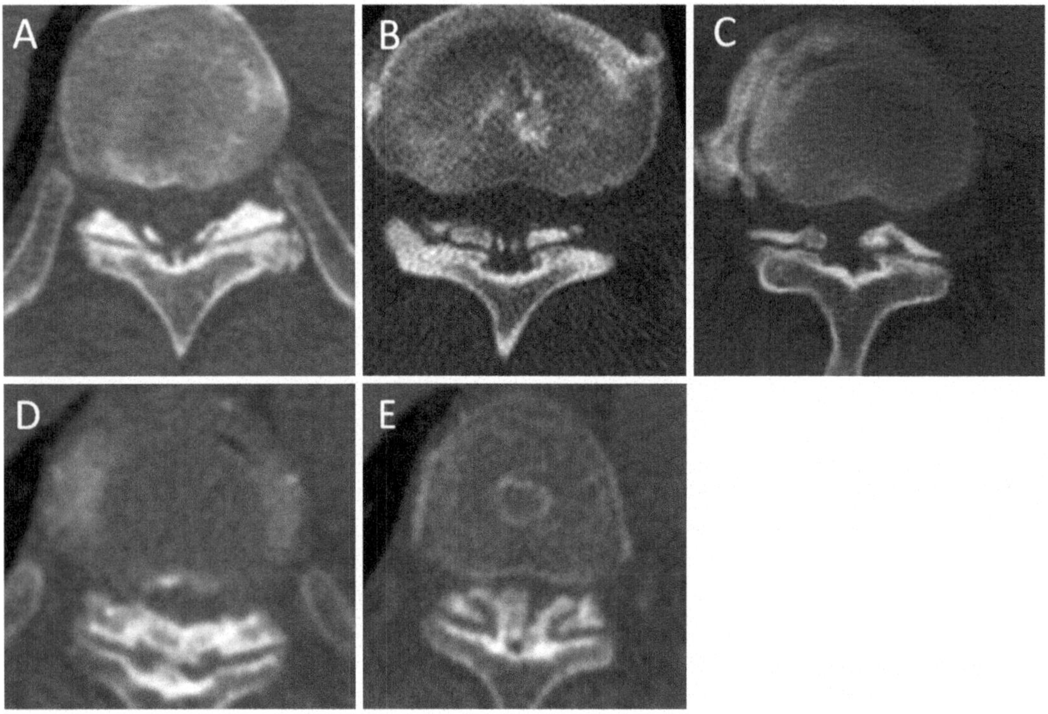

Fig. 31.1 Classification of ossification of the ligamentum flavum. (**a**) Lateral type, (**b**) extended type, (**c**) enlarged type, (**d**) fused type, and (**e**) tuberous type

may either occur separately on both sides or on one side in the early stages. As ossification progresses, it may extend ventrally with fusion of bilateral ossified ligaments in the midline. Five types of ossification have been reported based on axial CT scan images [7]: (1) lateral type: ossification exists only in the capsular portion of the ligamentum flavum, (2) extended type: thin ossification extends into the interlaminar portion of the ligamentum flavum, (3) enlarged type: the antero-posterior thickness of ossification increases without extending to the central part, (4) fused type: the size of ossification is not different from the enlarged type but the ossification on either side fuses in the middle of the lamina, and (5) tuberous type: central fused portion enlarges to form a tuberous mass and protrudes anteriorly (Fig. 31.1).

31.3 Radiographic Prediction of Dural Ossification

The existence of dural ossification (DO) has a negative impact on surgical outcomes and may lead to a high incidence of complications. Therefore, the preoperative diagnosis of DO is of considerable value in helping surgeons prepare for possible complications [8, 9]. One of the CT findings suggestive of DO is the "tram track" sign, which is a low-signal line between the parallel bony plates [8] (Fig. 31.2). Another CT finding suggestive of DO is a cross-sectional area occupying a ratio of >55% in the lower thoracic spine [9]. Other reported radiographic indicators include the presence of a fused or tuberous type of OLF (large OLF) and OLF in the lower thoracic spine [10, 11].

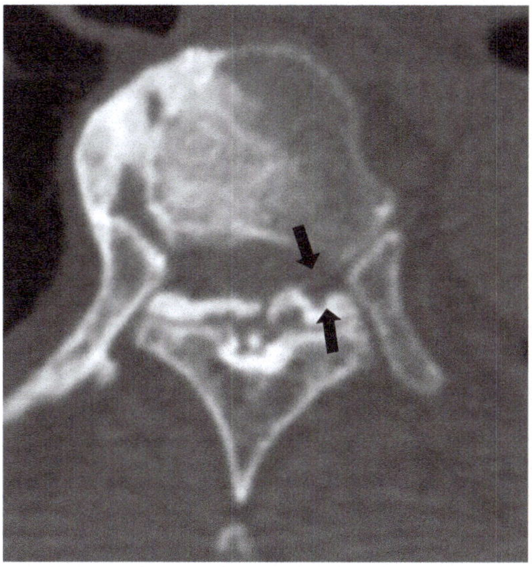

Fig. 31.2 The tram track sign of dural ossification. Arrows indicate "the tram track sign," which is defined as a hyper dense bony protrusion into the canal with a central area of hypodensity

31.4 Surgical Techniques

Surgical resection for OLF involves two techniques, based on the type of ossification observed after resection or division and thinning of the laminae (Fig. 31.3).

31.4.1 Double Open-DoorResection of OLF

In cases of ossification without bony fusion in the middle of the laminae, double open-door resection is employed. After the thinning or division of the superior articular processes, and thinning of the ossified ligaments, they are elevated bilaterally to allow release of the adhesions between their ventral aspect and the dura mater. This technique is also employed for fused types of OLF when the fused ossified ligaments at the central

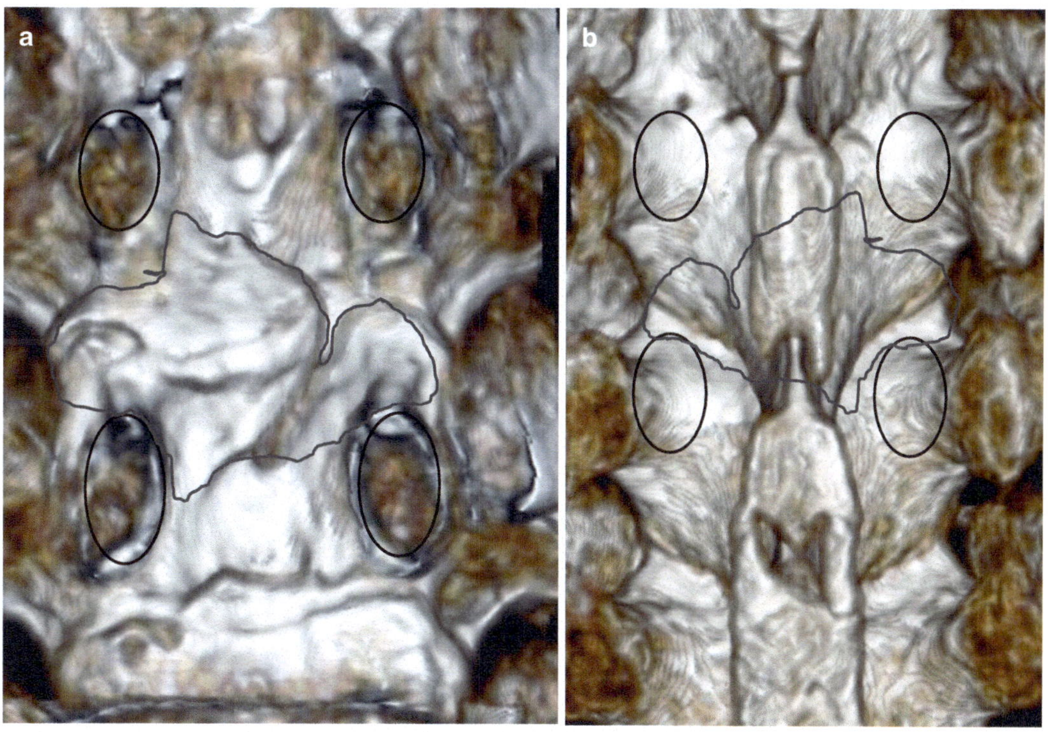

Fig. 31.3 3D CT images of ossification of the ligamentum flavum. (**a**) Ventral side and (**b**) and dorsal side of the laminae in the thoracic spine with ossification of the ligamentum flavum. The dotted line delineates the OLF

laminae are thin, and the right and left sides are separable on dividing the central fused portion (Fig. 31.4).

31.4.2 En Block Resection of OLF

In cases where the ossification fuses at the central part of the laminae, en block resection of OLF is employed. After the thinning and removal of the laminae, bilateral ossified ligaments and superior articular processes are thinned and divided at the lateral ends. The floating section of OLF is then elevated from all directions, taking particular care that the see-saw movement of the floating segment does not push the dura mater. In cases with DO, a partial or total layer of dura is resected leaving the arachnoid mater intact (Fig. 31.5).

Resection of a significant portion of bony and ligamentous structures may potentially cause spinal instability. However, the overall mean increase in kyphosis is usually slight. In a study, which compared the progression of kyphosis between the fusion and non-fusion groups, the difference in progression of kyphosis was less than three degrees [12]. Although there is presently no consensus on the issue of additional fusion with decompression, current evidence does not favor the routine use of posterior fixation. In addition to the impact of additional fixation, the negative impact of posterior fusion, which includes loss of spinal mobility and cost-effectiveness, needs to be validated.

31.5 Surgical Outcomes

The modified Japanese Orthopaedic Association (JOA) scoring system, which excludes the upper limb scores and includes a total of 11 points, is generally used to evaluate neurological status. The recovery rate according to the modified JOA score, which is calculated by the formula: (postoperative JOA score − preoperative JOA score)/(11 − preoperative JOA score) × 100, is reported to be 30–63% [12–14]. However, the recovery rate of OLF in the middle thoracic spine is reported to be low. Since the middle thoracic spine is less dynamic compared to the lower thoracic spine, prolonged compression of the spinal cord prior to surgery may cause irreversible damage [12].

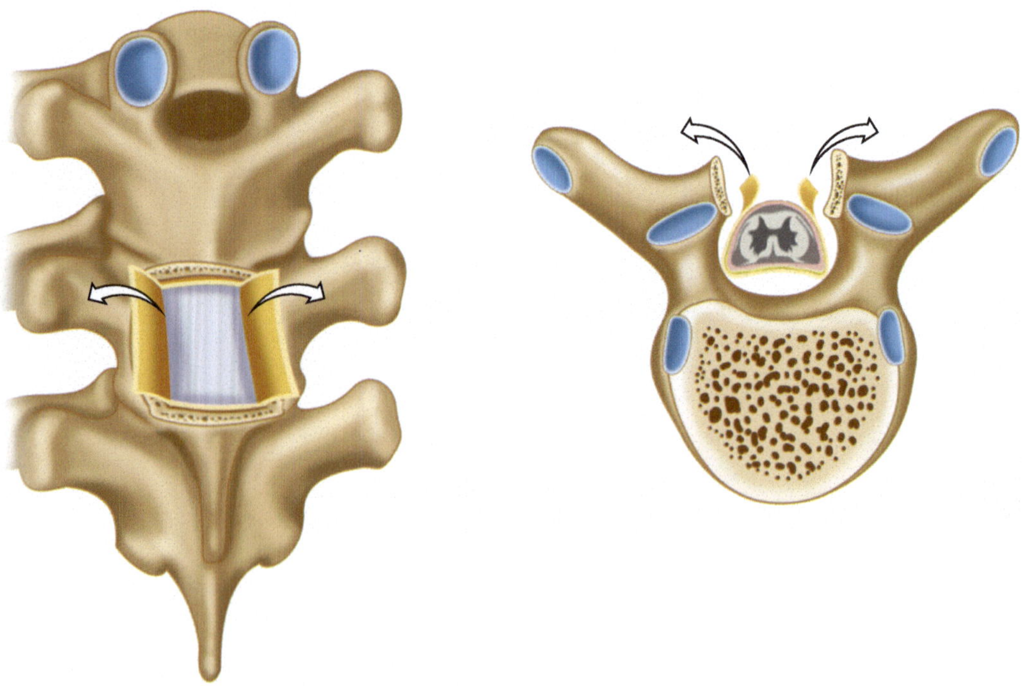

Fig. 31.4 Double open-door resection of ossification of the ligamentum flavum

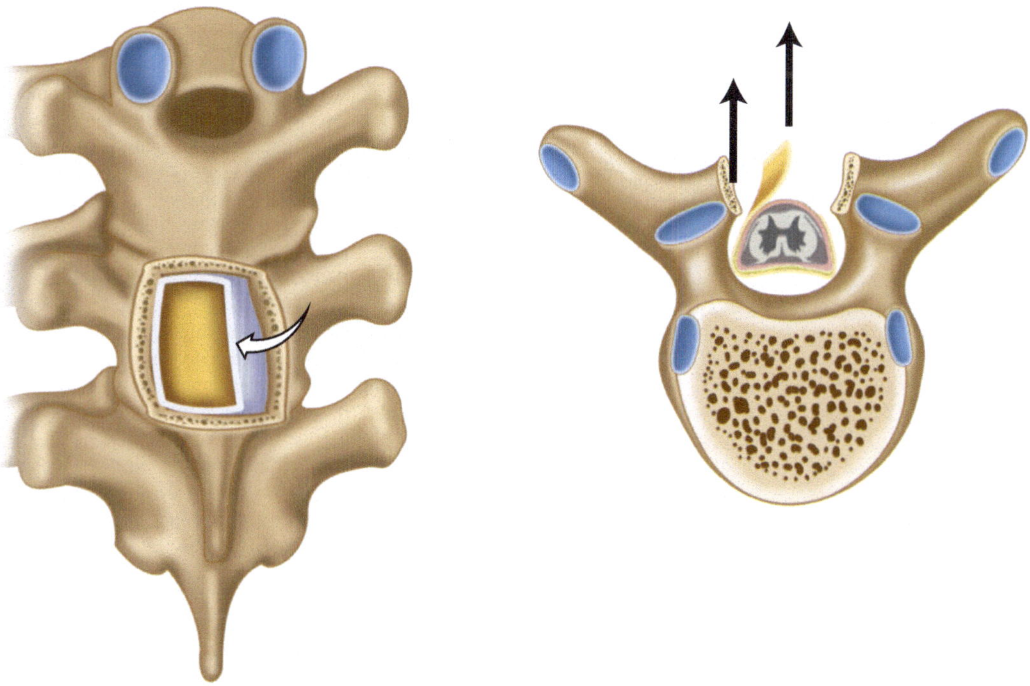

Fig. 31.5 En block resection of ossification of the ligamentum flavum

31.6 Surgical Complications

The most frequent complication during surgery for OLF is dural tear, with a reported incidence of 7–32% [8, 13–18]. Dural tear generally occurs during the removal of DO; concurrent damage to the arachnoid mater may lead to leakage of cerebrospinal fluid. Neurological deterioration after surgery is reported to be 0–18%; hematomas, reperfusion injuries, and surgical maneuvers are known related causes. In many cases, the neurological deterioration recovers early in the postoperative period [13, 17].

31.7 Predictive Factors for Neurological Recovery

Increased intramedullary signals on T2-weighted magnetic resonance imaging (MRI) [19], duration of disease, existence of non-fused ossification of the anterior longitudinal ligament at the same level, spinal ossification, DO [20], OLF in the middle thoracic spine [3], and low preoperative JOA scores [21] are the reported risk factors for poor surgical outcome. However, the association of these prognostic factors are inconsistent across reports.

31.8 Conclusions

Thoracic OLF is one of the major causes of thoracic myelopathy. After the symptoms of myelopathy appear, surgical decompression is the only effective treatment. It is essential to consider OLF in the differential diagnosis, even in patients who exhibit typical symptoms of lumbar degenerative disease, since this may have a bearing on prognosis. The preoperative diagnosis or prediction of DO is of considerable value, as it may help surgeons develop appropriate surgical strategies and prepare for complications related to dural injury.

References

1. Kudo S, Ono M, Russell WJ. Ossification of thoracic ligamenta flava. AJR Am J Roentgenol. 1983;141(1):117–21.

2. Williams DM, Gabrielsen TO, Latack JT, Martel W, Knake JE. Ossification in the cephalic attachment of the ligamentum flavum. An anatomical and CT study. Radiology. 1984;150:423–6.
3. Guo JJ, Luk KD, Karppinen J, Yang H, Cheung KM. Prevalence, distribution, and morphology of ossification of the ligamentum flavum: a population study of one thousand seven hundred thirty-six magnetic resonance imaging scans. Spine. 2010;25:51–6.
4. Mori K, Kasahara T, Mimura T, Nishizawa K, Murakami Y, Matsusue Y, Imai S. Prevalence, distribution, and morphology of thoracic ossification of the yellow ligament in Japanese: results of CT-based cross-sectional study. Spine (Phila Pa 1976). 2013;38(19):E1216–22.
5. Fujimori T, Watabe T, Iwamoto Y, Hamada S, Iwasaki M, Oda T. Prevalence, concomitance, and distribution of ossification of the spinal ligaments: results of whole spine CT scans in 1500 Japanese patients. Spine (Phila Pa 1976). 2016;41(21):1668–76.
6. Otani K, Aihara T, Tanaka A, Shibasaki K. Ossification of the ligamentum flavum of the thoracic spine in adult kyphosis. Int Orthop. 1986;10(2):135–9.
7. Aizawa T, Sato T, Sasaki H, Kusakabe T, Morozumi N, Kokubun S. Thoracic myelopathy caused by ossification of the ligamentum flavum: clinical features and surgical results in the Japanese population. J Neurosurg Spine. 2006;5(6):514–9.
8. Ju JH, Kim SJ, Kim KH, Ryu DS, Park JY, Chin DK, Kim KS, Cho YE, Kuh SU. Clinical relation among dural adhesion, dural ossification, and dural laceration in the removal of ossification of the ligamentum flavum. Spine J. 2018;18(5):747–54.
9. Yu L, Li B, Yu Y, Li W, Qiu G, Zhao Y. The relationship between dural ossification and spinal stenosis in thoracic ossification of the ligamentum flavum. J Bone Joint Surg Am. 2019;107(7):606–12.
10. Muthukumar N. Dural ossification in ossification of the ligamentum flavum: a preliminary report. Spine. 2009;34:2654–61.
11. Sato T, Kokubun S, Ishii Y. Choice of operative method for ossification of ligamentum flavum based on CT findings. Rinshoseikeigeka. 1996;31(4):541–5. Japanese.
12. Yu S, Wu D, Li F, Hou T. Surgical results and prognostic factors for thoracic myelopathy caused by ossification of ligamentum flavum: posterior surgery by laminectomy. Acta Neurochir (Wien). 2013;155(7):1169–77.
13. Li Z, Ren D, Zhao Y, Hou S, Li L, Yu S, Hou T. Clinical characteristics and surgical outcome of thoracic myelopathy caused by ossification of the ligamentum flavum: a retrospective analysis of 85 cases. Spinal Cord. 2016;54(3):188–96.
14. Onishi E, Yasuda T, Yamamoto H, Iwaki K, Ota S. Outcomes of surgical treatment for thoracic myelopathy: a single-institutional study of 73 patients. Spine (Phila Pa 1976). 2016;41(22):E1356–63.
15. Kawaguchi Y, Yasuda T, Seki S, Nakano M, Kanamori M, Sumi S, Kimura T. Variables affecting postsurgical prognosis of thoracic myelopathy caused by ossification of the ligamentum flavum. Spine J. 2013;13(9):1095–107.
16. Tang CYK, Cheung JPY, Samartzis D, Leung KH, Wong YW, Luk KDK, Cheung KMC. Predictive factors for neurological deterioration after surgical decompression for thoracic ossified yellow ligament. Eur Spine J. 2017;26(10):2598–605.
17. Wang H, Wei F, Long H, Han G, Sribastav SS, Li Z, Huang Y, Zhu R, Liang C. Surgical outcome of thoracic myelopathy caused by ossification of ligamentum flavum. J Clin Neurosci. 2017;45:83–8.
18. Sun X, Sun C, Liu X, Liu Z, Qi Q, Guo Z, Leng H, Chen Z. The frequency and treatment of dural tears and cerebrospinal fluid leakage in 266 patients with thoracic myelopathy caused by ossification of the ligamentum flavum. Spine (Phila Pa 1976). 2012;37(12):E702–7.
19. Zhang J, Wang L, Li J, Yang P, Shen Y. Predictors of surgical outcome in thoracic ossification of the ligamentum flavum: focusing on the quantitative signal intensity. Sci Rep. 2016;6:23019. https://doi.org/10.1038/srep23019.
20. Ando K, Imagama S, Ito Z, Hirano K, Muarmoto A, Kato F, Yukawa Y, Kawakami N, Sato K, Matsubara Y, Kanemyura T, Matsuyama Y, Ishiguro N. Predictive factors for a poor surgical outcome with thoracic ossification of the ligamentum flavum by multivariate analysis: a multicenter study. Spine. 2013;38(129):E748–54.
21. Kang KC, Lee CS, Shin SK, Park SJ, Chung CH, Chung SS. Ossification of the ligamentum flavum of the thoracic spine in the Korean population. J Neurosurg Spine. 2011;14(4):513–9.

Computer-Aided Surgery for Ossification of the Spinal Ligaments

32

Kenichiro Sakai

Abstract

Among the surgical treatments of ossification of the spinal ligaments, the anterior surgery for ossification of the posterior longitudinal ligament (OPLL) is especially difficult and various complications have been reported. Nowadays, intraoperative imaging modalities, such as fluoroscopic three-dimensional images, mobile helical computed tomography, and cone-beam computed tomography, are available in many institutions. The mobile intraoperative imaging system "O-arm," which is an operation support tool, enables three-dimensional imaging in a surgical position and also enables real-time navigation by linking with a navigation system. We introduce the procedure of anterior decompression and fusion for cervical OPLL and thoracic OPLL with the support of the O-arm and navigation system. This system is a helpful method to improve the accuracy and safety of anterior surgical procedures for OPLL.

Keywords

Ossification of the posterior longitudinal ligament · Anterior surgery · Anterior decompression · O-arm · Navigation Intraoperative image

K. Sakai (✉)
Department of Orthopedic Surgery, Saiseikai Kawaguchi General Hospital, Saitama, Japan

32.1 Introduction

Among the surgical treatments of ossification of the spinal ligaments, the anterior surgery for ossification of the posterior longitudinal ligament (OPLL) is especially difficult and various complications have been reported [1–5].

Anterior decompression and fusion (ADF) for OPLL is an ideal surgical procedure because OPLL is an anterior lesion and results in good neurological recovery [1, 4, 6]. However, it has a large learning curve and some specific complications, such as an insufficient decompression due to impingement between the floating OPLL and the residual vertebral body [7] (Fig. 32.1) or massive hemorrhage from epidural venous plexus around the OPLL lesion.

Nowadays, intraoperative imaging modalities, such as fluoroscopic three-dimensional (3D) images, mobile helical computed tomography (CT), and cone-beam CT, are available in many institutions. Previously, there were reports that intraoperative fluoroscopic 3D images were useful for adequate decompression in anterior cervical discectomy and fusion (ACDF) for cervical spondylosis patients [8] and mobile helical CT images in the anterior cervical corpectomy and fusion (ACCF) for C-OPLL patients [7].

The mobile intraoperative imaging system "O-arm" (O-arm™ Surgical Imaging System, Medtronic Navigation Inc., MA, USA) (Fig. 32.2), which is an operation support tool,

A. Okawa et al. (eds.), *OPLL*, https://doi.org/10.1007/978-981-15-3855-1_32

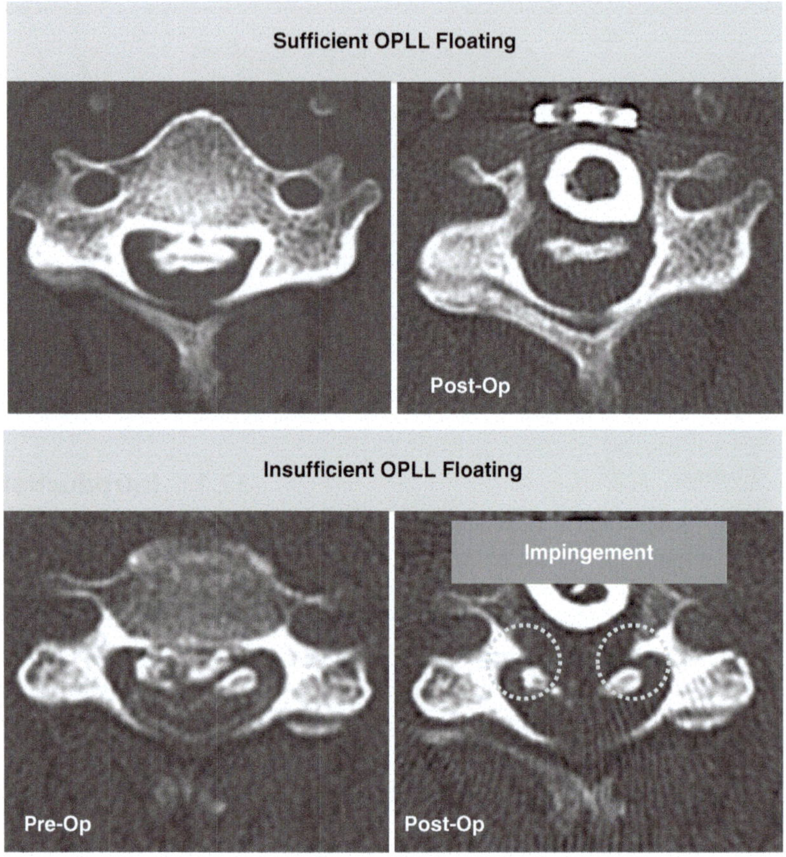

Fig. 32.1 CT images before and after anterior decompression and fusion with floating method in sufficient decompression case (upper part) and insufficient case, which has an impingement between the floating OPLL and the residual vertebral body (lower part)

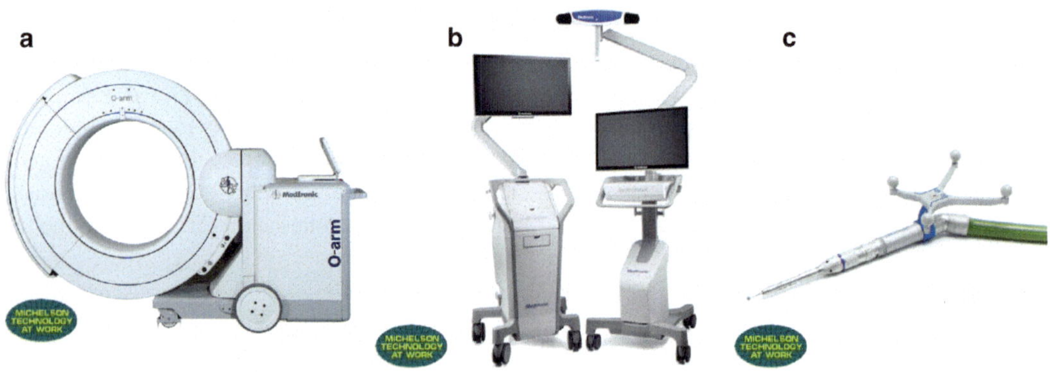

Fig. 32.2 (**a**) The mobile intraoperative imaging system "O-arm." (**b**) Navigation system. (**c**) Navigation-synchronized high-speed drill. (Source of photo: Medtronic Inc.)

enables 3D imaging in a surgical position and also enables real-time navigation by linking with a navigation system.

Here, we introduce the procedure of ADF with the floating method for cervical OPLL (C-OPLL) and thoracic OPLL (T-OPLL) with the support of the O-arm and navigation system.

32.2 Anterior Surgery for C-OPLL Assisted by O-Arm and Navigation System

We apply the anterior OPLL floating technique described by Yamaura et al. [6, 9]. A radiolucent operating table made of carbon is used. In a supine with neck sniffing position, we fix the patient's skull by carbon Mayfield cramp and attach a reference frame to the cramp (Fig. 32.3).

Operated cervical vertebral bodies are exposed by a standard Smith–Robinson approach [10]. After confirmation and exposure of the appropriate vertebral levels, we place a retractor on the cervical spine. After careful draping, we take the O-arm image. After we confirmed that the region for imaging was appropriately scanned, the scanned image is automatically synchronized to the navigation system (StealthStation™ System, Medtronic Navigation Inc., CO, USA) (Fig. 32.2). This process usually takes approximately 10 min from the draping to completing the review of the 3D image-linked navigation system.

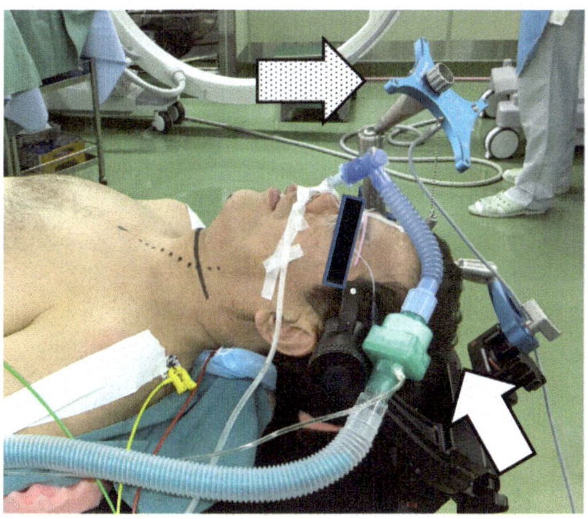

Fig. 32.3 In a supine with neck sniffing position, we fix the patient's skull by carbon Mayfield cramp (white arrow) and attach a reference frame to the cramp (dot arrow)

We performed the corpectomy and OPLL floating using a navigation-synchronized high-speed drill (Stealth-Midas™, Medtronic Powered Surgical Solutions, TX, USA) (Fig. 32.2). After corpectomy was performed by removing discs and vertebral bodies, the OPLL was cut very thin and allowed to float away from the dural sac without removal. This procedure is basically done by looking at the surgical field under a microscope, and we check the monitor when necessary. We can confirm the approach angle, decompression width, position of the vertebral artery and pedicle, and the OPLL lesion in 3D and real-time image (Fig. 32.4). When the thinned OPLL appear to be like a board floating on water, the decompression of the entire spinal cord is complete. The O-arm image is sometimes taken again to confirm the final decompression (Fig. 32.5).

The cervical spine was reconstructed using an autologous fibula, a local bone in metal cage, or a hydroxyapatite block with an anterior plate and screw system.

32.3 Clinical Outcomes of Anterior Surgery Assisted by O-Arm and Navigation System

We started to use O-arm and navigation system for this procedure from 2017. The surgical results of this technique were compared with a historical

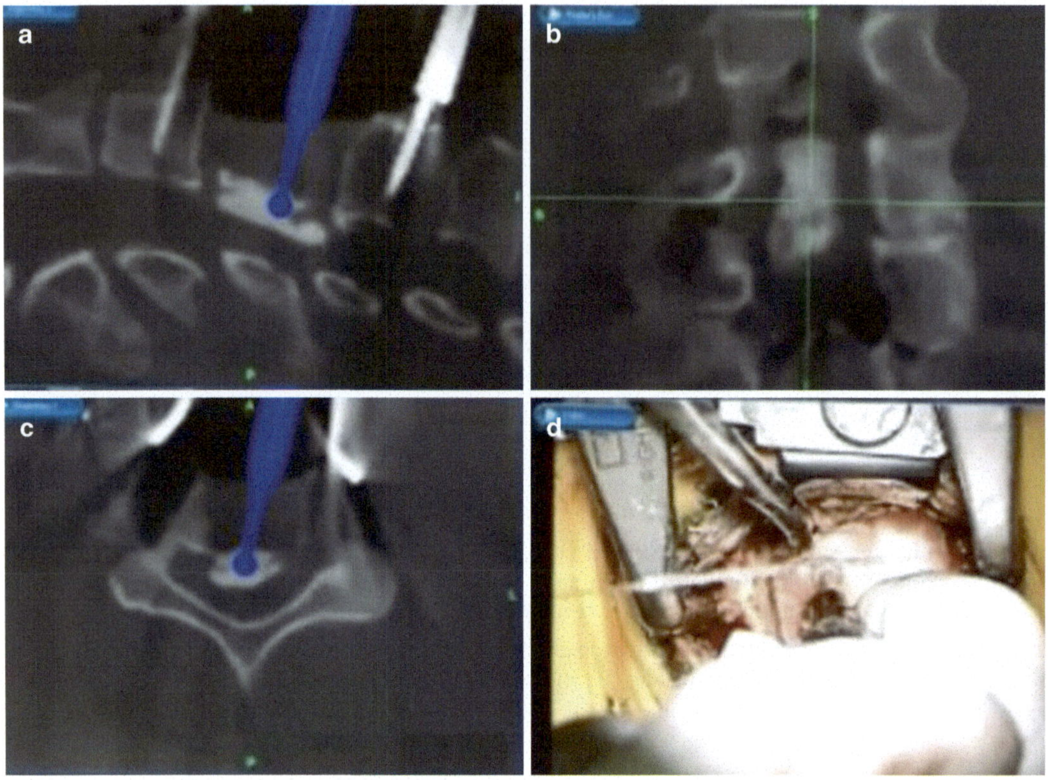

Fig. 32.4 Navigation monitor in anterior surgery for cervical OPLL. (**a**) Sagittal view. (**b**) Coronal view. (**c**) Axial view. (**d**) Microscope image in the operative field

control of OPLL cases that underwent anterior surgery without the use of this system.

The survey included a total of 26 consecutive patients who underwent anterior surgery with O-arm and navigation system for C-OPLL (O group). We compared 69 patients without O-arm and navigation system as a historical control (C group). Operative time, intraoperative bleeding, postoperative radiological impingement of the floating OPLL at CT, revision surgery, and neurological complications were evaluated.

There were no significant differences in patients' baseline data (age, gender, canal narrowing ratio of the OPLL, C2–7 lordotic angle, cervical sagittal vertical axis, and C7 tilt) between the two groups. There was no difference in the operative time between the two groups; however, the average intraoperative hemorrhage in O group was about half of that in the C group (O group: 127 mL, C group: 248 mL) (Fig. 32.7), and massive hemorrhage bleeding (>1000 mL) was not observed in the O group (O group: 0%, C group: 4.4%). Incidence of the postoperative radiological impingement of the floating OPLL in the O group was about one-fifth of that in the C group (O group: 3.8%, C group: 20.3%) and revision surgery due to the postoperative impingement of the floating OPLL in the O group could be reduced to about one-third of that in the C group (O group: 3.8%, C group: 11.6%) (Fig. 32.6). The postoperative neurological deterioration of lower-extremity was not observed in the O group (O group: 0%, C group: 4.4%).

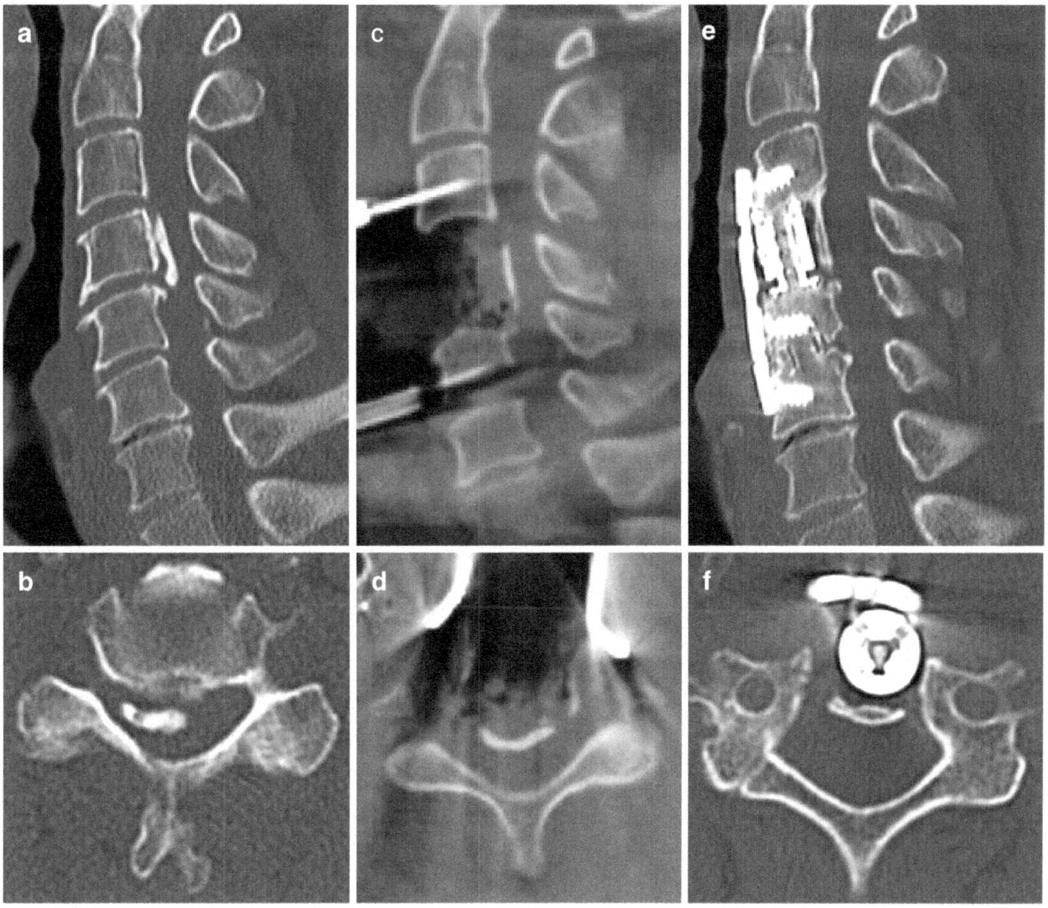

Fig. 32.5 Anterior surgery with floating method for cervical OPLL. (**a**, **b**) Preoperative CT images. (**c**, **d**) Intraoperative O-arm images after decompression. (**e**, **f**) Postoperative CT images at 1-year follow-up period

32.4 Anterior Surgery for T-OPLL Assisted by O-Arm and Navigation System

We apply the anterior decompression technique for thoracic OPLL described by Kurosa et al. [11]. We use the carbon bed, and fix it firmly so that the posture does not change during surgery. The reference frame is placed on the ilium of the patient. After an anterolateral standard approach to the thoracic spine, the lateral aspect of the vertebral body is exposed. After placing a retractor and careful draping, we take the O-arm image. The scanned image is synchronized to the navigation system. We carefully perform the OPLL decompression while checking with the navigation monitor as well as the cervical spine (Fig. 32.7). The thoracic spine was reconstructed using an autologous bone or a local bone in cage with an anterior screw system (Fig. 32.8).

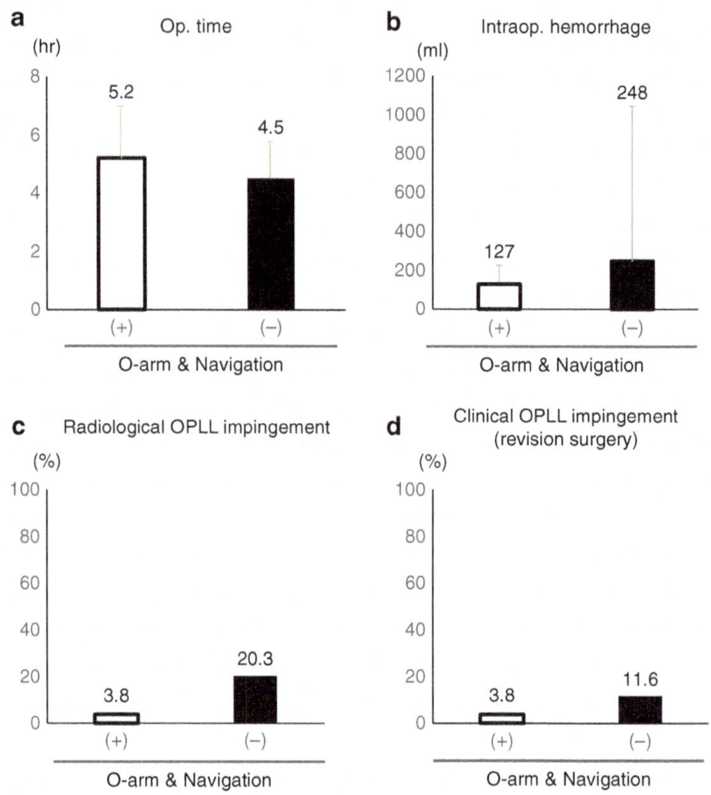

Fig. 32.6 Clinical results of comparison with and without O-arm and navigation. (**a**) Operative time. (**b**) Intraoperative hemorrhage. (**c**) Incidence of the postoperative radiological impingement of the floating OPLL. (**d**) Incidence of revision surgery due to the postoperative impingement of the floating OPLL

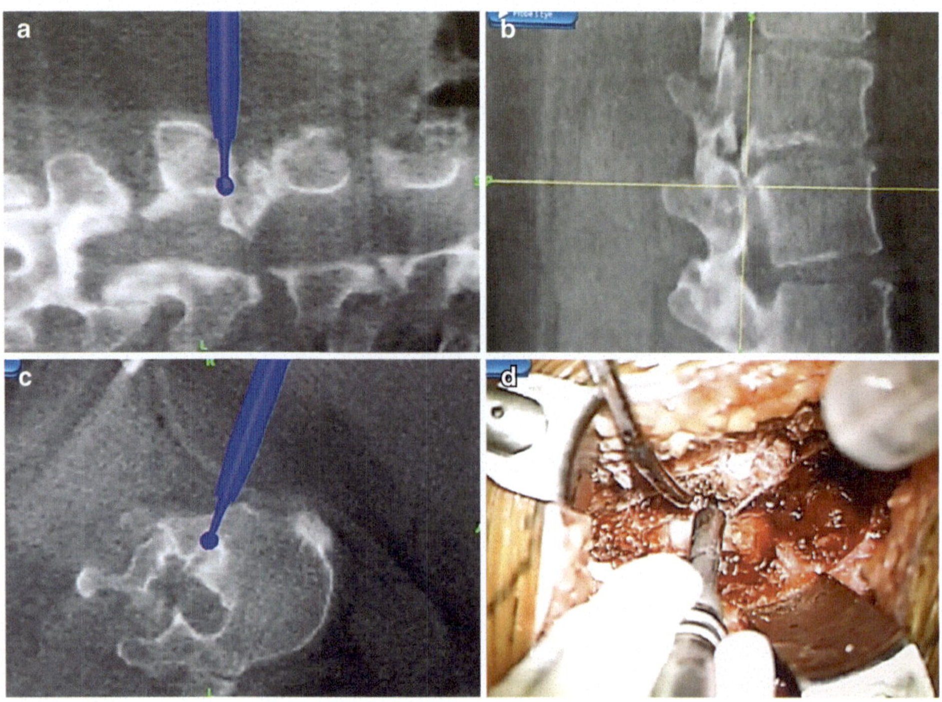

Fig. 32.7 Navigation monitor in anterior surgery for thoracic OPLL. (**a**) Sagittal view. (**b**) Coronal view. (**c**) Axial view. (**d**) Microscope image in the operative field

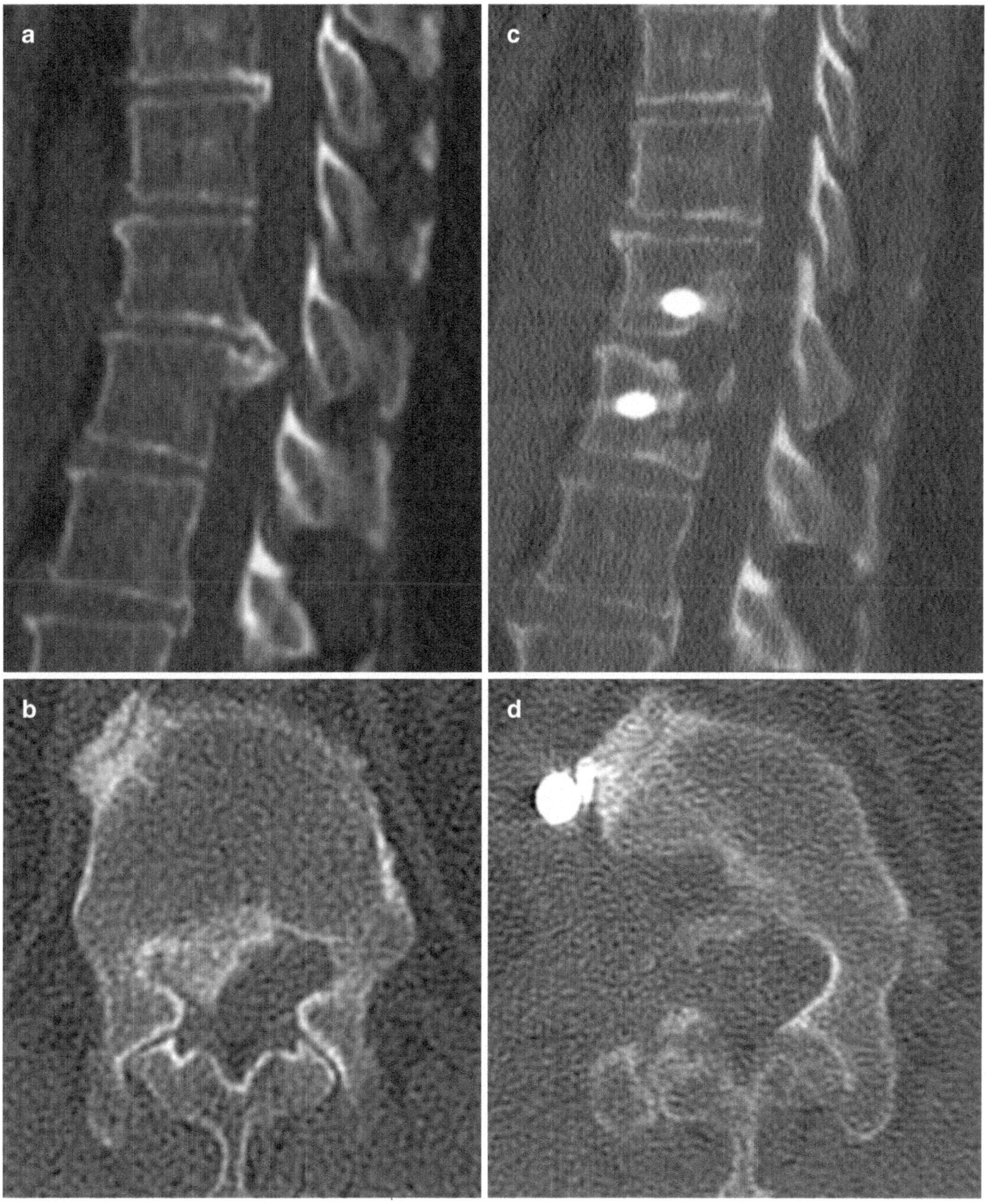

Fig. 32.8 Anterior surgery for thoracic OPLL. (**a**, **b**) Preoperative CT images. (**c**, **d**) Postoperative CT images at 1-year follow-up period

32.5 Conclusions

Anterior surgeries for cervical or thoracic OPLL assisted by O-arm and navigation system are helpful methods to improve the accuracy and safety of surgical procedures.

Acknowledgments Japanese Health, Labour and Welfare Sciences Research Grant.

References

1. Fujimura Y, et al. Long-term follow-up study of anterior decompression and fusion for thoracic myelopathy resulting from ossification of the posterior longitudinal ligament. Spine (Phila Pa 1976). 1997;22(3):305–11.
2. Imagama S, et al. Perioperative complications after surgery for thoracic ossification of posterior longitudinal ligament: a nationwide multicenter prospective study. Spine (Phila Pa 1976). 2018;43(23):E1389–97. https://doi.org/10.1097/BRS.0000000000002703.
3. Kimura A, et al. Perioperative complications of anterior cervical decompression with fusion in patients with ossification of the posterior longitudinal ligament: a retrospective, multi-institutional study. J Orthop Sci. 2012;17(6):667–72. https://doi.org/10.1007/s00776-012-0271-3.
4. Liu W, et al. Comparison of anterior decompression and fusion versus laminoplasty in the treatment of multilevel cervical ossification of the posterior longitudinal ligament: a systematic review and meta-analysis. Ther Clin Risk Manag. 2016;12:675–85. https://doi.org/10.2147/TCRM.S100046.
5. Matsumoto M, et al. Surgical results and related factors for ossification of posterior longitudinal ligament of the thoracic spine: a multi-institutional retrospective study. Spine (Phila Pa 1976). 2008;33(9):1034–41. https://doi.org/10.1097/BRS.0b013e31816c913b.
6. Matsuoka T, et al. Long-term results of the anterior floating method for cervical myelopathy caused by ossification of the posterior longitudinal ligament. Spine (Phila Pa 1976). 2001;26(3):241–8.
7. Yoshii T, et al. Intraoperative evaluation using mobile computed tomography in anterior cervical decompression with floating method for massive ossification of the posterior longitudinal ligament. J Orthop Surg Res. 2017;12(1):12. https://doi.org/10.1186/s13018-017-0515-1.
8. Deinsberger R, et al. Intraoperative evaluation of bone decompression in anterior cervical spine surgery by three-dimensional fluoroscopy. Eur Spine J. 2005;14(7):671–6.
9. Yamaura I, et al. Anterior floating method for cervical myelopathy caused by ossification of the posterior longitudinal ligament. Clin Orthop Relat Res. 1999;(359):27–34.
10. Smith GW, Robinson RA. The treatment of certain cervical-spine disorders by anterior removal of the intervertebral disc and interbody fusion. J Bone Joint Surg Am. 1958;40-A(3):607–24.
11. Kurosa Y. Selecting a surgical method for thoracic myelopathy caused by ossification of the posterior longitudinal ligament. Spine (Phila Pa 1976). 1996;21(12):1458–66.

33 Surgical Treatment of Thoracic Ossification of the Posterior Longitudinal Ligament: Intraoperative Spinal Cord Monitoring

Go Yoshida, Tomohiro Banno, and Yukihiro Matsuyama

Abstract

Surgical management of OPLL is challenging because of high neurological complication rate. Intraoperative spinal neuromonitoring (IONM) can reduce neurological deterioration and provide increased accuracy in the detection of spinal cord injury. In this chapter, we report the efficacy, limitations, and the possibility for prevention neurological complication during OPLL surgery.

Keywords

Ossification of the posterior longitudinal ligament · Intraoperative spinal neuromonitoring · Transcranial electrical stimulation motor-evoked potentials · Neurological complications · Decompression Neurological rescue · Anterior spinal artery

33.1 Introduction

Ossification of the posterior longitudinal ligament (OPLL) surgery is challenging and technically demanding because of its pathological feature and complicated surgical procedure [1–4]. The reason for the poor surgical outcomes may be the presence of physiological kyphosis and poor vascular supply in the thoracic spine, which does not exist in the cervical or lumbar spine. Therefore, the effect of spinal cord decompression via a posterior approach is not sufficient. In addition, anterior procedures are technically demanding because of adhesion of the dura mater to ossified ligaments or small visualization of surgical field. Neurological complications in both anterior and posterior OPLL surgery are relatively high and unfortunate events associated with increased rates of morbidity, mortality, and increased health care costs. The rate of neurological complications of T-OPLL was reported to be up to 28.9% in Japanese national wide multicenter survey in 2011 [2]. Recently, spinal monitoring working group of the Japanese Society for Spine Surgery and Related Research (JSSR) reported that the incidence of neurological complications C-OPLL and T-OPLL were 6.3% and 20.1%, respectively, in 2018 [5].

Intraoperative spinal neuromonitoring (IONM) can reduce neurological deterioration and provide increased accuracy in the detection of spinal cord injury [6, 7]. Transcranial electrical stimulation motor-evoked potentials (Tc(E)-MEPs) are widely used for intraoperative spinal cord monitoring and have become the gold standard due to their high sensitivity and to the

G. Yoshida (✉) · T. Banno · Y. Matsuyama
Hamamatsu University School of medicine, Hamamatsu, Shizuoka, Japan
e-mail: goy@hama-med.ac.jp

A. Okawa et al. (eds.), *OPLL*, https://doi.org/10.1007/978-981-15-3855-1_33

importance of motor function [8–10]. Recently, the efficacy of multimodal IONM methods such as Tc(E)-MEPs coupled with somatosensory-evoked potential (SEP) [11], cord-evoked potential after stimulation to the brain (D-wave) [12–15], free running wave (continuous EMG) [16], or triggered EMG (stimulated EMG) [17] compared to single modal IONM was demonstrated. Thus, the purpose of IONM is to *"prevent"* the irreversible neural damage by facilitating proper intervention after the IOMM alert rather than *"predict"* neurological complications.

33.2 Surgical Procedure for Thoracic OPLL

Posterior decompression is indicated for many cases of thoracic OPLL because of the frequent combination of OPLL with ossification of the yellow ligament (OYL). We routinely perform a posterior decompression and corrective fusion. De-kyphotic correction was performed after decompression because thoracic spine is usually kyphotic alignment. Our procedures are (1) position change to prone (2) exposure (3) pedicle screwing (4) in situ temporary rodding (5) decompression (6) de-kyphotic correction and (7) clousure. In cases of postoperative newly occurred neurological complication or insufficient neurological recovery, an additional decompression procedure via an anterior or posterior approach is performed as two stages [18].

33.3 Protocol of Intraoperative Spinal Neuromonitoring (IONM)

Total intravenous anesthesia (TIVA) was administered during IONM. Systolic blood pressure was controlled more than 90 mmHg. The drugs administered were propofol (3–4 μg/mL), fentanyl (2 μg/kg), and vecuronium (0.12–0.16 mg/kg). Anesthesia was maintained using propofol (100–150 μg/kg/min with target-controlled infusion technique), remifentanyl (1 μg/kg/h), and vecuronium (0–0.04 mg/kg/h). The transcranial stimulus conditions comprised 5–10 train stimuli, a stimulus interval of 2 ms, a stimulus of 100–200 A, a stimulus duration of 500 μs, a filter of 50–1000 Hz, a recording time of 100 ms, and a total of fewer than 20 stimuli. Corkscrew-type stimulating electrodes (Nihon Kohden, Inc., Tokyo, Japan) were inserted bilaterally and symmetrically 5 cm lateral and 2 cm anterior to Cz (international 10–20 system of electrode placement). The Tc(E)-MEPs were recorded from the peripheral limbs via needle or surface electrodes and from the anus via plug-type electrodes. The evoked muscles, depending on the site of surgery, were selected from some or all of the deltoid, biceps, triceps, abductor pollicis brevis, quadriceps femoris, hamstrings, tibialis anterior, gastrocnemius, abductor hallucis, and sphincter muscles. We measured the amplitudes of the Tc(E)-MEPs using baseline-to-first negative peak voltages. The amplitudes prior to the invasive procedures were regarded as the control values. We set a 70% decrease in amplitude as the alarm threshold for Tc(E)-MEPs.

33.4 Clinical Practice of IONM in OPLL Cases

In out multicenter study of JSSR monitoring working group, we analyzed 871 continuous patients including 622 cervical OPLL cases and 249 thoracic OPLL cases [5]. Newly occurred neurological deficit was observed in seven patients with cervical OPLL and 30 patients with thoracic OPLL. Therefore, the motor deficit rate was 1.1% for cervical OPLL and 12.0% for thoracic OPLL. On the other hand, the rescue cases were found in 32 patients with cervical OPLL and 20 patients with thoracic OPLL. Therefore, the potential neurological deficit rate was 6.3% for cervical OPLL and 20.1% for thoracic OPLL. For cervical OPLL, alerts occurred at lamina opening for laminoplasty in 24 (61.5%) cases, corpectomy in 6 (15.4%) cases, and were unrelated to surgery in 7 (17.9%) cases. For thoracic OPLL, alerts occurred during decompression in 27 (54.0%) cases, dekyphosis in 5 (10.0%)

cases, exposure in 4 (8.0%) cases, rodding in 4 (8.0%) cases, and were unrelated to surgery in 4 (8.0%) cases [5]. After the monitoring alert, adequate interventions were implemented by the surgeons, anesthesiologists, and electrophysiologists according to the individual situation. Adjustment of blood pressure, heart rate, body temperature, and depth of anesthesia was performed by the anesthesiologist after an impedance check by the electrophysiologist. In cervical OPLL, most of the alerts (61.5%) occurred during lamina opening for laminoplasty. Among these patients, 73.3% were rescued by suspension surgery, irrigation, or additional decompression/foraminotomy after the monitoring alarm. However, suspension surgery and waiting in corpectomy cases were mostly ineffective. In thoracic OPLL, most alerts (54.0%) occurred during posterior decompression for OPLL. For these patients, suspension surgery and steroid injection after the monitoring alarm were also ineffective. However, posture change, bilateral rodding, or additional dekyphosis after the monitoring alarm were effective [5]. We determined *the rescue rate*, defined as the ratio of rescued patients with potential neurological deficits, as follows: the number of rescued patients/(the number of rescued patients + paralysis cases). The rescue rates were 82.1% for cervical OPLL and 40.0% for thoracic OPLL.

33.5 Case Presentation

Case 1 A 47-year-old female with cervico-thoracic OPLL planned to treat by posterior dekyphotic decompression and fusion (Fig. 33.1). After intubation on supine position, MEP monitoring showed enough amplitude as controls. However, after position change to prone, MEP amplitudes of lower extremities were deteriorated (Fig. 33.2). Therefore, operation was canceled and postponed to 2 months later using halo-vest fixation.

Case 2 A 48-year-old female treated by T5–10 laminectomy and T2-L1 dekyphotic posterior fusion (Fig. 33.3). When performing posterior decompression at OPLL compression area, MEP was deteriorated to almost flat (Fig. 33.4).

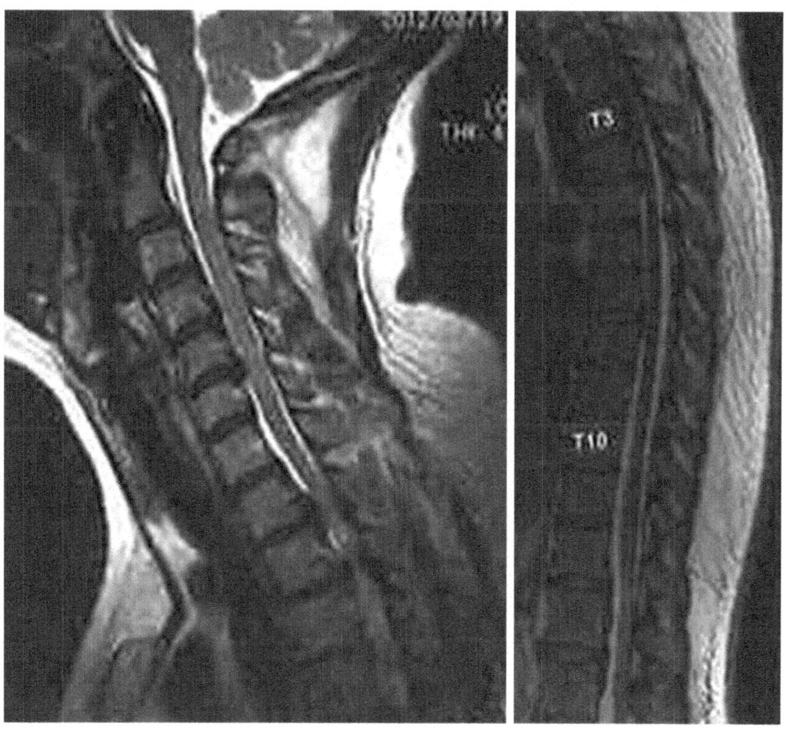

Fig. 33.1 MRI findings in patient with cervico-thoracic OPLL. We planned cervical laminoplasty and thoracic posterior decompression and dekyphotic fusion

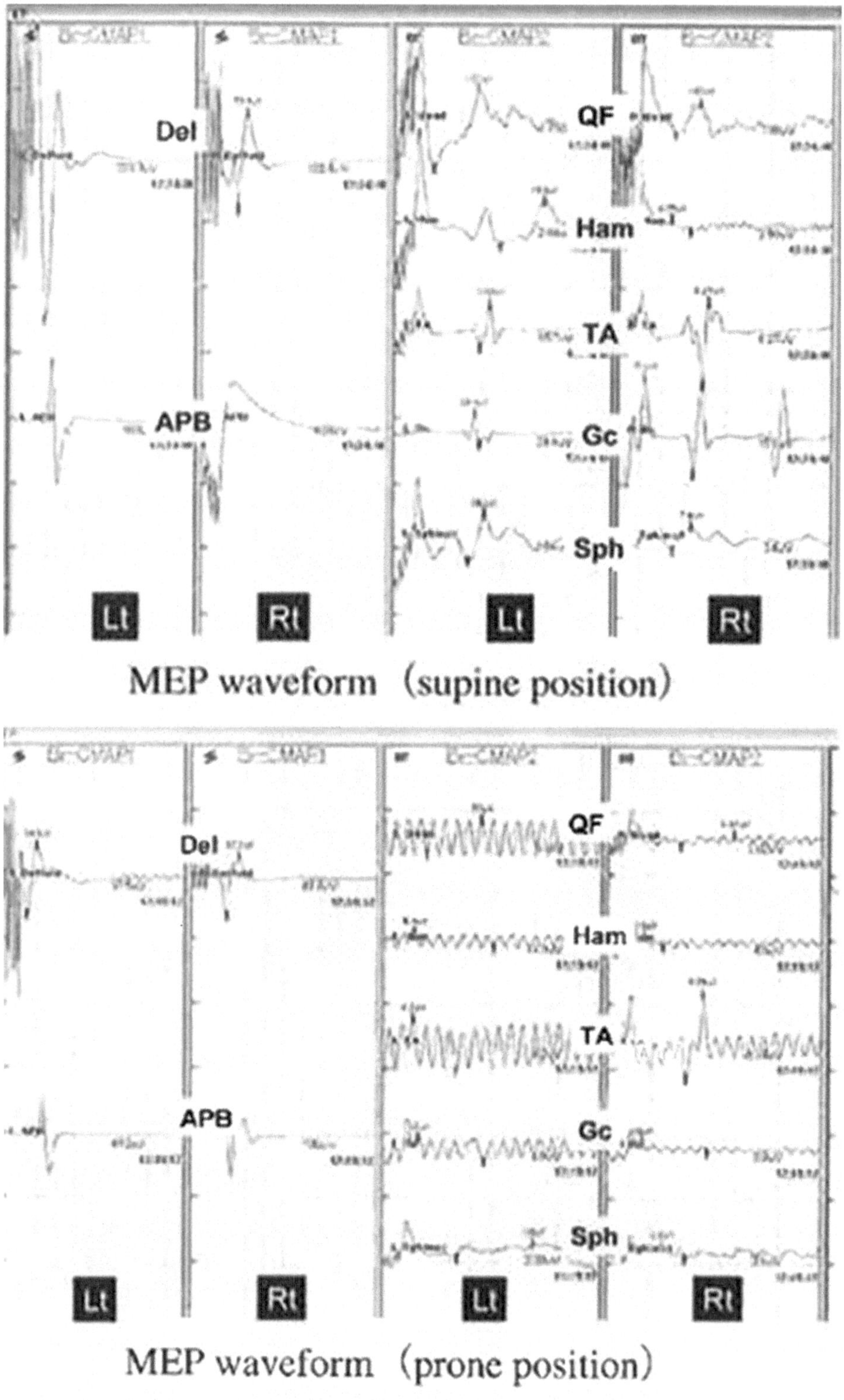

Fig. 33.2 MEP waveform before and after position change. After position change to prone, MEP amplitudes of lower extremities were deteriorated

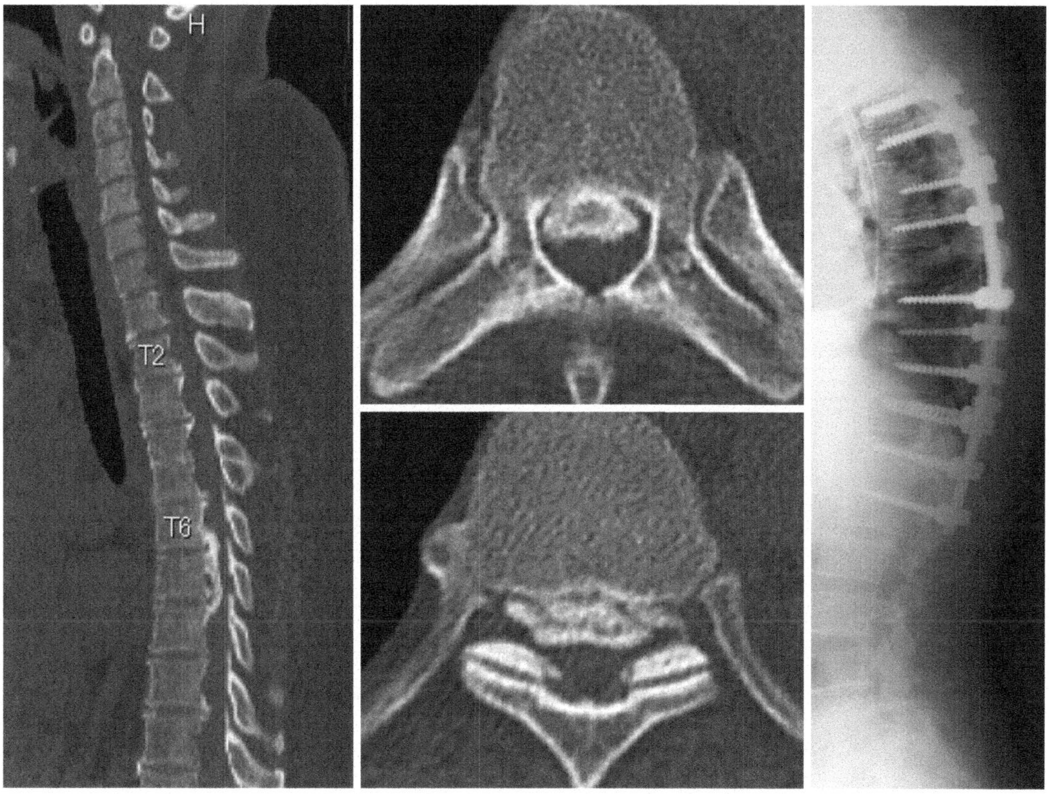

Fig. 33.3 Thoracic OPLL case treated by posterior decompression and dekyphotic fusion. Main lesion was T6–T8

Intervention of steroid injection and suspension surgery was not effective. Postoperatively, temporary motor weakness of lower extremities (MMT 3) was observed until 3 months. This was considered as the true positive case.

33.6 Discussion

Among various types of spinal surgery, OPLL decompression has high neurological deficit rates due to long operative times, complicated procedures, and pathologically critical situations. Tc(E)-MEPs during these high-risk spinal surgeries are indispensable for predicting neurological deterioration and have been proven to have high sensitivity and specificity. In cervical OPLL, most alarms occurred during lamina opening for laminoplasty and were rescued by additional laminectomy or foraminotomy, although corpectomy for cervical OPLL is a high risk factor for neurological deficit. In thoracic OPLL, the total rescue rate remained at only 40% in our prospective study [5]. Additionally, decompression for the stricture of OPLL was particularly risky and ineffective. In this situation, suspension of the surgery and administration of steroids were ineffective, and the rescue rate was relatively low. The thoracic spinal cord has a low blood supply from the radiculomedullary artery and is located in an ischemic area. In severe thoracic OPLL cases, thoracic spinal cord ischemia and ischemia–reperfusion injury upon decompression may aggravate irreversible cord damage. Thus, interventions after the monitoring alarm may not be meaningful for protecting the spinal cord. Therefore, interventions (e.g., steroid or prostaglandin E1 injection, stable blood pressure) before a monitoring alert may be essential to avoid aggravated cord damage from spinal cord edema or ischemia. Alerts also occurred at posture change, dekyphosis, and rodding as well as exposure and PS insertion. These

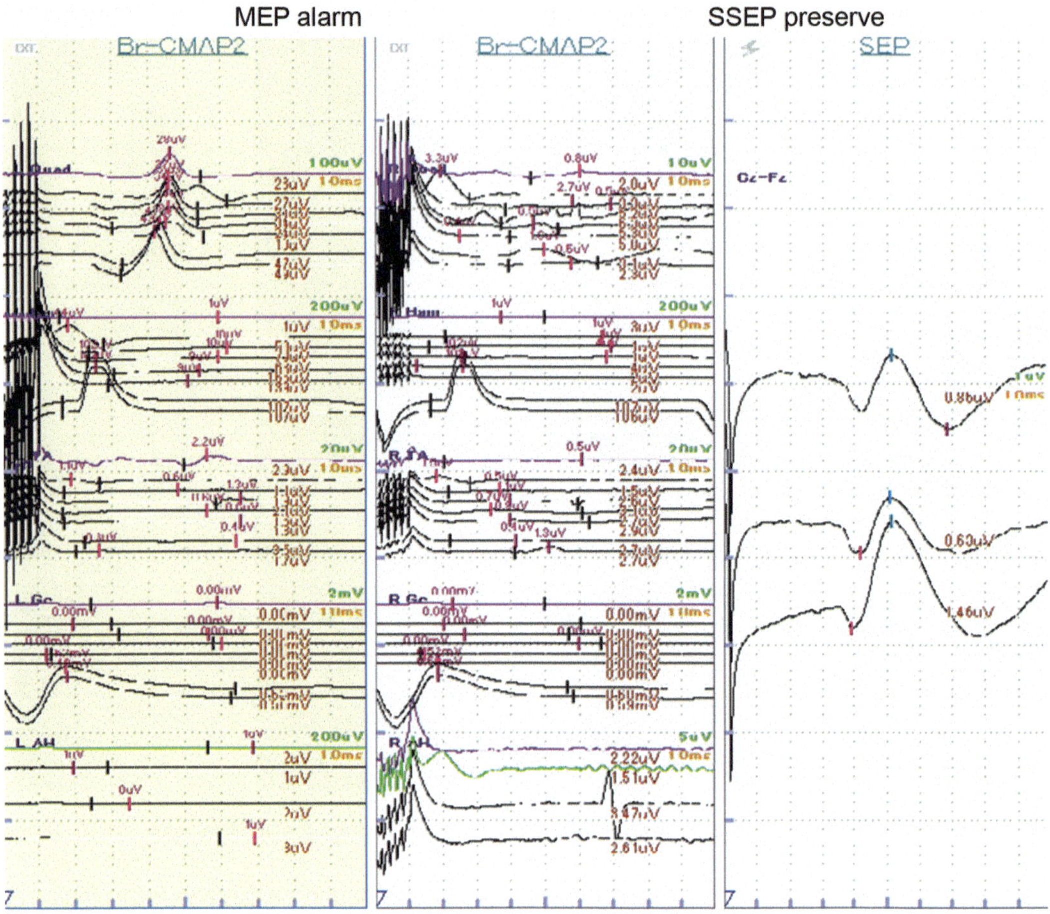

Fig. 33.4 MEP waveform after posterior decompression at T6 to T8, MEP was deteriorated

maneuvers may change the spinal alignment before and during surgery. Even in the thoracic spine, there is a limited range of motion in the sagittal plane. The sagittal alignment of patients with thoracic OPLL may also change at posture change or during surgical maneuvers. In these situations, adequate interventions were effective with realignment or posterior shifting of the spinal cord.

33.7 Limitations of Tc(E)-MEPs

Macdonald et al. [7] reported that Tc-MEPs tend to exhibit gradually falling amplitudes and rising thresholds during surgery, despite stable anesthesia, and called this phenomenon "anesthetic fade." Recognition of such false-positive alerts is important for intraoperative decision-making when the surgeon is faced with a potentially unexplainable TcMEP alert. To rule out false-positive alerts and to recognize risk factors for false-positive alerts might be most important for surgeons, anesthesiologists, and neurophysiologists.

Ushirozako et al. [19] reported that an intraoperative total propofol dose >1550 mg, length of surgery >300 min, and greater blood loss are independently associated with false-positive Tc-MEP alerts during spinal surgery. Surgical procedures for thoracic OPLL were complicated, long length of surgery and relatively large blood loss. Therefore, awareness of such risk factors may prepare surgical teams for the possibility of false-positive Tc-MEP alerts and help in deciding how to appropriately respond to such intraoperative alerts.

33.8 Conclusions

Neurological deficit after thoracic OPLL surgery was high because of physiological kyphosis, poor vascular supply, and complicated surgical procedures for thoracic lesion. There were typical timings for Tc(E)-MEPs deteriorate MEP amplitude regarding to surgical procedures. Therefore, appropriate intervention for protecting the spinal cord and blood supply immediately after IOMN alert was effective even in high-risk OPLL surgery.

References

1. Matsuyama Y, Goto M, Kawakami H, et al. Surgical outcome of ossification of the posterior longitudinal ligament (OPLL) of the thoracic spine: implication of the type of ossification and surgical options. J Spinal Disord Tech. 2005;18(6):492–7.
2. Matsumoto M, Toyama Y, Chikuda H, et al. Outcomes of fusion surgery for ossification of the posterior longitudinal ligament of the thoracic spine: a multicenter retrospective survey. J Neurosurg Spine. 2011;15:380–5.
3. Matsunaga S, Nakamura K, Seichi A, et al. Radiographic predictors for the development of myelopathy in patients with ossification of the posterior longitudinal ligament: a multicenter cohort study. Spine. 2008;15(24):2648–50.
4. Kawahara N, Tomita K, Murakami H, et al. Circumspinal decompression with dekyphosis stabilization for thoracic myelopathy due to ossification of the posterior longitudinal ligament. Spine. 2008;33(1):39–46.
5. Yoshida G, Ando M, Imagama S, et al. Alert timing and corresponding intervention with intraoperative spinal cord monitoring for high risk spinal surgery. Spine. 2019;44(8):E470–9.
6. Fehlings MG, Brodke DS, Norvell DC, et al. The evidence for intraoperative neurophysiological monitoring in spine surgery: does it make a difference? Spine. 2010;35:S37–46.
7. Macdonald DB, Skinner S, Shils J, et al; American Society of Neurophysiological Monitoring. Intraoperative motor evoked potential monitoring—a position statement by the American Society of Neurophysiological Monitoring. Clin Neurophysiol. 2013;124:2291–2316.
8. Bartley K, Woodforth IJ, Stephen JP, et al. Corticospinal volleys and compound muscle action potentials produced by repetitive transcranial stimulation during spinal surgery. Clin Neurophysiol. 2002;113:78–90.
9. Langeloo DD, Lelivelt A, Louis Journée H, et al. Transcranial electrical motor-evoked potential monitoring during surgery for spinal deformity. Spine. 2003;28:1043–50.
10. Luk KD, Hu Y, Wong YW, et al. Evaluation of various evoked potential techniques for spinal cord monitoring during scoliosis surgery. Spine. 2001;26:1772–7.
11. Pelosi L, Lamb J, Grevitt M, et al. Combined monitoring of motor and somatosensory evoked potentials in orthopaedic spinal surgery. Clin Neurophysiol. 2002;113(7):1082–91.
12. Ando M, Tamaki T, Yoshida M, et al. Intraoperative spinal cord monitoring using combined motor and sensory evoked potentials recorded from the spinal cord during surgery for intramedullary spinal cord tumor. Clin Neurol Neurosurg. 2015;133:18–23.
13. Fujiki M, Furukawa Y, Kamida T, et al. Intraoperative corticomuscular motor evoked potentials for evaluation of motor function: a comparison with corticospinal D and I waves. J Neurosurg. 2006;104:85–92.
14. Kothbauer KF, Deletis V, Epstein FJ. Motor-evoked potential monitoring for intramedullary spinal cord tumor surgery: correlation of clinical and neurophysiological data in a series of 100 consecutive procedures. Neurosurg Focus. 1998;4:e1.
15. Ulkatan S, Neuwirth M, Bitan F, et al. Monitoring of scoliosis surgery with epidurally recorded motor evoked potentials (D wave) revealed false results. Clin Neurosurg. 2006;117:2093–101.
16. Thorsteinn G, Andrei VK, Roger S, et al. Real time continuous intraoperative electromyographic and somatosensory evoked potential recordings in spinal surgery: correlation of clinical and electrophysiologic findings in a prospective, consecutive series of 213 cases. Spine. 2004;29:677–84.
17. Raynor BL, Lenke LG, Bridwell KH, et al. Correlation between low triggered electromyographic thresholds and lumbar pedicle screw malposition: analysis of 4857 screws. Spine. 2007;32:2673–8.
18. Imagama S, Ando K, Ito Z, et al. Risk factors for ineffectiveness of posterior decompression and dekyphotic corrective fusion with instrumentation for beak-type thoracic ossification of the posterior longitudinal ligament: a single institute study. Neurosurgery. 2017;80:800–8.
19. Ushirozako H, Yoshida G, Kobayashi S, et al. Impact of total propofol dose during spinal surgery: anesthetic fade on transcranial motor evoked potentials. J Neurosurg Spine. 2019;8:1–9.

34 Intraoperative Ultrasonography for Patients with Ossification of the Posterior Longitudinal Ligament

Tomohiro Banno and Yukihiro Matsuyama

Abstract

Intraoperative ultrasonography (IOUS) is a non-invasive and simple tool to assess the real-time anatomic data of the spinal cord during a surgical procedure. The normal anatomical landmarks and pathological lesions can be obtained accurately through IOUS images that can help to shorten the duration of surgical procedures and improve surgical results. In cases of ossification of the posterior longitudinal ligament (OPLL), the relationship between OPLL and the spinal cord can be easily visualized using IOUS. It is important to confirm an echo-free space between OPLL and the ventral side of the spinal cord to achieve adequate decompression. If IOUS shows no echo-free space on the ventral side of the spinal cord from OPLL, additional procedures to decompress the spinal cord would be required. This chapter describes the suitable application of IOUS for OPLL surgery.

Keywords

Ossification of the posterior longitudinal ligament · Intraoperative ultrasonography Echo · Spine surgery · Posterior decompression Dekyphosis

34.1 Introduction

Intraoperative ultrasonography (IOUS) is a non-invasive and simple technique to depict real-time anatomic data during a surgical procedure. Normal anatomical landmarks and pathological lesions can be obtained accurately through IOUS images that can help to shorten the duration of surgical procedures and improve surgical results.

The use of IOUS in neurosurgical procedures was first reported by Tanaka et al. [1] who observed that A-mode ultrasound was useful for detecting brain tumors. After systematic reports of more specifically designed probes by Rubin et al. [2] in 1982, IOUS has been widely used in neurosurgical fields.

Multiple applications for IOUS have been described, including evaluation of the extent of decompression, location of intradural or intramedullary tumors, confirmation of tumor resection, and evaluation of adequate decompression in Chiari malformation [3, 4].

In spinal surgery, IOUS enables confirmation of the subarachnoid space, spinal shape, and spinal cord palpation, thus facilitating dynamic and morphological assessment of the spinal cord by the surgeons. Certainly, IOUS is also valid in cases of ossification of the posterior longitudinal ligament (OPLL).

T. Banno (✉) · Y. Matsuyama
Department of Orthopaedic Surgery, Hamamatsu University School of Medicine, Hamamatsu, Japan

A. Okawa et al. (eds.), *OPLL*, https://doi.org/10.1007/978-981-15-3855-1_34

34.2 Application of IOUS in Spinal Surgery

For the preparation of IOUS, bony tissue should be resected completely above the region of interest so that an appropriate level of ultrasound can pass and reflect.

The IOUS probes and cords must be maintained in a sterile state by direct sterilization of the IOUS probes or by applying sterile probe covers. The surgical field is then filled with sterile degassed saline. Special care is taken to ensure that the microbubbles and blood clots are removed to limit artifacts.

The transducer is set at the highest frequency (7–15 MHz) and deepest penetration possible for reliable identification of the anatomic landmarks [5]. The higher the transducer frequency, the greater is the axial resolution of the image and the poorer the depth of penetration of the sound beam. We usually use a linear probe at 7.0–13.0 MHz for IOUS in spine surgery (Fig. 34.1a). The transducer is then gently placed onto the dura matter (Fig. 34.1b).

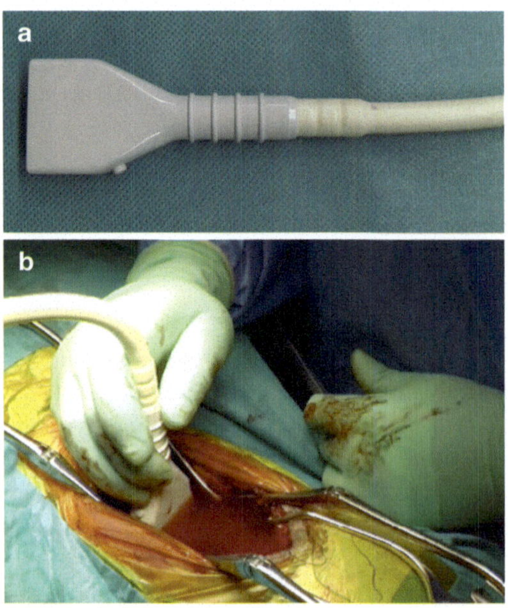

Fig. 34.1 (**a**) Echo probe (linear-type). (**b**) Intraoperative scanning by ultrasonography. During scanning, the surgical field is filled with an adequate amount of sterile degassed saline

The patient is imaged in the prone position, and the cord is assessed in the longitudinal and transverse planes. It is important to place the probe perpendicular to the target area of the spinal cord. Image is provided with cranial on the left in the longitudinal plane, and the left side of the patient on the left in the transverse image.

34.3 Normal Spine

The spinal cord is identified through the dura matter, which appears as an echogenic ring. Within the dura matter, the spinal cord is surrounded by hypoechoic cerebrospinal fluid (CSF) and suspended from the dura by the dentate ligament, which is seen as echogenic linear structures attached bilaterally. The spinal cord is seen as homogeneous and hypoechoic, covered by a bright echogenic line. The central canal, which is identified as an echogenic structure, is located slightly ventral to the central point of the spinal cord (Fig. 34.2a).

Ventral and dorsal roots are seen as linear echogenic structures within the subarachnoid space running along the ventrolateral and dorsolateral surface of the spinal cord, respectively (Fig. 34.2b).

The surrounding nerve routes are echogenic and become particularly prominent at the level of the conus medullaris, appearing as bright linear echoes in the longitudinal axis.

The normal pulsatile movement of the dural sac during breathing and cardiac cycle can be observed in real-time. Color and power Doppler techniques are useful to evaluate the surrounding normal vasculature [6].

34.4 Application of IOUS for OPLL

34.4.1 Evaluation of Spinal Cord Decompression

Posterior spinal cord decompression is usually achieved by multilevel laminoplasty or laminectomy using a surgical air drill. Wide decompression is essential for adequate decompression and spinal cord floating. Following adequate decom-

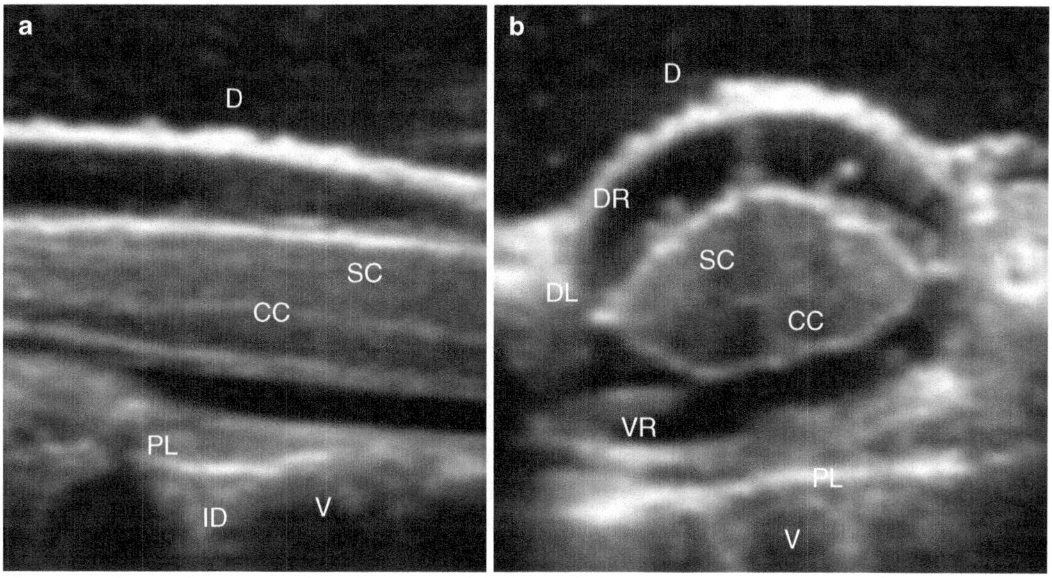

Fig. 34.2 Images of posterior scanning by ultrasonography. (**a**) Long-axis image of the spinal cord at the C5 and C6 levels. Dura matter (D), surface of the spinal cord (SC), and posterior ligament (PL) are visualized as hyperechoic. The spinal cord is surrounded by hypoechoic cerebrospinal fluid. The central canal is visualized as a hyperechoic linear structure located slightly ventral to the central point of the spinal cord. Vertebral body (V) shows acoustic shadow and intervertebral disc (ID) is visualized as longitudinally linear and hyperechoic. (**b**) Short-axis image of the spinal cord at the C6 levels. The spinal cord is surrounded by cerebrospinal fluid and suspended from the dura by bilateral dentate ligament (DL) imaged as echogenic linear structures. The dorsal root (DR) and ventral root (VR) arise from the dorsal and ventral surface of the spinal cord

pression, the spinal cord can be evaluated using the sagittal and axial images of IOUS. In ultrasonographic images, OPLL is provided a thick echogenic layer compressing the spinal cord from the front. Sagittal ultra-sonographic images are useful to evaluate the extent of OPLL and confirm the range of laminectomy in multilevel OPLL cases. On the other hand, axial images are useful to evaluate the degree of spinal cord compression by OPLL and the shape of the spinal cord. Moreover, restoration of the spinal cord shape can be confirmed with the posterior shift of the spinal cord. IOUS is useful to provide real-time information regarding the degree of the spinal cord compression. If the laminectomy range is considered to be insufficient based on IOUS imaging, additional decompression can be performed at once. When the subarachnoid space is confirmed between OPLL and the anterior aspect of the spinal cord, sufficient decompression is achieved [7–9]. Tokuhashi et al. [8] reported that the restoration of the anterior subarachnoid space was important for neurologic improvement following posterior cervical decompression surgery.

It should be noted that IOUS cannot evaluate the dynamic factor caused by spinal instability; therefore, the preoperative assessment of spinal instability using functional radiographs is crucial. Moreover, the necessity of spinal fusion should be discussed preoperatively.

34.5 Evaluation of Spinal Cord Decompression via Posterior Approach for Thoracic OPLL

In cases with thoracic OPLL, gentle pedicle screw insertion and placement of temporary rod on one side is important before decompression to prevent intraoperative spinal cord damage.

Sufficient spinal cord decompression often cannot be achieved by laminectomy and in situ fixation; thus, indirect decompression by dekyphosis [10] or direct decompression by circumferential decompression [11] is needed. We have been performing indirect decompression by laminectomy and dekyphosis using instruments via a posterior approach, because this procedure is less technically demanding and associated with a lower risk of neurological complications [12]. The damaged spinal cord could be protected and restored after fusion surgery.

If IOUS shows no echo-free space on the ventral side the spinal cord from OPLL, additional dekyphosis with in situ rod bending or Ponte osteotomy would be needed [13]. Ando et al. [13] reported that the recovery rate of patients with echo-free space on the ventral side of the spinal cord after decompression and dekyphosis procedure was 66.0%, while that of the patients with no echo-free space was 33.4%. Imagama et al. [14] reported that the residual spinal cord compression by beak-type OPLL in IOUS is significantly related to reoperation for OPLL resection. Therefore, surgeons should evaluate spinal cord decompression using IOUS in every case.

34.6 Case Series

34.6.1 Cervical OPLL

34.6.1.1 Case 1 (Fig. 34.3)

The patient, a 48-year-old woman with OPLL in the cervical spine, exhibited finger dyscoordination and gait disturbance. Imaging studies demonstrated OPLL at C3–C7, and intramedul-

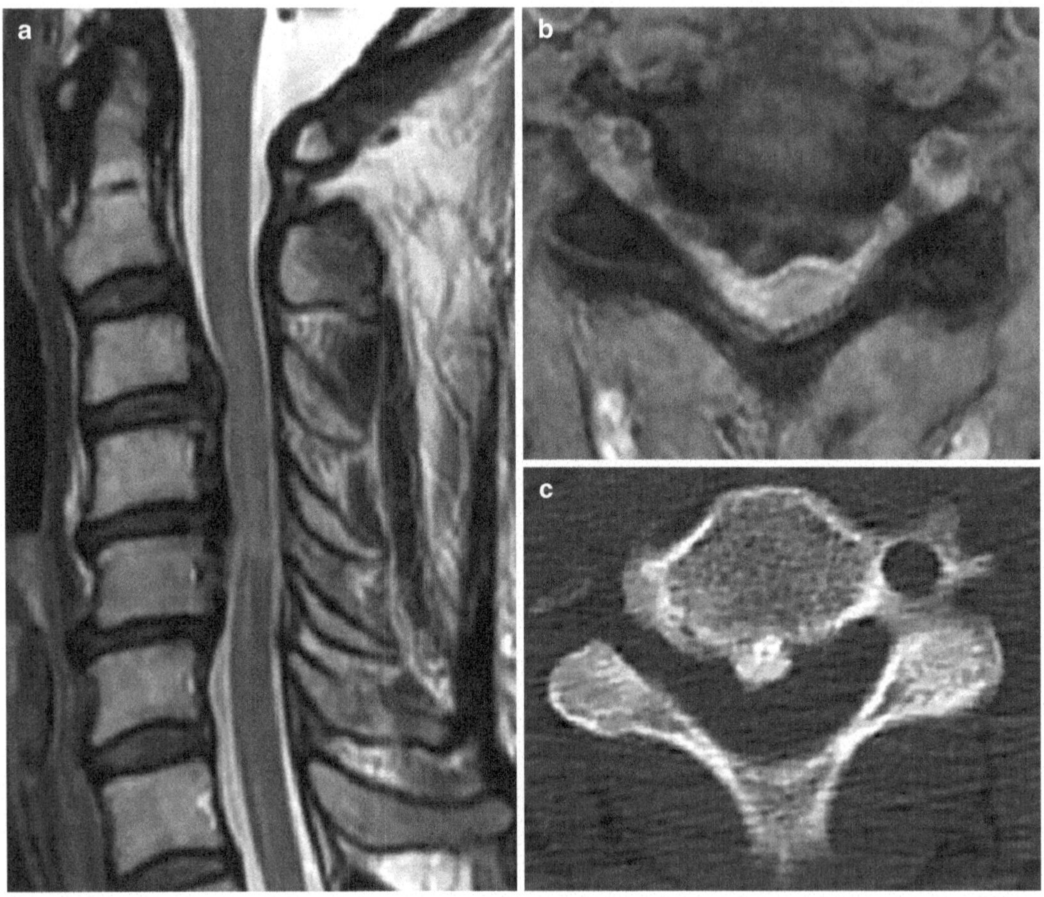

Fig. 34.3 A 48-year-old woman with cervical ossification of the posterior longitudinal ligament (OPLL). (**a**) Sagittal magnetic resonance imaging (MRI). Spinal cord compression at C3–6 and intramedullary high signal intensity changes are observed. (**b**, **c**) Axial MRI and CT at C4/5. Spinal cord is compressed by OPLL. (**d**, **e**) Intraoperative ultrasonography (IOUS). After laminectomy, spinal cord has shifted posteriorly and echo-free space is confirmed in front of spinal cord (white arrow). (**e**) Postoperative radiograph. Posterior decompression and fusion at C3–6 is performed using lateral mass screw

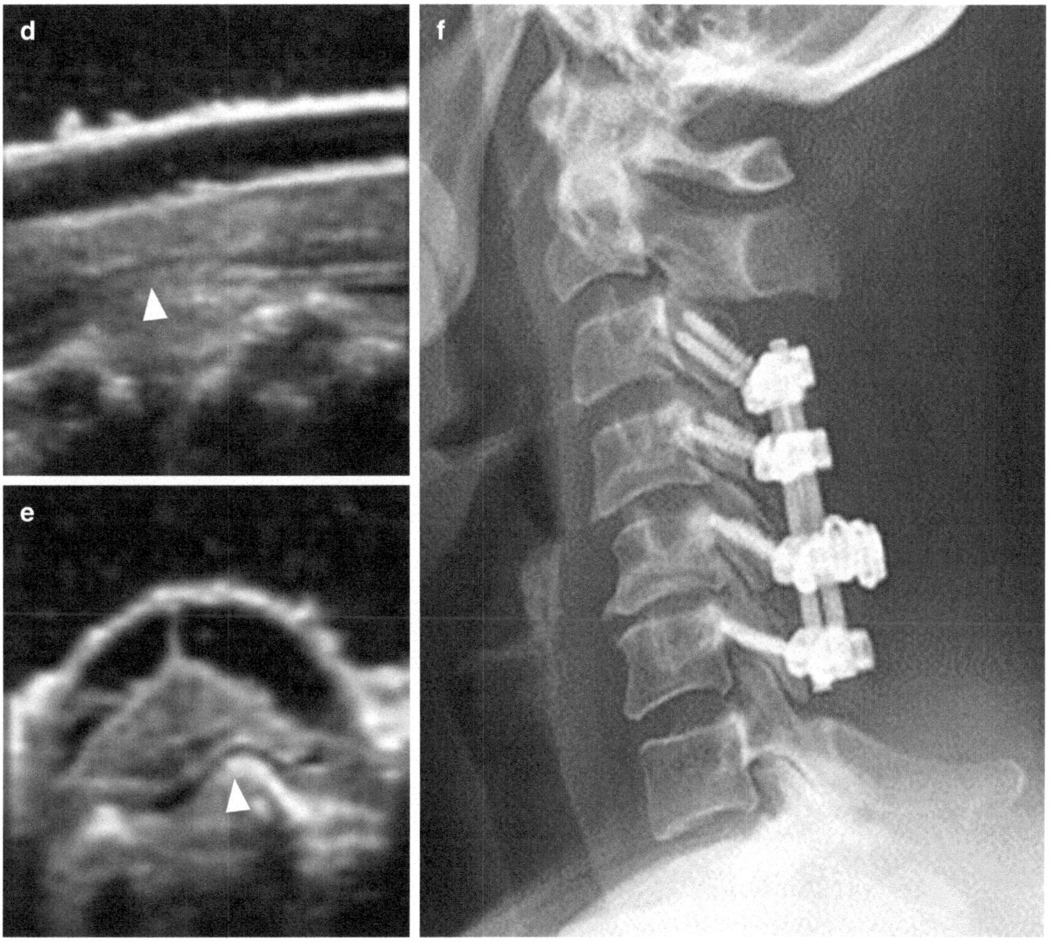

Fig. 34.3 (continued)

lary high signal intensity change on T2-weighted image was observed at C4–5. The patient underwent posterior decompression and fusion surgery at C3–7. After laminectomy, the morphological findings of the spinal cord and positional relations with OPLL were evaluated using IOUS. The ultrasound images demonstrated that deformation of the spinal cord by OPLL still remained; however, an echo-free space was detected on the ventral side of the spinal cord.

34.6.1.2 Case 2 (Fig. 34.4)

The patient, a 78-year-old man with OPLL in the cervical spine, exhibited finger dyscoordination and gait disturbance. Muscle motor weakness was also observed in the right upper extremity. Imaging studies demonstrated OPLL at C3–C6 and intramedullary high signal intensity change in the T2-weighted image at C3–5. The patient underwent posterior decompression and fusion surgery at C2–5 and French door laminoplasty at C6. After decompression and fusion, IOUS demonstrated that the spinal cord was still compressed by OPLL; however, the shape of the spinal cord was restored, and an echo-free space was detected on the ventral side of the spinal cord.

34.6.2 Thoracic OPLL

34.6.2.1 Case 3 (Fig. 34.5)

The patient, a 58-year-old man with OPLL in the thoracic spine, exhibited gait disturbance with

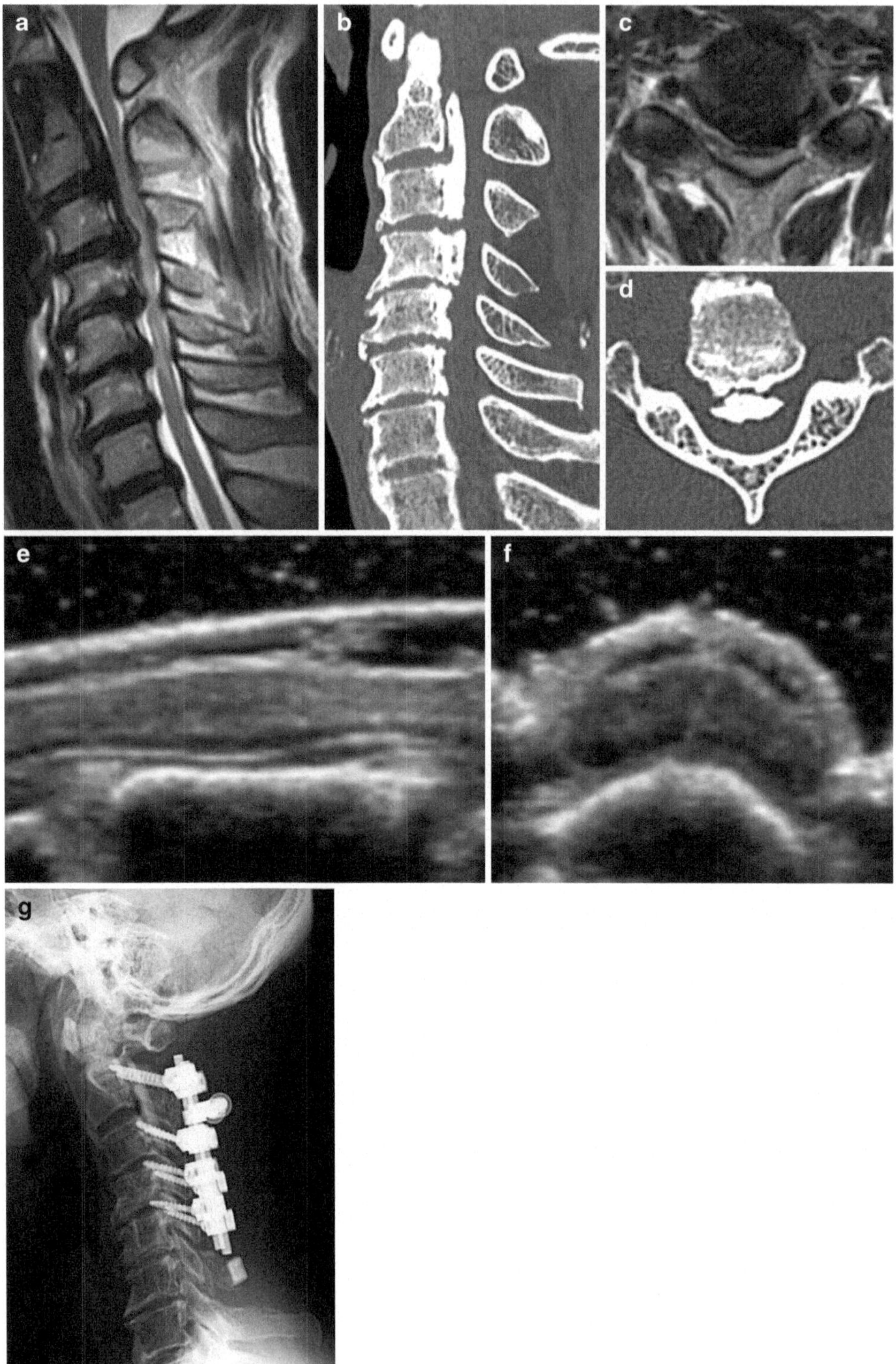

Fig. 34.4 A 78-year-old woman with cervical ossification of the posterior longitudinal ligament (OPLL). (**a**, **b**) Sagittal magnetic resonance imaging (MRI) and computed tomography (CT). MRI demonstrates multi-segmental spinal cord compression at C2–6. CT demonstrates mixed-type OPLL. (**c**, **d**) Axial MRI and CT at C3/4. Spinal cord is severely compressed by OPLL. (**e**, **f**) Intraoperative ultrasonography (IOUS). After laminectomy, spinal cord from OPLL and restoration of the spinal cord shape are confirmed. (**g**) Postoperative radiograph. Posterior decompression and fusion surgery at C2–5 and French door laminoplasty at C6 are performed

muscle motor weakness in the lower extremity. Imaging studies demonstrated that mixed-type OPLL was observed at T5–T9, and severe spinal cord compression was observed at the T5/6 and T8/9 levels. The patient underwent thoracic posterior decompression and fusion surgery. Before laminectomy, the patients underwent in situ unilateral temporal fixation using pedicle screw at T3–T11 to prevent spinal cord injury owing to progression of spinal kyphosis during laminectomy. After laminectomy at T5–9, IOUS demonstrated that the spinal cord was compressed by OPLL, and no echo-free space was confirmed on the ventral side of the spinal cord. The anterior

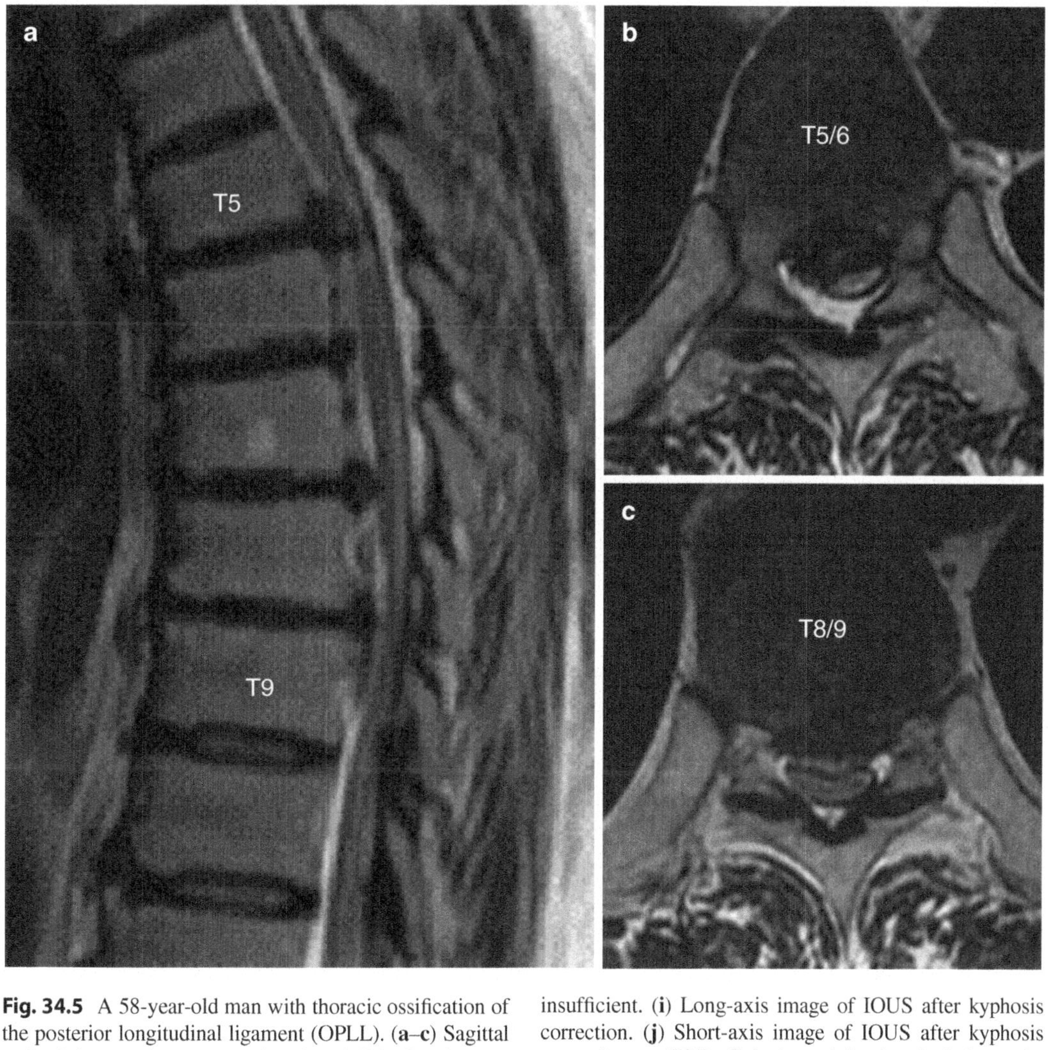

Fig. 34.5 A 58-year-old man with thoracic ossification of the posterior longitudinal ligament (OPLL). (**a–c**) Sagittal and axial magnetic resonance imaging (MRI). Canal stenosis observed at T5–9 with severe spinal cord compression at T5/6 and T8/9. (**d–f**) Sagittal and axial computed tomography (CT). Mixed-type OPLL observed at T5–9, and ossification of yellow ligament (OYL) was also observed at T8/9. (**g**) Long-axis image of intraoperative ultrasonography (IOUS) after laminectomy. (**h**) Short-axis image of IOUS after laminectomy at T8/9. Spinal cord is still compressed by OPLL, and no echo-free space was confirmed between OPLL and spinal cord; thus, spinal cord decompression is insufficient. (**i**) Long-axis image of IOUS after kyphosis correction. (**j**) Short-axis image of IOUS after kyphosis correction at T8/9. Spinal cord is detached from the OPLL. Echo-free space between OPLL and spinal cord and restoration of the spinal cord shape is confirmed. (**k, l**) Sagittal and axial IOUS images of color and power Doppler. Blood flow of anterior spinal artery is interrupted around the stenosis site. (**m**) Postoperative radiograph. Posterior decompression at T5–9 and fusion surgery at T3–11 is performed. (**n, o**) Sagittal CT before and after posterior corrective fusion surgery. Local kyphosis angle at T5–9 has decreased from 25° to 22°

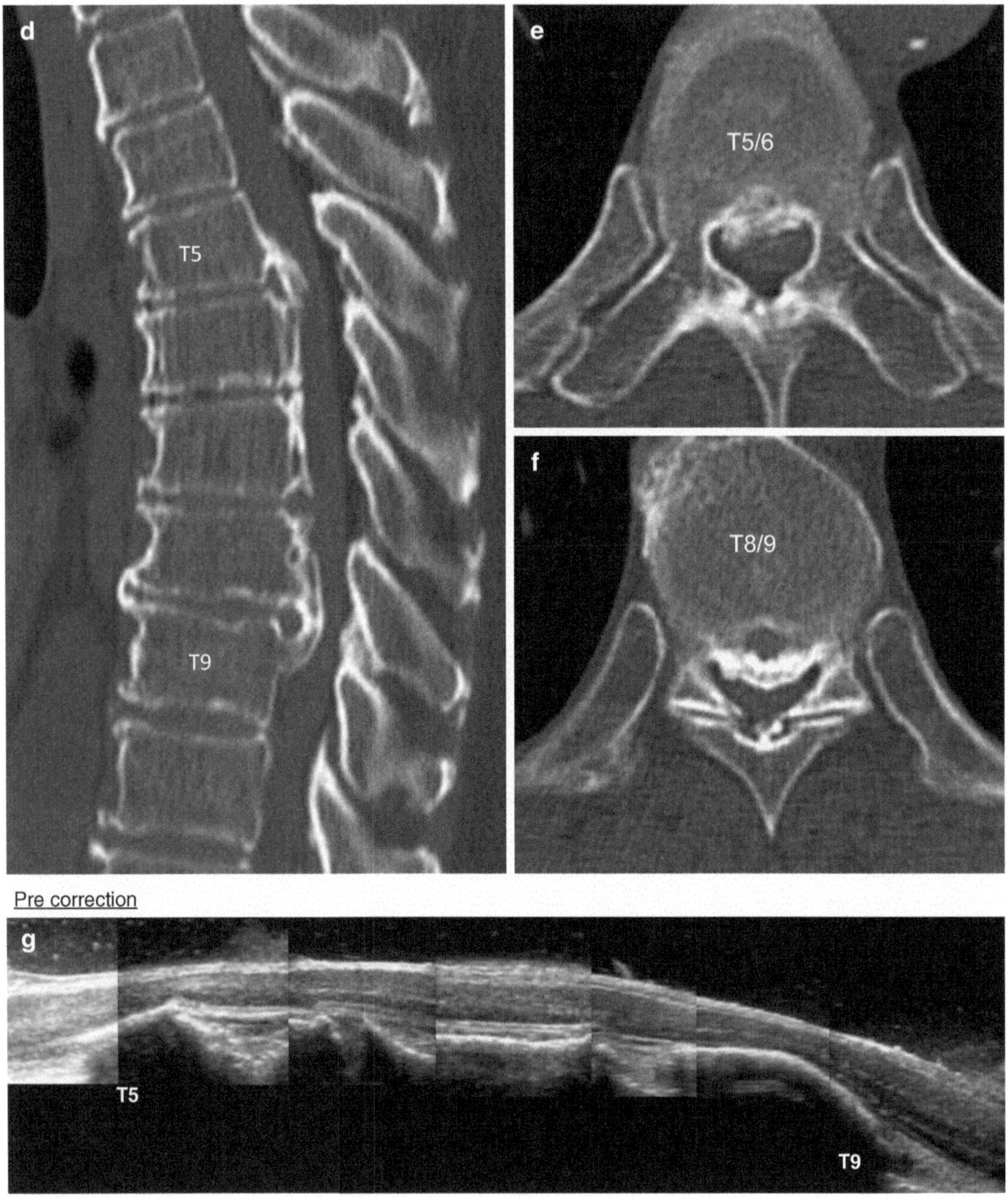

Fig. 34.5 (continued)

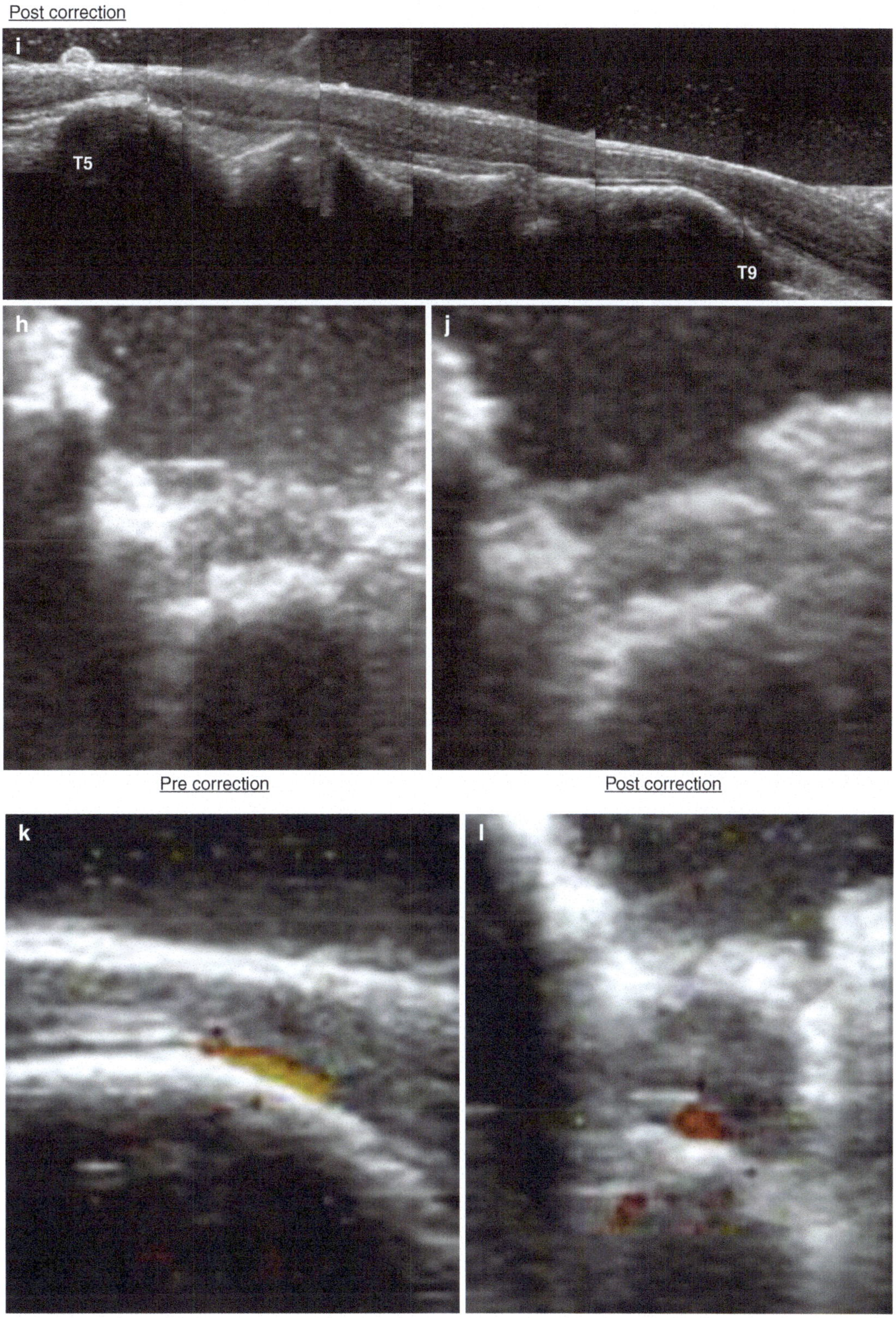

Fig. 34.5 (continued)

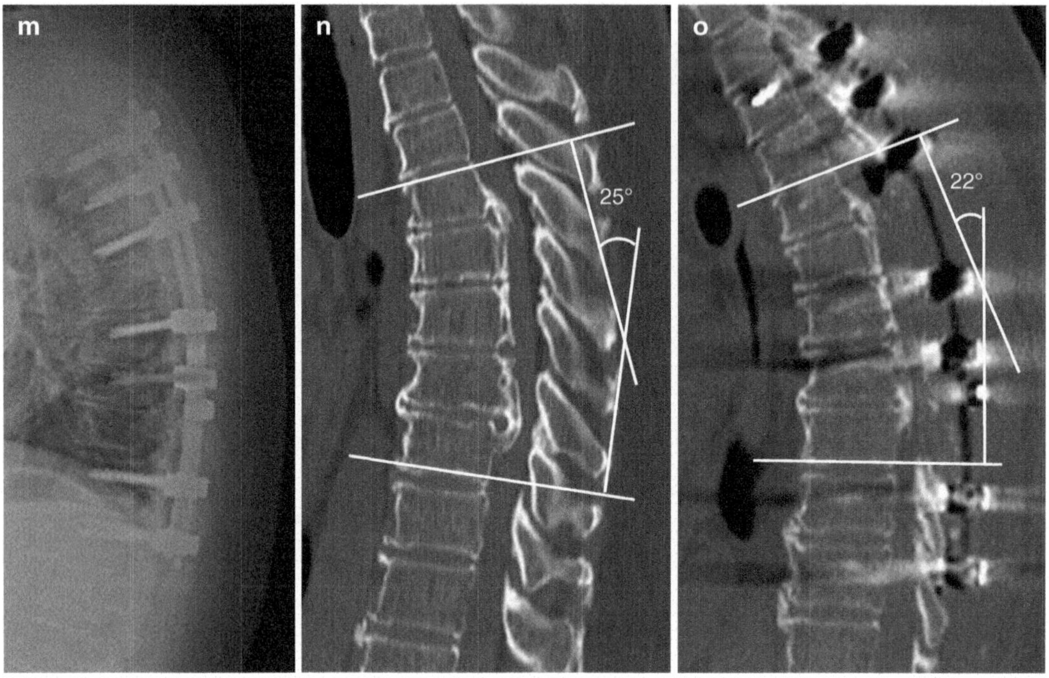

Fig. 34.5 (continued)

spinal artery could be evaluated using color and power Doppler images. Blood flow was interrupted around the site of the stenosis. Therefore, indirect decompression was achieved by kyphosis correction using fixation of a bent rod with cantilever force, following which sufficient decompression of the spinal cord could be confirmed by IOUS.

34.6.2.2 Case 4 (Fig. 34.6)

The patient, a 62-year-old man with OPLL in the cervical and thoracic spine, who had undergone cervical laminoplasty in another hospital, exhibited gait disturbance and bilateral lower extremity numbness. Imaging studies demonstrated continuous-type OPLL at T1–3 and segmental-type OPLL at T6–9. Severe spinal cord compression was observed at the T6/7, T7/8, and T9/10 levels. The patient underwent posterior decompression and fusion surgery. Before laminectomy, the patients underwent in situ unilateral temporal fixation using pedicle screw at T5–T11 to prevent spinal cord injury due to progression of spinal kyphosis during laminectomy. After laminectomy at T6–10, IOUS demonstrated no echo-free space associated with the spinal cord, and OPLL suggested insufficient decompression of the spinal cord. Following kyphosis correction, IOUS demonstrated echo-free space, and the OPLL indicated sufficient decompression of the spinal cord.

34.7 Limitations of IOUS Evaluation

IOUS is useful for assessing the subarachnoid space between the spinal cord and the OPLL, and restoration of the anterior subarachnoid space was considered to be a significant factor for neurologic improvement following posterior decompression surgery [7, 8, 10]. When no anterior subarachnoid space is available after posterior decompression and dekyphotic corrective fusion, additional surgical procedures, such as direct OPLL resection,

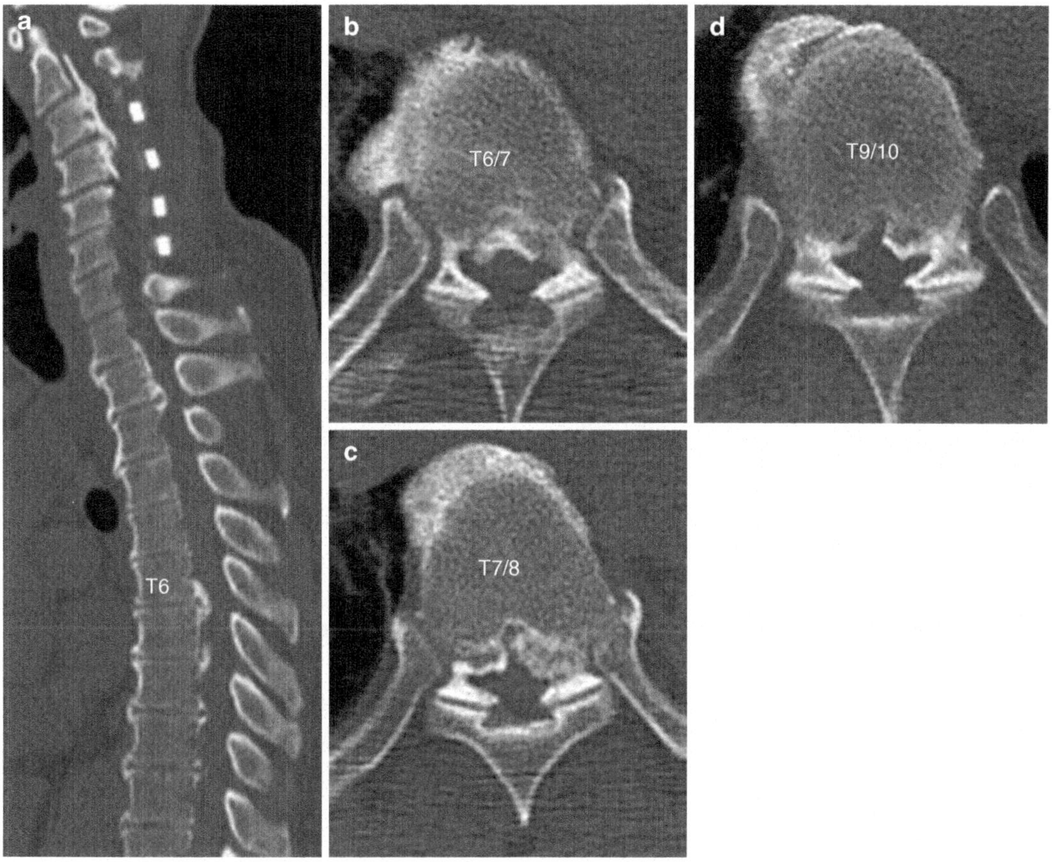

Fig. 34.6 A 62-year-old man with cervico-thoracic ossification of the posterior longitudinal ligament (OPLL). (**a–d**) Sagittal and axial computed tomography (CT). Laminoplasty had already been performed for cervical OPLL. Segmental type OPLL observed at T1–3 and T6–10. (**e–h**) Sagittal and axial magnetic resonance imaging (MRI). Canal stenosis observed at T6–10 and severe spinal cord compression observed at T6/7, T7/8, and T9/10. (**i**) Long-axis image of Intraoperative ultrasonography (IOUS) after laminectomy. (**j**) Short-axis image of IOUS after laminectomy at T6/7. Spinal cord is still compressed by OPLL, and no echo-free space is confirmed between OPLL and spinal cord; thus, spinal cord decompression is insufficient. (**k**) Long-axis image of IOUS after kyphosis correction. (**l**) Short-axis image of IOUS after kyphosis correction at T6/7. Spinal cord detached from OPLL. Echo-free space between OPLL and spinal cord, and restoration of spinal cord shape is confirmed. (**m**) Postoperative radiograph. Posterior decompression is seen at T6–10, and fusion surgery at T5–11 is performed. (**n**, **o**) Sagittal CT before and after posterior corrective fusion surgery. Local kyphosis angle at T6–10 decreased from 18° to 10°

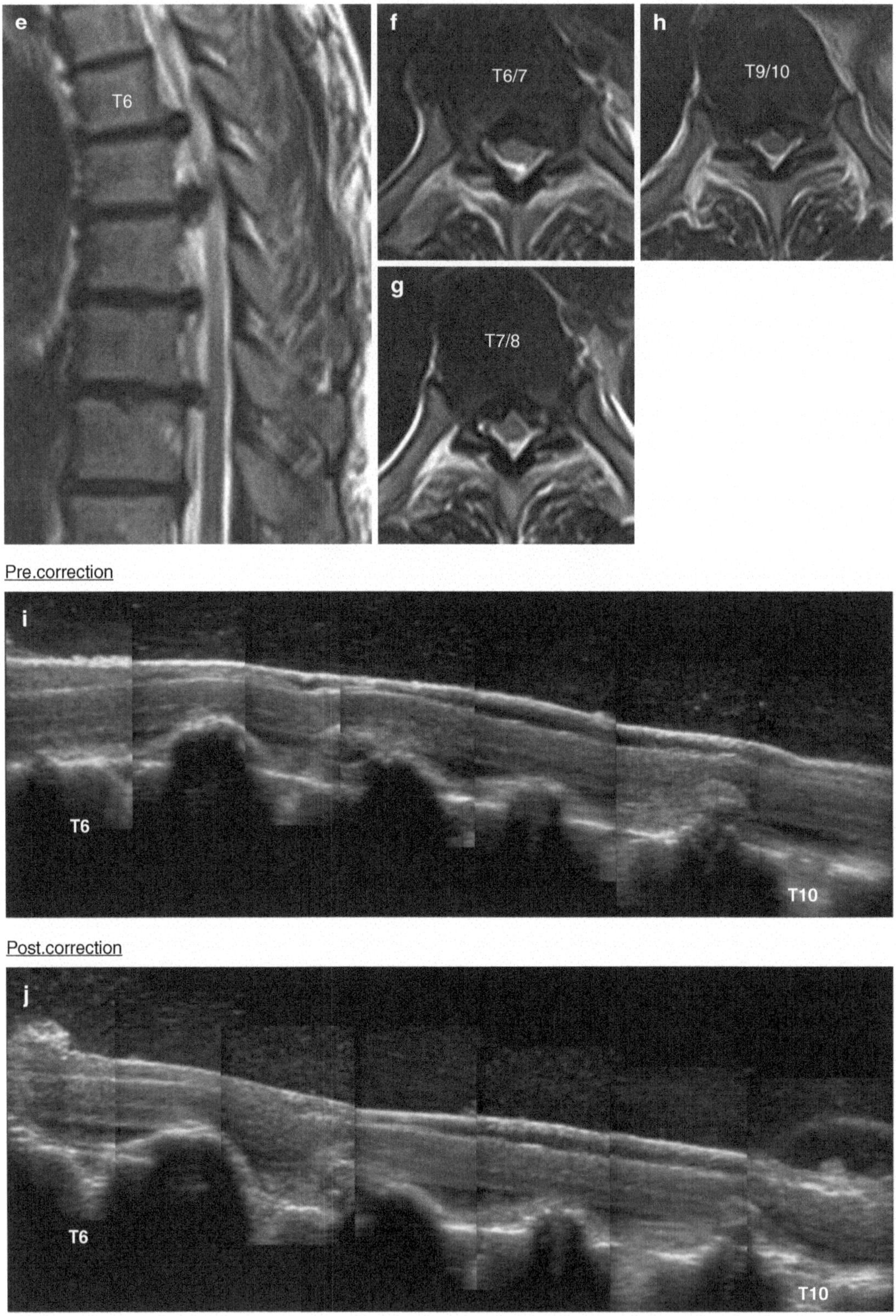

Fig. 34.6 (continued)

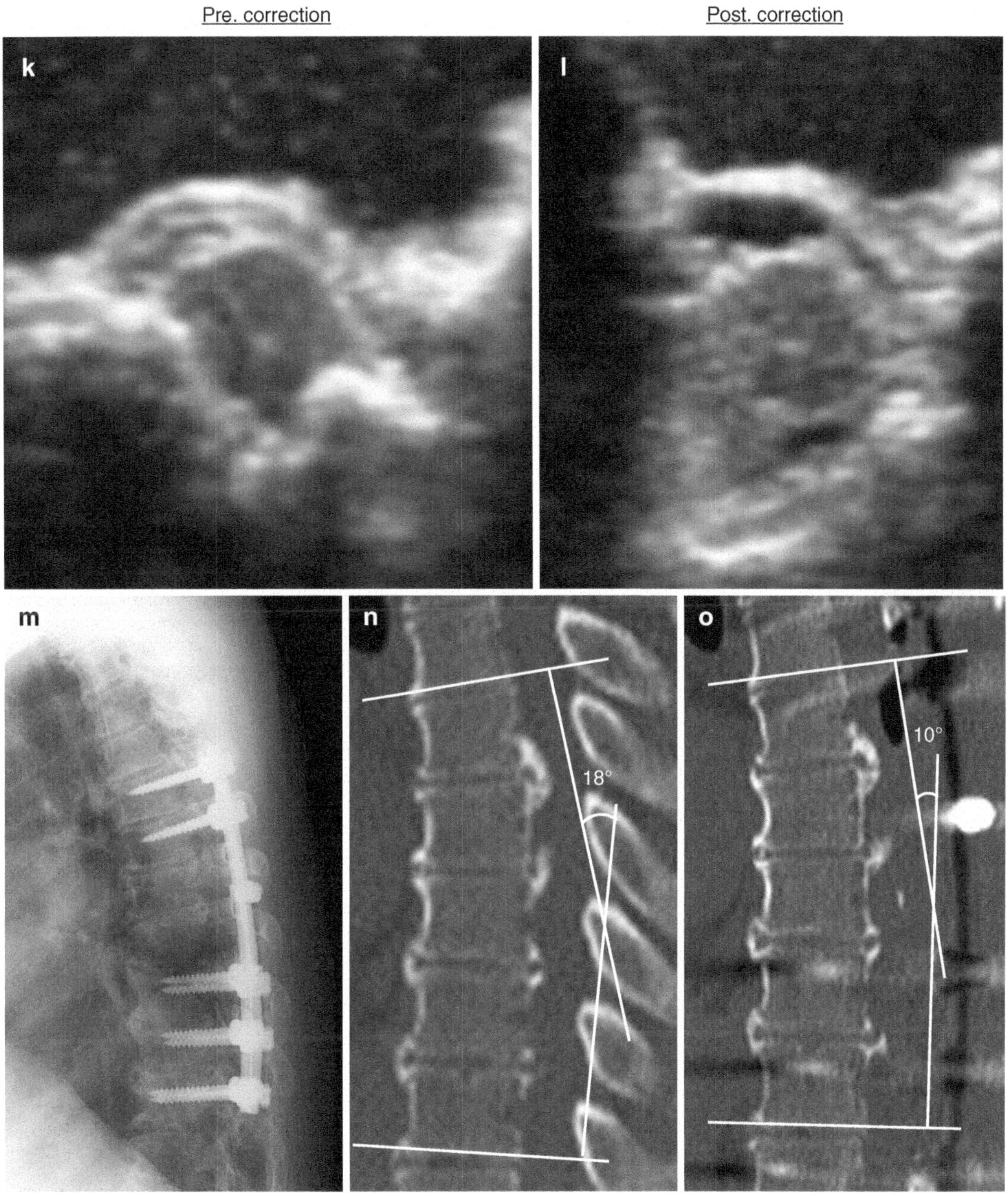

Fig. 34.6 (continued)

should be considered. However, there have been no controlled studies about the necessity of additional surgical procedures in such occasions.

Moreover, it is sometimes difficult to judge whether restoration of the anterior subarachnoid space is required during surgery because IOUS assessment depends on the skill and experience of the inspector. Thus, IOUS assessment should not be an absolute diagnostic tool, but an assisted tool for surgical decision.

34.8 Conclusions

IOUS is a simple, noninvasive tool for assessing the anatomical features in real-time. In OPLL surgery, the surgeon can evaluate the condition of the spinal cord and the relative positions with OPLL using IOUS. Additionally, color and power Doppler techniques are effective tools to evaluate the surrounding vasculature in the spinal cord. Little is known about the relationship between blood flow in the spinal cord and clinical outcome in patients with OPLL; however, blood flow assessment of the spinal cord is expected to be established in the future.

References

1. Tanaka K, Ito K, Wagai T. The localization of brain tumors by ultrasonic techniques. A clinical review of 111 cases. J Neurosurg. 1965;23(2):135–47.
2. Rubin JM, Dohrmann GJ. Use of ultrasonically guided probes and catheters in neurosurgery. Surg Neurol. 1982;18(2):143–8.
3. Schabel AB, Shah LM. Intraoperative ultrasound of the spine. Neurographics. 2015;5(1):28–35.
4. Alvarado E, Leach J, Care M, Mangano F, Hara SO. Pediatric spinal ultrasound: neonatal and intraoperative applications. Semin Ultrasound CT MR. 2017;38(2):126–42.
5. Sosna J, Barth MM, Kruskal JB, Kane RA. Intraoperative sonography for neurosurgery. J Ultrasound Med. 2005;24(12):1671–82.
6. Kane RA, Kruskal JB. Intraoperative ultrasonography of the brain and spine. Ultrasound Q. 2007;23(1):23–39.
7. Seichi A, Chikuda H, Kimura A, Takeshita K, Sugita S, Hoshino Y, et al. Intraoperative ultrasonographic evaluation of posterior decompression via laminoplasty in patients with cervical ossification of the posterior longitudinal ligament: correlation with 2-year follow-up results. J Neurosurg Spine. 2010;13(1):47–51.
8. Tokuhashi Y, Matsuzaki H, Oda H, Uei H. Effectiveness of posterior decompression for patients with ossification of the posterior longitudinal ligament in the thoracic spine: usefulness of the ossification-kyphosis angle on MRI. Spine. 2006;31(1):E26–30.
9. Matsuyama Y, Kawakami N, Yanase M, Yoshihara H, Ishiguro N, Kameyama T, et al. Cervical myelopathy due to OPLL: clinical evaluation by MRI and intraoperative spinal sonography. J Spinal Disord Tech. 2004;17(5):401–4.
10. Matsuyama Y, Sakai Y, Katayama Y, Imagama S, Ito Z, Wakao N, et al. Indirect posterior decompression with corrective fusion for ossification of the posterior longitudinal ligament of the thoracic spine: is it possible to predict the surgical results? Eur Spine J. 2009;18(7):943–8.
11. Wang YQ, Liu XG, Jiang L, Jiang L, Wei F, Yu M, et al. Intraoperative ultrasonography in "cave-in" 360 degrees circumferential decompression for thoracic spinal stenosis. Chin Med J. 2011;124(23):3879–85.
12. Matsumoto M, Toyama Y, Chikuda H, Takeshita K, Kato T, Shindo S, et al. Outcomes of fusion surgery for ossification of the posterior longitudinal ligament of the thoracic spine: a multicenter retrospective survey: clinical article. J Neurosurg Spine. 2011;15(4):380–5.
13. Ando K, Imagama S, Ito Z, Kobayashi K, Ukai J, Muramoto A, et al. Ponte osteotomy during Dekyphosis for indirect posterior decompression with ossification of the posterior longitudinal ligament of the thoracic spine. Clin Spine Surg. 2017;30(4):E358–e62.
14. Imagama S, Ando K, Ito Z, Kobayashi K, Hida T, Ito K, et al. Risk factors for ineffectiveness of posterior decompression and Dekyphotic corrective fusion with instrumentation for beak-type thoracic ossification of the posterior longitudinal ligament: a single institute study. Neurosurgery. 2017;80(5):800–8.

The manufacturer's authorised representative in the EU is Springer Nature Customer Service Centre GmbH, Europaplatz 3, 69115 Heidelberg, Germany. If you have any concerns regarding our products, please contact ProductSafety@springernature.com

Printed and bound by CPI Group (UK) Ltd, Croydon, CR0 4YY
30/09/2026
02225241-0019